Illness and healing among the Sakhalin Ainu

Illness and healing among the Sakhalin Ainu

A *symbolic interpretation*

EMIKO OHNUKI-TIERNEY
Department of Anthropology
University of Wisconsin, Madison

CAMBRIDGE UNIVERSITY PRESS

Cambridge
London   New York   New Rochelle
Melbourne   Sydney

Published by the Press Syndicate of the University of Cambridge
The Pitt Building, Trumpington Street, Cambridge CB2 1RP
32 East 57th Street, New York, NY 10022, USA
296 Beaconsfield Parade, Middle Park, Melbourne 3206, Australia

First published 1981

Printed in the United States of America
Typeset by The Composing Room of Michigan, Inc., Grand Rapids, Michigan
Printed and bound by The Murray Printing Co., Westford, Massachusetts

Library of Congress Cataloging in Publication Data
Ohnuki-Tierney, Emiko.
Illness and healing among the Sakhalin Ainu.
Includes bibliographical references and index.
1. Ainu – Medicine. I. Title.
DS832.034 306'.4 80-24268
ISBN 0 521 23636 3

In memory and with love to Husko

In gratitude to Jan Vansina

*With love and gratitude to my parents, Kozaburo and Taka Ohnuki,
and to my family members, Tim, Alan, and Roderic*

Contents

Preface   *page* xi

Ainu phonemes   xiv

1   Introduction: aims and scope of the book   1

2   The Ainu   19
    The Ainu   19
    The Sakhalin Ainu   22
    The Ainu way on the northwest coast of southern
        Sakhalin   25

3   The ethnomedical approach in anthropology and the
        Ainu domain of illness   31
    Ethnomedicine   31
    The Ainu domain of illness   34

4   Habitual illnesses   39
    General characteristics of habitual illnesses   39
    Healing of habitual illnesses   44
    Summary   47

5   Classification of body-part and skin illnesses   49
    Taxonomy of headaches and boils   49
    Wet–dry opposition in the classification of other illnesses   56
    The nature of pain as a classificatory principle   60
    Illness classification and grammatical structure   60
    Summary   62

6   Metaphysical illnesses and their healing rituals   63
    Epidemics   63
    Somatic illnesses afflicting individuals   65
    Mental illnesses   69
    Shamanistic healing rites   73

Spirits and deities involved in shamanistic rites   76
Sorcery   78
Summary   80

7   A symbolic interpretation of metaphysical illnesses and
    healing rituals   82
    Deities and humans in Ainu symbolic classification   82
    Demons in Ainu symbolic classification   87
    Illness and health in Ainu symbolic classification   88
    Symbols in medical rituals   90
    The power of anomalous symbols   92
    *Anarchic anomaly and creative anomaly: demons and other
       anomalous symbols*   96
    The use of senses in Ainu symbolic perception   97
    /Sacred:profane::nature:culture/   98
    Multiplicity of belief systems   100
    Summary   103

8   Theories in symbolic studies and the Ainu data   105
    Interpretation of symbols   105
    /Sacred:profane/ opposition   108
    /Sacred:profane::nature:culture/   110
    /Nature:culture::men:women/, or its inversion?   111
    Anomaly: problem of definition   119
    Anomaly and power   124
    Multiple symbolic systems: /public:domestic::men:women/   129
    Summary   131

9   Modes of perception and the classification of illnesses: a
    synthesis   133
    *The domain of illness: problems of codification and
       subdivision*   134
    *Contrasts between habitual illnesses and metaphysical
       illnesses*   135
    Degrees of subclassification   140
    Modes of perception   141
    Emotive and sensory patterns of perception   147
    Summary   149

10 Language and cognition: theoretical and methodological
    problems in arriving at perceptual categories   151
    Ethnosemantics   151
    Sapir–Whorf hypothesis   156

	Meaning of conceptual forms	157
	Summary	160
11	Illness, the individual, and society	161
	Shamans and their power: a description	162
	Multiple roles of Ainu shamans: an interpretation	166
	Shamans as healers of social ills and as covert politicians	169
	The politically peripheral, nonformalized power,	
	and shamans	172
	Shamans in other Ainu societies	173
	Individual personality: imu: *and shamans*	175
	Symbolic power and sociopolitical power	179
	Summary	181

Appendixes
A	Details of Ainu habitual illnesses	183
B	Beings and objects used in the cures of habitual illnesses	196
C	*Imu:*	198
D	Biological, cultural, and linguistic identity of the Ainu	204
E	The history of the Sakhalin Ainu	213

Notes	218
References	226
Index	239

Preface

This book is an outgrowth of my fifteen-year attempt to understand Ainu culture and of my quest to determine the role of culture in the ordering and, in particular, the classification of one's universe.

The Ainu discussed in this book are a group of Sakhalin Ainu who during the first half of the twentieth century inhabited the northwest coast of southern Sakhalin, a region that stretches north of Rayčiska (Japanese call the place "Raichishika") to the former Russo-Japanese border. My fieldwork (1965–6, 1969, 1973) was carried out among the Sakhalin Ainu, who have been relocated on Hokkaido since the Russian occupation of southern Sakhalin in 1945.

I am most grateful to the National Science Foundation (GS 817), which supported my first field research (1965–6). Much of the research on anthropological theories presented in this book was accomplished during a leave in 1978 supported by the National Science Foundation (BNS77-12988). The Research Committee of the University of Wisconsin Graduate School has been most supportive of my research, and I thank the committee members.

There are too many individuals to mention in this Preface who have contributed to my growth, both professionally and personally. I must, however, mention a few. First, my deepest appreciation and affection go to Husko. Husko, which is her nickname, meaning "ancient," was born in 1900 in a winter settlement near Esituri and spent most of her life on the northwest coast of southern Sakhalin. Both her paternal and maternal ancestors had lived for many generations in the area. She was very shy when young and preferred to be with her parents and elderly people, from whom she learned the Ainu way more thoroughly than her contemporaries did. During her late teens, she married an Ainu who later became headman of Rayčiska, one of the largest settlements on the northwest coast. She had five children by him. After World War II, she moved to Tokoro, Hokkaido, where she lived until her death in 1974 with two of her remaining daughters and their families. Any fieldworker realizes that only a few individuals are able to explain their own culture well, especially when the investigation involves such complex matters as world view. Husko was one of those few precious individuals. Without her patience and genuine interest in the purpose of my work, this book, or, for that matter, any of my work on the Ainu, would not have been possible. I cherish our relationship, however, not simply because of my anthropological interests but because it was a most fulfilling experience for me to get to know her – a brilliant and warm woman who shared her joys and sufferings of life with me. Although this book, I am sure, falls short of the expectations of this woman who held an unshakable pride in her own culture, it is dedicated to her memory.

My other Ainu friends at Tokoro are also gratefully remembered. Either individually or often during our fireside group discussions, they supplied me with rich ethnographic information. My deep appreciation also goes to my many Ainu friends at Wakasakunai. I thank Miharu Fumio, the head of the local community, who, without hesitation, took the entire responsibility for my presence even at the beginning when others were not certain of the purposes of my work. Emiko Kawamura, who let me stay with her and has since extended a close and enduring friendship to me, is also affectionately acknowledged here. Her daughter, then four years of age, taught me the beauty of sharing when wealth is not plentiful. I will never forget her face when she pulled a piece of candy from her mouth and asked me if I wanted to suck on it for a while. I also thank Shirayama no Baba, as she was fondly called in the community, who taught me much about Ainu religion and other matters.

Numerous scholars in Japan, the United States, and elsewhere have contributed either directly or indirectly to this book. My indebtedness to Professor Jan Vansina of the University of Wisconsin, my former professor, is long-standing as well as multifaceted. When I was a student, he first introduced me to the field of symbolic anthropology, and since then he has painstakingly read almost every paper I wrote and generously offered me his suggestions. As I grow in my profession, I am even more amazed at his generosity in imparting to me his most original ideas and analyses, many of which I "stole" and attempted to develop. His review and criticism of Chapters 1, 7, and 8 were most helpful. I dedicate this book to him as a small token of my appreciation for his guidance and personal encouragement through the years.

I am most grateful to Professor Toshi Yamamoto, former director of the Sakhalin Museum. The superb quality of his ethnographic work among the east coast Sakhalin Ainu has been a source of inspiration. In 1972, he hand-carried from Japan to Madison, Wisconsin, many illustrations, which he originally prepared for his publication, and various Sakhalin Ainu ethnographic specimens. My long hours of discussion with him about the northwest coast Ainu whom he had visited while in Sakhalin were most instructive as well as inspirational to me.

Somehow, I have been lucky in my anthropological career in that some of the established scholars, with whom I originally had no personal connections, have opted to encourage me in my research endeavors. Professor Robert J. Smith of Cornell University, in particular, has generously extended his help and encouragement. Others include Professors Alfonso Ortiz, John J. Stephan, Shinichiro Takakura, Shiro Hattori, and Chester S. Chard. I have learned from them how to give to my students and young scholars.

My warmest personal appreciation goes to my parents, Kozaburo and Taka Ohnuki, whose unconditional love has been the source of strength in my life. They have also helped me in my research in many practical ways. I thank my husband Tim and our sons Alan Ohnuki and Roderic Kenji for teaching me the meaning, beauty, and joy of life. They have been most generous in letting me be obsessed with writing, especially during the summer of 1979, when they even had to go on vacation without me. I dedicate this book to my family members with profound gratitude and affection.

EMIKO OHNUKI-TIERNEY

Madison, Wisconsin
February 1981

Ainu phonemes

Ainu spoken on the northwest coast and used in this book is one of the six Sakhalin Ainu dialects investigated by linguists and is labeled the *Raichishika dialect* (Hattori, ed., 1964:18).

Phonemes
vowel – /i, e, a, o, u/
length – /:/
consonants – /p, t, k, č, s, m, n, r, h/
semivowels – /w, y/

Syllabic patterns
V   – as in /oha/ "empty"
VC_2 – as in /ah/ "Japanese wych elm." S. Hattori does not include this
           pattern (Hattori, ed., 1964:34).
C_1V – as in /kačo/ "drum"
C_1VC_2 – as in /kimun/ "mountain"
         Where C_1 = p, t, k, č, s, m, n, r, h, w, y
         Where C_2 = s, m, n, h, w, y

Vowels

	Front	Central	Back	English approximation
High	i		u	/i/ as in s*i*t
Mid	e		o	/e/ as in b*e*t
Low		a		/a/ as in r*o*d
				/o/ as in *o*bey
				/u/ as in p*u*t

/i/ – A high front unrounded vowel
/e/ – A mid front unrounded vowel
/a/ – A central low unrounded vowel
/o/ – A mid back rounded vowel
/u/ – A high back rounded vowel

Length

I heard a clear contrast between short and long vowels. Hattori also interprets length as phonemic in the Raichishika dialect (Hattori, ed., 1964:42). Chiri, however, claims that length is not phonemic in all the Ainu dialects (Chiri 1956:123).

Consonants

/p, t, k/ – Bilabial, alveolar, and velar stops. They have both voiced and voiceless allophones.

   In my analysis, the stops at the initial position are more often voiceless, but this is merely a tendency. By usage, in some words they are pronounced usually as voiceless and in others as voiced regardless of the position. For example, /kahkemah/ "wife of a great person," was always [gahkemah], and /putuhka/ (a personal name) as [butuhka], whereas /kaama/ "to set a trap" as [kaama] and /pu:ri/ "custom" as [pu:ri]. There are also words pronounced either with a voiceless stop or a voiced stop. For example, /tonkori/ is pronounced sometimes as [tonkori] and other times as [donkori]. On the whole, words with a voiceless stop at any position outnumber those with a voiced stop.

   Chiri states that the voiceless allophones are the more standard pronunciation and that the voiced ones are used more often by Japanized Ainu (Chiri 1956:124–5). Hattori claims that the stops are usually voiceless at the initial position, especially at the beginning of an utterance (Hattori, ed., 1964:34). According to Tae Okada, in the Hidaka dialect of Hokkaido, the voiceless are used at the initial position, but are in "free variation" elsewhere (cited in Raun et al. 1965:124).

/č/ – A predorsal affricate, with [j] as a voiced allophone.

/s/ – Voiceless alveolar spirant, with an alveopalatal spirant as an allophone. /s/ is more frequent. It is highly palatalized before or after /i/, as in /sis/ "eye."

/m/ & /n/ – Bilabial and alveolar nasal resonants, respectively.

/r/ – A short voiced alveolar flap.

/h/ – A voiceless glottal fricative. At the final position, it is a very soft voiceless fricative with the same articulation as that of the preceding vowel, e.g., /ahkas/ "to walk" = [aạkas], /ohkayo/ "man" = [oọkayo].

Semivowels

/w/ & /y/ – Bilabial and alveopalatal resonants, respectively.

In my analysis, accent is not phonemic in the Raichishika dialect used in this book. Hattori considers accent as nonphonemic in the Bihoro and

Raichishika dialects but phonemic in all the other Hokkaido dialects (Hattori, ed., 1964:35). Chiri, however, argues that accent is phonemic in all the Ainu dialects, including all the Sakhalin Ainu dialects (Chiri 1956:142–56).

Hattori includes /'/, which is [?] at the initial position and simply a tension in the throat between two vowels (Hattori, ed., 1964:34). I did not hear such a sound. Moreover, in Hattori's notation it is predictable, appearing either at the beginning of a word when the next (in his interpretation) phoneme is a vowel, or between two successive vowels when the vowels are different (Hattori, ed., 1964). Therefore I do not consider it necessary to postulate the existence of this phoneme.

Both [ŋ] and [l] may be phonemic. Each was heard only in one word, however. [ŋ] was in the Ainu pronunciation of a Gilyak personal name [koyŋahte] and [l] in onomatopoeia of the cry of a crow [holowlowlow] with the same pronunciation as the English dark /l/.

The most important works by linguists on Sakhalin Ainu include Kindaichi (1960:337–62), Chiri (1942, 1953, 1954, 1956, 1962), Hattori (1957, 1961; Hattori, ed., 1964), and Pilsudski (1912). Works by Pilsudski and Kindaichi are based on the dialects on the east coast of southern Sakhalin. Chiri's works include dialects as far north as Ustomonaypo but do not include the Raichishika dialect. Hattori worked intensively with my key informant, Husko, and his analysis of the Raichishika dialect is of high scholarly quality.

1

Introduction: aims and scope of the book

The major objective of this book is a critical evaluation of theories in symbolic anthropology, structuralism, linguistic anthropology, and medical anthropology and to suggest possible directions for theoretical development of these fields. In so doing, the book also makes a contribution to the field of ethnomedicine (the study of people's view of health and illness) by suggesting ways in which this field can contribute to anthropological theory and by adding to the existing body of ethnographic data. The third objective of the book is to contribute to the study of the Ainu – hunter-gatherers known by most of us yet little understood – by describing their views of illness.

I will begin in reverse order, with a brief discussion of the second and third objectives, and then devote the rest of the Introduction to theoretical issues – the major objectives of this book.

Hunter-gatherers, whose mode of subsistence represents 99% of our evolutionary past, are currently in the anthropological limelight. As the pendulum has once again swung back from an extreme form of cultural relativism, anthropologists are now more eager to accept not only the biochemical basis of our personality and social behavior but also the idea of long-range genetic programming. A famous statement by Washburn and Lancaster (1972:293) is, "In a very real sense our intellect, interest, emotions, and basic social life – all are evolutionary products of the success of the hunting adaptation." For those who concur, the swing in anthropological opinion means focusing on foraging populations not only to find the range of human variability but also to understand them in order to understand ourselves.

Whatever their position on sociobiology may be (see Sahlins 1976b), the intensive examination of foraging populations is an important task for anthropologists. Together with Tasmanians, Australians, and a few others, the Ainu rank among the "classic" peoples in anthropological literature; yet even such simple facts as their racial, linguistic, and cultural identity are still not known, especially in the English-speaking world. This lack of information about the Ainu is partially due to historical and linguistic factors. World War II cut off access to the Ainu by outside scholars. Also,

1

because most of the literature on the Ainu is written in Japanese, with a few studies in Russian and other European languages, the dissemination of information on the Ainu into the English-speaking world has been severely curtailed. Furthermore, the majority of publications on the subject deal with the Hokkaido Ainu. This book, then, provides ethnographic information about the little-known Sakhalin Ainu – specifically, those on the northwest coast of southern Sakhalin, about whom no other anthropologist has systematically written.

Although anthropological literature abounds in information about non-Western medicine, during the first half of the twentieth century ethnographic data on illness and healing were often gathered and interpreted only as they related to subject matters central to anthropological interests of the time. Thus, shamanism and witchcraft, for example, drew attention from anthropologists more as magico/religious activities and methods of social control than as aspects of non-Western medical systems. This lack of focus on non-Western medicine is peculiar, because most anthropologists experience severe cases of illness in the field; many spend their first day lying down with a fever or dysentery. They also observe many cases of illness afflicting their informants and witness the subsequent curing procedures. Yet, as Carstairs (1977:1) notes, in the past "it was rare indeed for concepts of health, ill-health and cure to form the centre of inquiry" in anthropology.

How do we account for this glaring blind spot? The explanation, at least in part, comes from the major premise of this book: We look at our world from a cultural perspective – a theme soon to be elaborated. In other words, even anthropologists share with fellow members of Western societies an unconscious bias toward an unquestioning faith in Western scientific medicine. Indeed, the decline of interest during the first half of this century in indigenous concepts of illness in anthropology is paralleled by significant and rapid advances in Western medicine, especially in bacteriology and parasitology, during the same period. Might it be that, even for anthropologists, who often claim to be less culture-bound than other members of their society, the advancement of scientific medicine was "of such compelling importance that traditional concepts of illness seemed positively irrelevant" (Carstairs 1977:1)?

If anthropologists were influenced by their own society during the first half of the twentieth century, the recent resurgence of interest in non-Western medical systems is also a manifestation of this influence. After seeing some of the devastating effects of extreme technological development and realizing that human ailments may not simply be reduced to "biomedical thing" (Fabrega 1975), we have started to look for alternative ways of life and alternative medical systems. Holistic health, natural food, and the growing tendency of people to be personally responsible for their physical and mental health are only a few signs of this new direction in American society. As a consequence, ethnomedicine now receives considerable attention and is considered an indispensable starting point even in biomedical approaches within medical anthropology, a field that has rapidly become central to our discipline.

As a result, many studies of non-Western medical systems are now available. However, most of these studies concentrate on in-depth interpretations of certain aspects of non-Western medicine. Rarely do we find a discussion of the entire domain of a particular medical system. Yet in order to understand how a population deals with its problems of health and illness, one must examine the entire domain of illness, carefully codifying what phenomena are included and how the different parts are interrelated. This book is an attempt to fill this gap by examining the entirety of Ainu medicine. It therefore deals not only with serious illnesses in which the Ainu see the involvement of demons, deities, and other significant beings of the universe as pathogens, sources of healing power or etiologies but also with aches, boils, and other minor ailments, as well as the healing methods for all of these illnesses.

In so doing, this book demonstrates that an ethnomedical study can make a significant contribution to anthropological theories. Medical anthropology, including ethnomedicine, is still a new field. Hopper (1979) perceptively describes medical anthropology currently as experiencing "pre-paradigm crises" – a term Kuhn (1962) used to refer to periods of confusion and dissension in the physical sciences. Indeed, medical anthropology is growing almost too rapidly, and a number of approaches, with incompatible basic assumptions, are competing with each other (Hopper 1979:9). If the field is to remain viable or, better yet, to occupy a central place in anthropology in the future, it must make a unique and significant contribution to theoretical development. This book represents such an effort.

The remainder of the Introduction presents the theoretical issues raised in this book. I begin this task by stating the major premise of the book – the assumption that human beings must order their universe, and that to a large degree the ordering comes from cultural patterning, although age, sex, social position, individual experience, and many other factors are responsible for creating intracultural variations. In the introduction to the translation of *Primitive Classification* by Durkheim and Mauss, Needham (1963) eloquently illustrates this point with an analogy between a person born blind and anthropologists who are culturally blind in a society they attempt to understand. The physically blind must find order and sense in a painful chaos of forms, colors, and sounds, just as anthropologists must do in host societies.

This view was revealed to me early in my anthropological career. It was the first day of plant gathering during my first fieldwork among the Ainu. Early on a fine spring morning, my informant and I stepped out to gather plants in the field in front of her house. Not knowing what to look for, I felt totally lost, whereas my informant, despite her advanced age, spotted every edible and medicinal plant – even those well beyond the scope of my eyesight. She went directly to plants whose useful parts were well developed. The Ainu find different uses for the various parts of a plant. Thus they have different names for each part, often leaving nameless some parts, such as flowers, that are not useful to them. Needless to say, my training in both Japanese and American cultures enabled me to spot only colorful flowers, which are of little concern to the Ainu. It was indeed a startling realization that the highlights in her mental picture of the grass field and those in mine were entirely different. As my aesthetic elevation on a fine spring morning was transformed into a sad feeling of inadequacy as a student of a new culture, I recalled a statement by Whorf (1952:5): "The categories and types that we isolate from the world of phenomena we do not find there because they stare every observer in the face; on the contrary, the world is presented in a kaleidoscopic flux of impressions which is to be organized by our mind. . . ." I had favored this statement despite some fundamental difficulties I saw in the Whorfian hypothesis.

The purpose of my work is to arrive at the basic perceptual structure[1] that enables the Ainu to identify a certain swelling on the body as a "crab boil" and not a "fox boil" or any other type of boil – a distinction the non-Ainu are not equipped to make. I am searching for a model that generates concrete behaviors with their infinite varieties. As an outsider, I attempt to arrive at this model by interpreting the behavior of the Ainu, including their verbal statements. Methodologically, then, I am inductively interpreting Ainu behavior in order to arrive at the Ainu model for behavior. (Compare the now famous distinction between the "model of" and "model for" behavior by Goodenough [1957:167–8], and sharp criticism by Geertz [1973:11] of Goodenough and others.) Returning to the example above, to the extent that most Ainu would identify a certain boil as a crab boil, the perceptual structure I attempt to uncover is public.

Within the broad framework of perceptual structure, my major concern is the problem of classification. Taking Ainu culture as an illustrative example, I question what kind of classificatory system or systems we can find in a given culture. The domain of illness is an especially good area for this exploration. Although the cure of an illness is the major concern and goal of any medical system, this cure must necessarily be preceded by a proper identification of the illness. Therefore, in any society, an illness must be identified, immediately if not instantly, so that a proper cure may be administered. As Kleinman notes, "Classification of disease is, in fact, the first therapeutic act" (1974:209).

This process entails identifying an illness in relation to other illnesses and involves the entire classificatory schema. In other words, to classify a swelling as a crab boil, the Ainu must first identify it as a boil, rather than any other category of illness; second, they must recognize that it is not a fox boil or a lamprey boil but instead a crab boil.

To interpret the Ainu classification system, I examine the entire domain of Ainu illness. This starts with a brief introduction to the Ainu way of life on the northwest coast of Sakhalin, providing ethnographic background on the people. In Chapter 3, after outlining the field of ethnomedicine, I examine the problem of codifying the Ainu domain of illness and pose such questions as: Are all illness labeled as "illnesses" (*araka* in Ainu), or are some phenomena considered as departures from health but not commonly referred to as illnesses? Here the reader first encounters a theme that runs through the book – the problem of language and cognition or, more broadly, the problem of evidence for the presence of a conceptual form. In Chapter 4, I outline the major characteristics of minor ailments, such as the body-part illnesses and skin abnormalities, which I call *habitual illnesses;* details of each illness are found in Appendixes A and B. In contrast to a biomedical tradition in which we customarily look for the cause of a disease, Ainu habitual illnesses are minutely defined in terms of symptoms, but pathogens and etiologies are generally ignored. Furthermore, these minor illnesses are meticulously classified into a taxonomic system.

Chapter 5 attempts to reveal the taxonomic principles underlying the classification of these minor illnesses. I examine ten headaches, including four land animal headaches (e.g., the bear headache) and three sea animal headaches (e.g., the octopus headache), and nine boils, including five land animal boils and four sea animal boils. Most intriguing is the fact that the classificatory principles of these illnesses – which are seemingly uninteresting, at least for outsiders, and relatively unimportant even for the Ainu – parallel the principles that govern the spatial classification of the universe, one of the most basic perceptual structures.

In Chapter 6, I describe the more serious illnesses, which I call *metaphysical illnesses,* and their healing ritual. These metaphysical illnesses involve such spiritual beings as a spirit, a soul, a deity, or a demon either in the etiology, as a pathogen, or as the source of healing power. Causal factors are the defining characteristics of metaphysical illnesses for which symptoms are only broadly defined. Their identification rests upon the diagnosis of individual shamans, who also prescribe the cure.

Chapters 1 to 6 lay the groundwork for subsequent chapters in which I discuss broader aspects of Ainu symbolic structure and relate them to more general theoretical issues in symbolic, medical, and linguistic anthropology, as well as structuralism. In Chapter 7, I relate symbols in the

concepts of illness and healing rituals to the basic symbolic structure of
the Ainu, which consists of the /sacred: profane/ dyad. Negative symbolic
power, conceived as pathogens and etiological agents and personified as
demons, estranged souls, and so on, is seen to relate to a symbolic anomaly that threatens the Ainu symbolic system. In other words, the life–
death struggle in real life is a mirror image of a struggle between structure
and antistructure, or between order and disorder. On the other hand, the
positive power of healing seen in the symbols of healing and preventive
rituals represents the profane half of the /sacred:profane/dyad. These
symbols derive their power from their symbolic identification with the
Ainu way of life. Therefore, the task of fortifying the basic dyadic structure against the antistructural threat is assigned to the profane half of the
dyad.

Ainu data on symbolic anomalies as pathogens and etiologies of illness
suggest that symbolic analysis of illness necessitates a close scrutiny not
only of the classification system(s) of a people but, even more importantly,
of the "unclassifiable" – the area of investigation crucial for theoretical
advancement in symbolic classification and other structural approaches in
anthropology. If one takes the view that the human mind requires a
certain degree of ordering to perceive the environment, and that ordering
derives mainly from cultural patterning, what are clearly symbolic expressions of the unclassifiable demand explanation. Many scholars have
offered valuable interpretations (Beidelman 1963; Steiner 1967). Because
of an early and perceptive work by van Gennep (1961; originally 1909),
the problem of temporal liminality and the related problem of ritual
reversal have received particular attention by many scholars, including
Leach (1963) and Turner (1967, 1969).

Despite advances made by these scholars, the problem of symbolic
expressions of the unclassifiable, that is, anomaly, requires further clarification. First, conceptually, a better delineation of those unclassifiables
that receive further symbolic meaning as being abnormal, anomalous,
ambiguous, marginal, liminal, and so on is necessary. The range of
phenomena often labeled by these terms seems to include several distinct
types of classificatory inversions. I choose *anomaly* as a generic term
referring to symbolic expressions of the unclassifiable. Thus, we urgently
need a classification of anomaly, if I may use these terms in seeming contradiction to each other.

Second, statements about the unclassifiable in anthropological literature often switch too easily from a symbol of the unclassifiable in a particular culture to such phenomena as dirt or viscosity, which are seen to
symbolize the unclassifiable in the human mind. The juxtaposition of emic
and etic treatment often confuses the issue. It seems to me that at this
point in the development of the anthropology of folk classification, we

need a more meticulous analysis of a symbolic structure or structures in a particular culture. Only then would we be able to identify symbolic expressions of the unclassifiable within that system. For example, after the discovery of classificatory principles that order the domain of animals (which may include creatures not classified as animals in Western zoology and exclude those that are), a particular animal can be identified as unclassifiable. To those of us with a Western zoological orientation, the duck-billed platypus may be an apt symbol of the unclassifiable. However, in order to prove that it is so among an Australian population, their emic explanation must be clearly spelled out. This is particularly important because if one chooses to be arbitrary, most phenomena can be presented as unclassifiable. In addition, we must examine whether the platypus remains as a simple taxonomically aberrant form or becomes a symbol of classificatory inversions.

Third, a problem in symbolic classification that has hitherto received little attention is the relationship, if any, between the anomalous symbols and those of mediation. Turner (1969), Douglas (1966), and others have expounded upon a strong ritual power generated by an anomalous symbol that challenges an existing structure and that may indeed create a new one. At the same time, these scholars and others, notably Lévi-Strauss, point out that the lack of structural or classificatory constraints is also the basis for a certain being or object becoming a symbol of mediation; the act of mediation necessitates crossing categorical boundaries. Whereas anomaly poses an antistructural threat, mediation fortifies the structure by strengthening the relationships among categories within it. I have not encountered any scholar who has explored the relationship between anomaly and mediation – both sharing the structural feature of being nonclassifiable and yet having diametrically opposite effects. We must then attempt to discover when an unclassifiable element generates a negative power threatening the structure, when an antistructural power creates a new order, and when it generates a positive power of mediation.

In Chapter 7, I attempt to clarify these points about the anthropological understanding of symbolic anomaly in relation to symbolic structure by using Ainu data. In Chapter 8, my interpretations of Ainu data are placed against a broader theoretical background. The two chapters complement each other. In them I use two major analytical frameworks. First, to understand anomaly in a particular symbolic structure, I find it crucial to examine the relationship among such symbolic oppositions as /nature:culture/, /sacred:profane/, and /men:women/ as they are defined in that system. My major proposition here is that if animals are deified, nature is sacred in that symbolic system. If they are not, as in the Judeo-Christian religion, then nature is "beastly," and hence humans must sharply differentiate themselves from animals. The interrelationships among God or deities, animals, and humans is therefore crucial in determining the nature of symbolic oppositions of /nature:culture/, /sacred:profane/, and /men:women/.

Second, there is a clear analytical advantage in allowing multiple symbolic systems within a culture, or at least two sets: formalized and nonformalized. Only then can we unfold an intricate dialectic between the two sets. This dialectic, at least in the Ainu system, allows us to understand how a symbol with a negative meaning or power in one system receives a positive meaning and power in the other. A mystery such as the symbolic significance of menstrual blood becomes intelligible. It is assigned a negative meaning in the public domain, where the formalized symbolic system prevails, but it is endowed with strong positive power in the nonformalized symbolic system, which governs the domestic domain.

Another emphasis in Chapter 7 is a tripartite approach to the study of perception that recognizes the cognitive, emotive, and sensory dimensions of perception. A frequent diatribe against Lévi-Strauss – his focus on rationality or cognition – is now pointing the way to a new direction in anthropology. In the forefront of the attack is Geertz, who sees Lévi-Strauss as the direct descendant of the French Enlightenment, epitomized in Rousseau (Geertz 1973:356–8). Geertz urges us to bring together mind and emotion, or cognition with affection. He eloquently points out that a world view is "made emotionally acceptable" by an ethos, and an ethos is "made intellectually reasonable" by a world view (1973:127). The key to understanding the two is the sacred (religious) symbols that, according to Geertz, have "peculiar power... to identify fact with value at the most fundamental level" (1973:127).

The emphasis on the emotive dimensions of symbol perception is echoed in Turner's notion of "evocative symbols" and the "emotional resonance of symbols," as well as in works by Douglas, Beidelman, and many others. It should be remembered, however, that Durkheim and Mauss did give credit to emotion. In fact, they proclaimed that the "emotional value of notions... is the dominant characteristic in classification," although they excluded it from their treatment because "emotion... is something essentially fluid and inconsistent" (1963:86–7). In understanding symbol perception, anthropologists have now begun to stress the importance of the emotive dimension, but they have not successfully demonstrated how to deal with it. Medical symbols promise to be a fruitful area of investigation for this endeavor, because people in most societies react to illnesses with the strongest emotions.

The third dimension in symbolic perception, which has received virtually no systematic treatment by anthropologists, is the sensory one. Might it be that even chimpanzees can perceive a sign with their senses, and hence that our "symbolic perception" must be sharply differentiated from theirs? In perceiving the universe, we human beings not only think and feel with our emotions but also feel with our senses. To a large degree, the use of our senses is culturally patterned too. For example, in early infancy there is a stage when infants in any society start to perceive their social and behavioral environment largely through the use of their tactile sense. Every culture sooner or later instructs them as to where, when, what, and who to touch. Such scholars of communication as McLuhan (1964) and Hall (1969) have offered perceptive comments on the use of senses and its cultural patterning. Their observations and insights, however, have not been systematically incorporated in anthropological studies of symbol perception. Illness again is an excellent area for this investigation, because illnesses are often perceived through various senses. Even in the vision-dominated American culture, pain throbs and pounds; it is auditorily felt, or at least expressed as such. Ainu data are rich in information on the use of senses in illness perception. How the Ainu hear, touch, smell, and see their animals, plants, and other phenomena of the universe are translated into how they experience their illnesses. I therefore take a tripartite approach to the Ainu perception of medical symbols. My concern is with how the Ainu think and feel, with emotions and with senses, about their state of health and illness, although my data on the emotive dimension are not as rich as those on the cognitive and sensory dimensions.

It is in the matters of health and illness that any people most dramatically reveal the fusion of the cognitive, emotive, and sensory dimensions of their perception. Thus, the domain of illness is a uniquely rewarding field in which to investigate the three dimensions of our perception.

In Chapter 9, I return to the problem of classification. The purpose of discovering any classificatory schema is not just to pigeonhole all the members of a particular domain but ultimately to find classificatory principles. Binary opposition as a classificatory principle, for example, does not mean a simple division of the whole into two when the dichotomy is a natural way to divide. Sorting out red balls from yellow balls when a pile consists of only red and yellow balls is not evidence that the people or the individual who divided the balls used binary opposition. Furthermore, a particular feature(s) that distinguishes the items in category A from those in category B must be specified. In other words, the minimal distinctive feature must be determined, if possible (Jakobson, Fant, and Halle 1967:esp. 2–3). Instead of binary opposition, trinary or other kinds of classificatory principles may be at work; or the simultaneous presence of more than one system within a culture may be involved, as Needham suggests (1963:xix). In fact, so far there has been little ethnographic evidence to assure an equal degree of classificatory complexity in every part of even a single domain, especially when the domain is fairly broad and complex, such as illness. These are some of the issues addressed in Chapter 9. In this chapter, I again consider the problem of a tripartite approach to perception and its cultural patterning in order to place my interpretation of the Ainu case in Chapter 7 against the broader theoretical background.

Chapter 10, on language and cognition, focuses on the problem of evidence for the presence of a conceptual form. In part, the chapter is also an explanation of my methodology, which combines symbolic classification and ethnosemantics. Although the two approaches share an interest in arriving at folk classification, ethnosemantics differs sharply from symbolic classification in its basic premise that culturally significant categories must have lexical expressions – a basic problem in language and cognition. A comparison of ethnosemantics, the Whorfian hypothesis, and symbolic classification – three approaches in anthropology that attempt to arrive at conceptual forms – indicates that no particular linguistic or nonlinguistic structure can claim to be the only means of expressing a conceptual form. Furthermore, broad and complex conceptual forms tend to be only vaguely defined and are less amenable to a method of investigation such as ethnosemantics; a general ethnographic method seems to be more fruitful. I advocate a clear distinction between individual beliefs and culturally shared conceptual forms; it is only the latter that we anthropologists seek. I also hypothesize that this distinction is crucial in understanding that more complex ideas involve the beliefs of individuals and therefore must be quite broad and simple as collective representations.

The major part of Chapter 11 diverges from the issues involved in symbolic perception and classification and examines shamans as social personae in Ainu society. The chapter starts by describing who shamans are in Ainu society and then discusses the multiple roles of Ainu shamans. The next section examines in detail the relationships of the politically and socially marginal status of many shamans to the nonformalized power assigned to the shaman's role. I then briefly discuss whether some Ainu shamans are not only politically peripheral but also have major psychological difficulties. For this purpose, I introduce the psychobehavioral disorder known among the Ainu as *imu:*; its detailed description is presented in Appendix C. In the last section of Chapter 11 I return to the problem of symbolic system and explore the relationship between symbolic power assigned to the profane and marginal symbols in Ainu shamanistic rituals and the nonformalized sociopolitical power assigned to shamans.

Throughout the book, but especially in Chapters 4, 5, 6, and 7, I try to separate descriptions from my own interpretations. But this format contradicts the basic theme of the book – that we all look at our universe with cultural biases. Therefore, what I recorded as data may itself reveal my cultural perspective; I may have missed other types of data that are important, especially to the Ainu. Yet, in my anthropological research, I have used my theoretical orientations and anthropological curiosity as tools of data retrieval. When I found patterns and structures after laboriously combing through my data, I basked in warm rays of sunshine; perhaps I am obsessed with regularities. However, my aim has never been to find regularities when the data deny their presence. Nor has it been to reduce human behavior to the skeletal framework that anthropologists call patterns, structures, and so on. At the risk of making a hasty compromise between Geertz and the approaches he opposes, my aim in anthropology, as in this book, is to arrive at meaningful "thick description" (Geertz 1973), and thick description renders meaning when I discover its skeletal framework or structure. Furthermore, by presenting as much ethnographic data as possible, rather than simply data that support my interpretations, I can provide others with a chance to examine them and perhaps disagree with me. Hopefully those with different theoretical orientations or different problems may still find my work useful for their purposes.

An etic/emic comparison is a tradition in ethnosemantics, and some medical anthropologists are now urging cross-cultural comparisons. I attempt neither a comparison of biomedicine and Ainu medicine nor a comparison of Ainu medicine and another nonbiomedical medical tradition. As will be discussed in Chapter 3, biomedicine as developed in Western societies involves a great deal of Western cultural tradition that must be sifted out before it can be a candidate for an etic framework. Any cross-cultural comparison of illness categories in particular is a formidable task, especially if we focus upon classificatory principles rather than a simple pigeonholing of illness categories. For example, a category of cancer, defined in terms of etiology in biomedicine, simply does not exist in nonbiomedical traditions. A tuberculosis in biomedicine may be equivalent to several illnesses in another medical system. This is the case with the Ainu medical system. An illness called *kemasinke* (blood-vomiting illness) includes not only tuberculosis of the lung at its final stage, but it may also include other illnesses such as peptic ulcer and stomach cancer. Yet, other expressions of tuberculosis, such as tuberculosis of the bone, and their stages of development are not included in *kemasinke* because they are not accompanied by hemoptysis. Furthermore, tuberculosis, ulcer, and cancer with hemoptysis may not, after all, be classified as *kemasinke* because some cases of blood vomiting are interpreted as the work of sorcery. In general, most diseases during their incubation periods are excluded from Ainu illness categories because of the lack of symptoms. Yet, a group of Ainu illnesses discussed in Chapters 5 and 6 are defined primarily in terms of pathogens and etiologies, which are supernatural in nature, and symptoms are given only secondary importance. An even more striking illustration of Ainu concepts is the case of a scratch from a bear. Whereas cuts, bruises, and burns are normally not even illnesses, a cut inflicted by a bear, no matter how small, is not even a minor habitual illness but a grave metaphysical illness requiring an elaborate treatment. In short, the Ainu concepts of illness are basically so different from those involved in biomedicine that a comparison between biomedical categories and Ainu illness categories would be quite difficult.

Nor is a comparison of several nonbiomedical traditions an easy task, if we focus upon classificatory principles. Suppose one finds that in another medical system all the incidents of boils that the Ainu would classify as octopus boils are grouped in a single category. Even then, Ainu octopus boils are sorted according to a set of classificatory principles, and at this level of comparison the two categories may not be equivalent.

A brief discussion of the nature of the data used in this book is in order here. I have been able to abstract an extremely rich and complex perceptual structure of the Ainu, with its dynamics of formalized/nonformalized symbolic structures, through an in-depth study of information obtained from a limited number of individuals. This information has been checked thoroughly against available data gathered by other anthropologists and linguists, past and present. The concordances between my ethnographic data on illness and those gathered by others (Chiri 1953, 1954; Chiri and B. Wada 1943; B. Wada 1941, 1956; K. Wada 1964, 1965a) are truly striking. Consider, for example, the description of an Ainu illness called *hana* (not translatable; see Chapter 5). It has about eight symptoms, all of which are included both in my data and in the data collected in the 1940s by Chiri and Wada (1943). Needless to say, my key informant and others had no access to any of the recorded information; they could not read. Although a large number of informants would have been more desirable, an in-depth study such as this one can prove more valuable than a study consisting of a haphazardly construed common denominator of responses obtained from a large number of "unspecified informants" (see Ardener 1971:451).

Having delineated my basic approach, I further clarify my theoretical stance in the remainder of this Introduction by evaluating other approaches in symbolic and medical anthropology that are critical of the structural/symbolic approach. These include an emphasis on process, on behavior, on the individual as an actor, on transaction, and so on – all related to one another. To some anthropologists, the golden age of Lévi-Strauss and structural approaches is over. For them, anthropological emphasis is now upon behavior and ongoing processes, with a focus upon the individual as an actor – a person who can manipulate his or her environment, rather than a passive recipient and a robot in a structure. Thus, political anthropologists are now capitalizing upon political processes, in which individuals are involved in the manipulation of "spoils and strategems" (Bailey 1970). In symbolic studies, Geertz, Turner, and others now emphasize symbols in the "ritual process." For them, studies of native people's "models for perceiving, relating, and otherwise interpreting... things, people, behavior, or emotions" (Goodenough 1957:167) are no longer justifiable. Instead of "competence," we must study "situation" and "performance" themselves (Turner 1975:149), because anthropological interpretations must construct "a reading of what happens," and "it is through the flow of behavior – or more precisely, social action – that cultural forms find articulation" (Geertz 1973:18, 17). Turner (1975: 149–50) refers to this new direction in symbolic anthropology as "the processual symbology" and advocates "performance-analysis and event-analysis," which "involve symbols as agencies and foci of social mobilization, interaction, and styling of behavior."

Ethnomedicine, a field that includes many clinical specialists and scholars in the behavioral sciences, has most readily responded to this direction. It now seems to be one of the dominant approaches in medical anthropology in the United States. Kleinman, the author of a seminal article (1974) on the symbolic study of medicine, once urged the construction of "medemes" – symbolic categories of illness comparable to cognitive categories of ethnosemantics. However, his more recent writings indicate that he now sees little value in such an approach. Kleinman (1977:11) writes: "Lay and professional models of sickness, analyzed in the often exigent setting of sickness episodes, tend to be plural, fragmented, sometimes illogical, and even at times demonstrably contradictory when compared with detailed ethnoscientific reconstructions of 'emic' categories."

A new model in ethnomedicine may be found in a "semantic network" study by Good (1977). He is concerned not with illness categories as cognitive categories but with their instrumental value for the patient, an Iranian woman in this case, as an actor to "negotiate changes" in the behavior of others through "the rhetorical use of illness language" (1977:49).

Although these recent trends involve complex issues, I limit myself to two major themes here: emphasis on behavior and on the individual. Needless to say, anthropologists' raw data have always derived from people's behavior, verbal and nonverbal, in the broadest sense of the term. However, the emphasis on behavior as conceived by some, especially in medical anthropology, goes well beyond the contention that anthropologists must observe. It has a positivistic tenet that only behavior is important and that conceptual forms without evidence in the form of observable behavior are nonexistent or, at least, not worthy of scientific inquiry. This behavioral emphasis has an unfortunate consequence, as Chomsky (1968:58) describes the situation:

We live, after all, in the age of "behavioral science," not of "the science of mind"... But the term "behavioral science" suggests a not-so-subtle shift of emphasis toward the evidence itself and away from the deeper underlying principles and abstract mental structures that might be illuminated by the evidence of behavior. It is as if natural science were to be designated "the science of meter readings." What, in fact, would we expect of natural science in a culture that was satisfied to accept this designation for its activities?

The history of ethnosemantics, discussed in Chapter 10, is most illuminating in this respect. Ethnosemantics set out to locate observable evidence for conceptual forms and discovered "covert categories." To some, this was reason enough to abandon ethnosemantics; for others, it proved the futility of pursuing observable and concrete evidence for conceptual forms at all times.

Perceptual structure is not isomorphic with behavior. A major source of misunderstanding about the relationship between structure and behavior stems from the failure to realize that structure is an abstraction and hence does not correspond to any one specific incidence of behavior. In his spirited attack on the statistical approach "in the positivist West" (Ardener 1971:453), Ardener points out that a program – a concept equivalent to my use of the term *structure* – is "essentially *uncalibrated* to events" (1971:452). His explanation about the power of the program for prediction is also illuminating:

There is a great irony, for the only kind of prediction which has been accepted as "scientific" in positivist social science has been the statistical statement of probability... In contrast the programme is predictive rather of *kinds*... We might use a better terminology, and say that the programme is totally "generative" as to kind of event, but it is not necessarily predictive as to when the events will occur. (Ardener 1971:452)

In the quotation cited earlier, Kleinman raises a question about the relationship between illness categories and the actual diagnostic process. Actual cases of diagnosis are, in my view, the end result of a complex mental operation in which situational and other factors affect the classificatory decisions. The lack of precise illness classification in diagnosis, or the discrepancy between "clinical reality" and an explanatory model (Kleinman 1978a), is to be expected. It hardly constitutes evidence to negate the presence of classificatory structure.

Nor do illnesses falling between two categories deny the presence of a classificatory schema. The problem of "noncontiguous categories" with "intervening areas of low codability" is articulated by Walker (1965:268–9). He argues that "an ideal hierarchical taxonomy" with sharp demarcation lines between the color categories does not account for "the actual American English color taxonomy." In my view, what Walker refers to as an "ideal" taxonomy represents a conceptual structure, whereas his "taxonomy with noncontiguous categories" represents actual phenomena or behavior. Everyone knows that there are pinkish reds and reddish pinks, but the phenomena in no way deny the contrasting conceptual categories of red and pink. Similarly, a particular headache may rarely be typical. But, nonetheless, an octopus headache and a lamprey headache are two separate and contrasting conceptual categories.

What is important here is to clarify the objective of one's investigation. My interest in this book is the perceptual structure underlying behavior, verbal and nonverbal, but *not behavior itself*. To that extent, my objective is scientific:

The whole aim of theoretical science is to carry to the highest possible and conscious degree the perceptual reduction of chaos that began in so lowly and (in all probability) unconscious a way with the origin of life. In specific instances it can well be questioned whether the order so achieved is an objective characteristic of the phenomena or is an artifact constructed by the scientist. That question comes up time after time in animal taxonomy... Nevertheless, the most basic postulate of science is that nature itself is orderly. (Simpson 1961:5)

Although behavior and structure or performance and competence are two different entities, the relationship between them is worthy of scholarly investigation. It would require massive evidence to prove that there is no relationship whatsoever between cognitive or, more broadly, perceptual categories and actual behavior. Meanwhile, I join Ortiz, an eminent Third World anthropologist, who convincingly argues (1969:4–5):

While I concern myself primarily with thought rather than action, with the rules governing conduct rather than the conduct itself, there is such a goodness of fit between the two among the Tewa [the Eastern Pueblos in New Mexico] that such an approach does not serve to mislead. I believe, rather, that this approach serves to inform us in the most general and reliable terms possible about what holds Tewa society together and what gives it point and continuity. Nor do I ignore those instances in which there is not such a goodness of fit between thought and belief on the one hand and conduct on the other, for these instances often serve to lay bare some of the central concerns of Tewa life.

My interpretation of his last statement is that even when there is a misfit between thought and behavior, the misfit tells us something about both, just as the unclassifiable informs us of the structure in which it does not fit. In fact, these misfits must be carefully studied because they may hold the key to the dynamics of thought and behavior, perhaps revealing the force behind the dialectic between thought and behavior – how thought influences behavior and vice versa, thereby facilitating culture change.

As for the Ainu data, it is quite remarkable that, as noted earlier, statements obtained almost forty years ago by Chiri and Wada from Ainu informants regarding illness categories are almost identical to those I received, although during the interval the Ainu have gone through such drastic changes as their relocation to Hokkaido. Even if the Ainu do not precisely follow their cognitive categories when they diagnose illnesses, I find it quite intriguing and worthy of scholarly attention to understand their perceptual structure, which has been so enduring. Furthermore, I would seriously question whether, if their illness categories have had nothing to do with *their* clinical reality, they would have persisted this long.

The new emphasis on the individual complements the study of culture, just as Chapter 11 of this book, with its focus on the individual, complements the rest of the book, which focuses on structure and culture. Although the previously cited semantic network analysis of Good offers an interesting tool for description, the power of the Iranian woman to negotiate changes must be viewed not only from her standpoint but also from that of Iranian culture, in which women have no access to formalized power. Similarly, if I had limited my discussion to the power of an Ainu shaman or the symbolic power of menstrual blood, we would not understand the entire picture. Only when we see nonformalized power within the context of Ainu culture, with its public and domestic domain and its formalized and nonformalized power, do we understand the interplay between the individual and his or her culture or the dialectic between structure and antistructure.

A danger also lurks in the emphasis on the individual as an actor, however. For an individual, especially one outside the "structure" or the "establishment" of a society, to be able to maximize his or her resources in moving toward a goal is an attractive theme for many Americans, who cherish individualism and antistructural heroes and heroines (cf. a "system-beater" hero referred to by Hsu 1973:14). Furthermore, the individual in American society is, from a global point of view, unique, and American society differs basically from many other societies. Here "the economic symbolism is structurally determining," whereas in most other societies "the locus of symbolic differentiation remains social relations, principally kinship relations, and other spheres of activity are ordered by the operative distinctions of kinship" (Sahlins 1976a:211).[2] In interpreting the individual in other societies, we cannot reproduce the individual in American society, for whom relationships with other humans usually are temporary and not ascribed – to be terminated at will. In American society, it is much easier for individuals to maximize their goal, because they are much freer from involvement with other human beings.

An important corollary to this emphasis on the individual and behavior is the focus upon the instrumental values of symbols – how symbols "evoke sentiments and emotions and impel men to action" (Cohen 1974:ix). The emphasis by Geertz and Turner on the emotive dimension of symbols, which was discussed earlier, is partly related to this recent emphasis. In my view, it is very important to stress not only the emotive but also the sensory dimension of symbols and their power of evocation. It is the hypnotic sound of the drum, the aroma of burning plants, or the smell of filth that provokes such strong psychological reactions from the perceiver; it is the sensory appeals that evoke strong emotions. Our conceptual categorization of an item such as dirt may be last in the chain of reactions to the item, which starts with the sensory and is followed by the emotive reaction to its perception. Needless to say, however, these sensory stimuli are interpreted as such and have the power of evocation, not because of their objective properties but because perceivers have the culturally defined sensory image and concept in their minds.

A study of the instrumental value of symbols should not be confused with or replace the structural approach to symbols, which investigates what symbols are and what the perceptual structure behind them is; processual symbology studies, instead, how symbols are used.

This discussion of the function of symbols leads to my last point about the current trends in medical anthropology. One of the major approaches in medical anthropology today is a study of a medical system as an adaptive system in evolutionary perspective. Fabrega, whose emphases include ethnomedical approaches, also stresses the biocultural approach and believes that "disease . . . reflects broadly environmental adaptation" (Fabrega 1974:296). On this basis, he writes (1974:298): "In this light we should begin to see culture as only partially constraining this more generic biosocial dimension of disease and, on the other hand, as altering in only limited ways the outward appearance or morphology of the form in which disease is expressed in social groups." Again I stress that the adaptive function of a medical system must clearly be differentiated from its structure.

Let us hope that the brilliant statement by Sahlins (1976a:220) is an unnecessary precaution in our future investigations: "A praxis theory based on pragmatic interests and 'objective' conditions is the secondary form of a cultural illusion, and its elaborate empirical and statistical offspring, the 'etic' investigations of our social sciences, the intellectual titillation of an 'emic' mystification."

Used cautiously, however, the recent emphases in medical and symbolic anthropology serve to complement the structural approach. Together, these approaches can yield a better understanding of the human mind and behavior from the perspective of individuals and of the culture and society to which they belong. Neither approach should harden into stifling or stultifying dogma.

2

The Ainu

This chapter provides an ethnographic background of the Ainu people. After briefly introducing the Ainu people, and then the Sakhalin Ainu in particular, it outlines how the Ainu of the northwest coast of southern Sakhalin lived during the first half of the twentieth century. The primary emphasis is on their social, political, and economic activities and structures. This does not mean that their economic and political spheres are independent of the symbolic structure. On the contrary, I view culture as symbolic systems that express themselves in any of these activities, including what we call economic or political. Only for the purpose of presentation, I resort to these labels that express essentially etic views (see Sahlins 1976a).

The Ainu

The Ainu are a group of people in northeast Asia whose traditional way of life was based upon a hunting, fishing, and plant-gathering economy. Although only about 18,000 Ainu now live in Hokkaido, the northernmost island of Japan, this population used to be much larger and their homeland included southern Sakhalin, the Kurile islands, northern parts of Honshu (the main island of Japan), and adjacent areas (see Figure 2.1).

Not only was the hunting-gathering economy of the Ainu vastly different from that of their neighbors (the Japanese, Koreans, and Chinese), who had been agriculturalists for centuries, but they spoke a different language and bore different physical characteristics. The Ainu's most frequently cited distinguishing physical characteristic is abundant body and facial hair, which contrasts sharply to the lack or sparcity of hair in the neighboring Mongoloid populations. Some males even have hair on the shoulders and back, and their custom of growing long beards accentuates the abundance and waviness of their hair. Other features considered to distinguish the Ainu from other peoples in the area, especially the Japanese, are the tendency to dolichocephaly (long-headedness), a well-developed glabella, a deeply depressed nose root, widely projecting

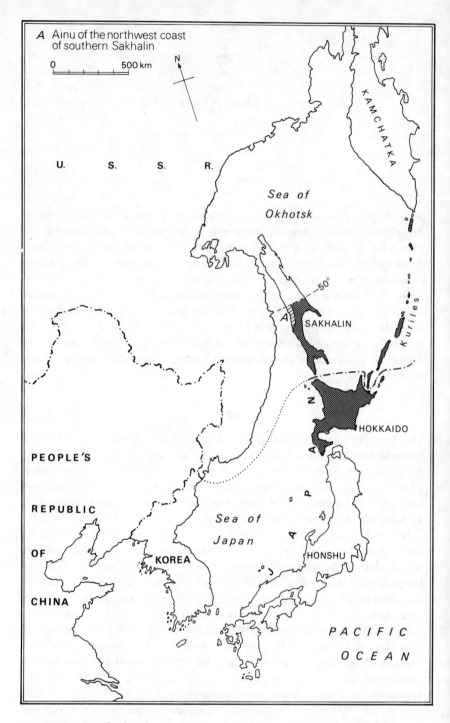

Figure 2.1.   Ainu land in the recent past and the location of the northwest coast Ainu.

cheek bones, a comparatively massive mandible (lower jaw), and an edge-to-edge bite.

The cultural, biological, and linguistic identity of the Ainu is not only intriguing in itself but also holds one of the keys to a broader anthropological problem – the peopling of the Old and New Worlds. The Ainu land is situated at a strategic location through which early migrants may have passed from the Old to the New World. Are the Ainu one of the peoples who stopped short of crossing the Bering Straits to the New World, when waves of big game hunters and gatherers were pushing their way through the Asian continent? Or do they represent a population that claimed the land before the ancestors of the native Americans passed through, as Birdsell (1951:19–20) maintains? Are they so-called genetic remnants like the Negritos, as Chard (1968) proposes? Also linked to the problem of Ainu identity is the relation of the prehistoric populations on the Japanese archipelago to the Ainu, on the one hand, and to the present-day Japanese, on the other. Who are the original inhabitants of the Japanese archipelago – the ancestors of the Ainu, those of the Japanese, both, or neither?

With all these pressing questions of interest and significance, scholars in various fields, including archaeology, human biology, genetics, linguistics, and sociocultural anthropology, have attempted to decipher the Ainu identity for over a century since outsiders first started to pay serious attention to the presence of the Ainu in the Far East corner. To put the conclusions first, we are still not certain of the Ainu identity and their relation to other peoples in the area, although we have a far better understanding of the Ainu people and their life as a result of endeavors by a number of scholars. Although the Ainu affiliation with the Caucasoid race was a prominent theory among early scholars, recent investigators favor Ainu affinity with other Mongoloid peoples in this part of the world. Also seen as probable is an interpretation that the Ainu are descendants of one segment of the Jomon people – a prehistoric hunting-gathering population who made the oldest known pottery in the world and who occupied the Japanese archipelago between 10,000 B.C. and 300 B.C. (Details of scholarly interpretations of the Ainu identity are found in Appendix D.)

Although the blanket term "Ainu" is often used by outsiders, as I have done above, Ainu culture is not monolithic but is rich in intracultural variation. Traditionally, the Ainu have been divided into the Hokkaido, Sakhalin, and Kurile Ainu. Although the designations "Hokkaido Ainu" and "Sakhalin Ainu" coincide with their residence, that is, Hokkaido and southern Sakhalin respectively, the label "Kurile Ainu" has been used in two ways. Some scholars include the Ainu on all of the Kuriles, whereas others include only the Ainu on the central and northern Kuriles. In the latter use, the Ainu on the southern Kuriles are excluded on the basis that they lead a life similar to that of the Hokkaido Ainu; Hokkaido and the southern Kuriles occupy the same ecological zone as well. The last of the Kurile Ainu died in 1941 (Kodama 1972a:17). The designations "Hokkaido Ainu," "Sakhalin Ainu," and "Kurile Ainu" do not simply represent a mechanical division of the Ainu on the basis of their geographical location; each reflects a distinctive way of life. In fact, even within each group, Ainu culture and society differed from region to region. Generally speaking, from the point of view of complexity in technology and social organization, the Kurile Ainu had the smallest and simplest society with the least-developed technological skills, whereas the Hokkaido Ainu formed the most complex society and culture, with the Sakhalin Ainu midway between them. Two major factors responsible for these regional differences are the adaptation to the local environment and the history of contact with outsiders. (For details of intracultural variation and the history of contact of each group, see Ohnuki-Tierney 1976a.)

The Sakhalin Ainu

Sakhalin is a small, long, narrow island located north of Japan and along the coast of the Eurasian continent, from which it is separated only by the narrow Tartar Strait (see Fig. 2.1). It is only 28,597 square miles in area, roughly comparable in size to Ireland. Southern Sakhalin is mountainous except for two sizable interior plains. Its climate is severely cold and humid during many months of the year, with an average temperature in the south of 17 degrees Fahrenheit in January and 63 degrees Fahrenheit in July.

The island is rich in natural resources. Its coasts, rivers, and lakes abound in salmon, trout, herring, cod, and king crab, as well as seals and other sea mammals. Whales, although abundant, come only to the more southern coasts. A diverse assortment of fauna and flora are found on the island. The bear is the largest animal as well as the most important to the Ainu, but there are also musk deer, reindeer, otter, marten, fox, and several other fur bearers. Out of a flora of 1,000 species, 95 are trees such as larch, fir, spruce, and birch. The island is also rich in coal, iron, gold, silver, and other metals, as well as oil and natural gas, although they were not utilized by the Ainu.

For the past several hundred years the Ainu have occupied the southern half of the island of Sakhalin, approximately south of 50 degrees north latitude, with the remainder in the hands of the Gilyaks. There is also a small number of other indigenous populations on the island, such as the Oroks and Nanays, as they are now called in the Soviet Union. We do not know when the Sakhalin Ainu first arrived in southern Sakhalin. The little information we do have on the prehistory of the island (see Ohnuki-

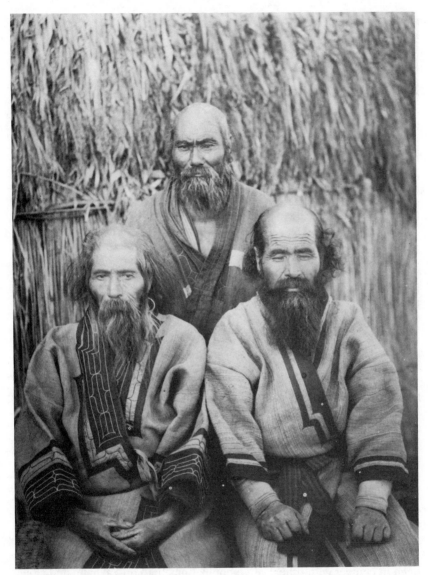

Three Sakhalin Ainu men (Kajima 1895).

Tierney 1968:384–91) is not helpful here. Chiri (1954:457), on the basis of
Ainu oral tradition, and Hattori (1956:130), applying the lexicostatistical
method to various Ainu dialects, both suggest 600 B.P. as the approxi-
mate date of separation of the Sakhalin Ainu from the Hokkaido Ainu.
However, other types of evidence point to a much earlier date. Our best

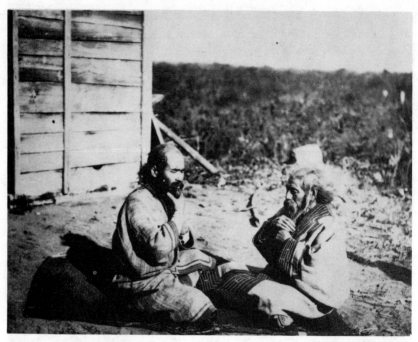

Greetings between two Sakhalin Ainu men (Kajima 1895).

guess is that they moved to the island from Hokkaido (Chard 1968) possibly as early as the beginning of the first millennium A.D. but definitely by the thirteenth century (Stephan 1971:20–1).

Censuses of the Sakhalin Ainu, taken at different times between the end of the nineteenth century and 1945, have given population estimates of 1,200 to 2,400 (the Hokkaido Ainu, by comparison, are estimated at between 15,000 and 17,000). These census figures include all who have any Ainu ancestry, no matter how little. Often, however, the counts fail to include those Ainu in remote areas, such as the settlements on the northwest coast, and thus are not reliable.

The Sakhalin Ainu have by no means been isolated. They have always been in contact with other native populations both on Sakhalin and along the Amur River. They also have been in contact with the Chinese, Russians, and Japanese, all of whom have exploited both the Ainu and their land. The northwest coast, however, was exempt from major agents of culture change, as seen in historical records as well as in personal observations by scholars. (Details of the history of contact of the Sakhalin Ainu and the assessment of its impact on the northwest coast Ainu are presented in Appendix E.)

The Ainu way on the northwest coast of southern Sakhalin

The basic pattern of movement of the northwest coast Ainu is a seasonal migration between a summer settlement on the shore and a winter settlement farther inland. In the winter settlement, the Ainu build semisubterranean pithouses, often against a hill.[1] Besides the seasonal movement, the Ainu in small communities at times abandon their settlements if an important fish, such as salmon, trout, or herring, ceases to be available in sufficient quantity. The Ainu settlements are located along the shore, with houses in a single file parallel to the shoreline.

The population is extremely sparse on the northwest coast, and many settlements house only a few families. However, there are a few larger settlements, such as Rayčiska, which has five to ten nuclear families. (For details of the population figures, see Ohnuki-Tierney 1976:309–10, footnote 3, and Tables 1, 2, and 3.)

The kinship organization is basically bilateral, with some tendency toward unilineality. Bilaterality is seen in the individual's status at birth, marriage exogamy, classification of kinsmen, and kinship terminology. Unilineality, on the other hand, is recognized in territoriality and the inheritance rule. Thus, although a settlement collectively owns the land and the adjacent water, its territory inherently belongs to the male agnates, who comprise the core members of the settlement. Important fur-bearing animals in a particular locale, such as martens in a river area, are sometimes even more explicitly owned by male agnates. Inheritance rules specify that the male's property is transmitted through the patrilineal line, whereas the female's property goes through the matrilineal line. In both cases, only members of one sex are involved; that is, the father bequeaths to sons and the mother to daughters. Exogamous rules are extended, as noted above, bilaterally to the first cousin. Often a mate is chosen from a related settlement, and it is preferred that the couple be related in some way, either consanguineally or affinally. A few of the more prominent and wealthier members of the society practice polygyny. For a secondary marriage, the levirate is strongly preferred and often practiced. The sororate is not culturally prescribed. The postmarital residence rule is matri-patrilocal for the first wife; a co-wife may either join her husband's household in his settlement or continue to live in her father's settlement.

The nuclear family is the basic social unit among these Ainu. In some cases elderly parents may live with a son's family, but they can also choose to live with a daughter's family. The family is the basic unit for most religious and economic activities, but some economic activities are carried out by members of more than one family or even more than one settlement.

Only the larger settlements have a formal political structure. Smaller settlements often belong politically to nearby large settlements. A large settlement is headed by a nonhereditary headman who is usually not an autocrat. Besides the headman, an assistant headman, official messenger, and/or "deity-headman" sometimes function in positions of responsibility. The messenger goes to related settlements in order to announce significant events such as weddings, funerals, and trials. He also plays an important role in legal cases that involve more than one settlement. Even more respected is a deity-headman, who is always a most revered elder and therefore called "deity" out of respect. If a headman is a revered elder, he can serve in both capacities at the same time. No position of authority represents full-time specialization; they are all held by widely respected men who hunt and fish or used to.

Even the larger settlements are politically autonomous only to a limited degree. Thus, for example, a headman of the Huroŏči settlement is respected for his capacity in handling mundane affairs such as legal cases, whereas the one at the Rayčiska settlement excels in the knowledge of religious matters. The latter often send advice on religious matters to the former, because these messages are considered to have been derived ultimately from the deities. On the other hand, the headman of the Huroŏči settlement gives directions in legal cases to the headman of the Rayčiska settlement. Furthermore, a man from a settlement geographically intermediate between the two serves as a messenger for all three settlements. Also, because the Ainu code requires that the consanguineal kinsmen of both the plaintiff and the defendant normally attend the resolution of a legal case, and because the Ainu in various settlements are often related through kinship ties, a legal case often means joint judgment by people from different settlements.

None of the settlements on the northwest coast is economically self-sufficient, for a settlement customarily depends on adjacent communities for certain foodstuffs. This is true even for the Rayčiska settlement, the largest on the northwest coast and the richest in natural resources; its inhabitants travel annually to the Ustomonaypo settlement for herring. Some economic activities are carried out regularly by people from more than one settlement. These activities include the spring seal hunt and other hunting activities by men, as well as important plant gathering by women. Even trout catching and smoking are frequently done, for example, by men and women from the Huroŏči and Ustomonaypo settlements. There are no regulations, kinship or otherwise, to restrict participation in these activities.

Therefore, the settlements on the northwest coast are closely related to each other through kinship ties, a high degree of mobility within the area, frequent contacts, and nonformalized economic and political interdependence.

Ainu men fish and hunt sea and land mammals, whereas women take the major responsibility for gathering plants and storing food. Large animals such as bears, musk deer, reindeer, and seals, and large fish such as trout and salmon, constitute important sources of food.

The men utilize individualistic techniques of hunting and fishing, although cooperation among a few persons does occur. They use the bow and arrow, the set-trap bow, the spear, and various kinds of traps for hunting land mammals, often combining the different methods. Sea mammals, especially seals, play an important role, providing food, oil, clothing, shoes, and stomachs for use as oil containers. Ainu fishing is characteristically confined to coastal waters, lakes, and rivers. Besides daytime fishing, nighttime fishing and ice fishing are also important. Even more crucial is the fishing of salmon and trout as they come upstream; they are caught in great quantity and smoked and dried for winter use. Some men also engage in trade with other peoples. (For a description of the trade, see Appendix D; for an analysis of the politicoeconomic nature of the trade, see Ohnuki-Tierney 1976a.)

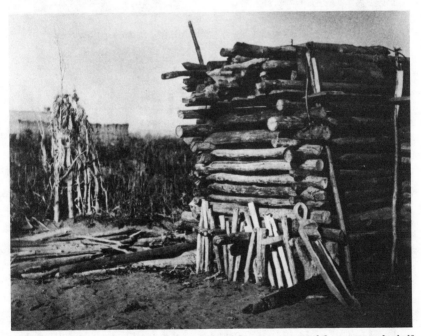

A bear house where a bear, the supreme deity of the Ainu, is raised for a year and a half (Kajima 1895).

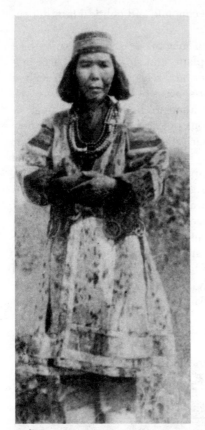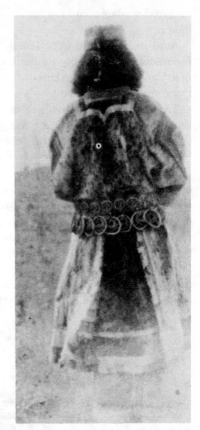

A Sakhalin Ainu woman from the east coast in a sealskin garment. (Courtesy of T. Yamamoto.)

Although the Sakhalin Ainu do not use hunting dogs, as do the Hokkaido Ainu, they use male dogs extensively for pulling sleds, which is the only means of transportation during their frozen winter; female dogs are important sources of meat and fur clothing. The Ainu practice selective breeding by castrating all male dogs except the leader of each sled.

Plant food, gathered by women, is of no less importance for the Ainu. Women ardently collect leeks, berries, and root crops such as lily bulbs, and preserve them for the winter supply. They also gather innumerable plants for both religious and medicinal uses. Women are highly skilled in basketry and weaving, although the techniques were originally introduced by the Japanese (Takakura 1960:13; Yamamoto 1970:215). They make garments and bags using fish skin and animal hides, as well as plant fibers such as elm bark and nettle.

The Ainu live in intimate and constant contact not only with their fellow

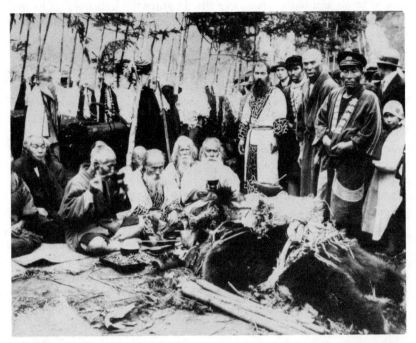

A Sakhalin Ainu bear ceremony. Some Ainu are wearing Japanese outfits (Fujita 1930).

Ainu but also with multitudes of beings of the universe. Soul owners, spirits, demons, and deities are all-important; Ainu welfare depends upon their good relationships with these beings, as we shall see in the remaining chapters. At the top of the hierarchy of these beings is their supreme deity – the bear. The most important religious ceremony of the Ainu is the bear ceremony, which is also the best-known aspect of Ainu life to outsiders. Bear ceremonialism starts in the spring, when men go to the mountains to catch either a newborn cub in the den or a cub strolling with its mother shortly after coming out of hibernation. The cub is referred to as "our deity-grandchild" and is regarded as a deity and a grandchild at the same time. The cub is raised inside the house of the host's family until its claws become too dangerous; then it is transferred to a "bear house," an outside cage. If the cub is newborn and requires nursing, a woman in the settlement who is nursing her baby will nurse the cub at the same time. (Since the introduction of dairy farming in the recent past, the bear is usually fed cow milk.)

Just before they move to their winter settlement, the Ainu slay the bear during an elaborate ritual for which they prepare for a long time. Although outsiders often misunderstand this ritual slaying as a cruel act, it is based upon the Ainu religious view that proper slaying of the bear and proper treatment of its carcass in a ritual ensure the transferral of its soul to the world of the deities, that is, bears. This act guarantees another visit to the Ainu by the bear, who brings gifts of meat and fur as an expression of goodwill, just as human guests would do. For this ceremony, many friends and relatives gather from both close and distant settlements to participate in the ceremony, which lasts for at least several days. (For ethnographic details of the bear ceremony, see Ohnuki-Tierney 1974a:90–7; for an analysis of its religious and political nature, see Ohnuki-Tierney 1976a.)

In addition to the bear, the Ainu pantheon includes the Goddess of Hearth, the Goddess of Sun-Moon, foxes (which are also raised and ritually killed), owls, and various other symbolically perceived fauna and natural phenomena of the land, sea, and sky. An important part of Ainu religion is shamanism, which receives major attention as a medical ritual in this book.

Ainu carving, weaving, embroidery, and music are all of high aesthetic quality, although they are part of daily life rather than isolated phenomena. Aesthetic sensitivity and intellectual sophistication are nowhere more evident than in the highly stylized epic poems of the Ainu, which also play an important role in their medical system, as we shall see.

3

The ethnomedical approach in anthropology and the Ainu domain of illness

Ethnomedicine

To explain how I attempt to understand Ainu concepts of illness, I begin with a brief characterization of the field of ethnomedicine. In the remainder of the chapter, I describe the domain of illness, identifying phenomena that are perceived by the Ainu as illnesses.

The ethnomedical approach is to study how a particular group of people perceives and deals with its health and illness. This approach thus includes the study of medical beliefs, healing techniques, and medical practitioners as these phenomena relate to the culture and society in which they are found. Expressions such as *emic* or *insider's view* are frequently associated with the ethnomedical approach; however, an emic view does not exclude interpretation by anthropologists, who are outsiders, even though these interpretations do not necessarily represent conscious formulations of the people themselves. For example, interpretation of medical symbols, such as those involved in healing rituals, is often part of an ethnomedical study. In attempting to arrive at a symbolic referent, an anthropologist must often engage in an extensive contextual analysis of particular medical symbols, unless the people under study is exceptionally articulate, as in the case of the Ndembu studies by V. Turner. In other words, even when the people themselves are not conscious of the meaning of a symbol or of a pattern underlying their behavior, as long as the anthropologist's interpretations represent abstractions from the people's words and behavior, they are referred to as emic in anthropological literature. (A detailed discussion of my method of interpretation is presented in Chapter 7.)

Another way of explaining the basic approach of ethnomedicine is to characterize it as viewing medical problems as sociocultural phenomena. Illnesses are seen as culturally definable. For anthropologists who regard a culture as a symbolic system, the people's view of illness is part of that system. Although his emphasis has changed in recent years, Kleinman in 1974 stated this symbolic approach to medicine: "any disease . . . is in part a cultural construct. Disease derives much of its form, the way it is

31

expressed, the value it is given, the meaning it possesses, and the therapy appropriate to it in large measure from the governing system of symbolic meaning" (Kleinman 1974:209).

Further understanding of this sociocultural approach to illness in ethnomedicine may be gained by contrasting the concept of illness in ethnomedicine with the concept of disease. In a celebrated distinction between the two, Fabrega (1972:213; 1975) emphasizes that, whereas the criteria used by nonprofessionals in identifying illness are social and psychological, disease in biomedicine is "an abnormality in the structure and/or function of any system of the body, and evidences of biological system malfunction serve as indicators of disease" (1972:168). Fabrega stresses that disease therefore "signifies an abstract biological 'thing'" (Fabrega 1975:969). This biomedical or disease framework is referred to by some anthropologists as the *etic* approach. It is seen as being culture-free, like the color spectrum, which is used to code and compare various emic divisions and definitions of color terms (cf. Berlin and Kay 1969).

In this book, I follow basically the terminological and conceptual distinctions proposed by Fabrega. However, these distinctions can be misleading unless they are carefully qualified and delineated. It is debatable whether or not science or scientific medicine as developed in the West is in part a product of Western culture and thus is not strictly culture-free. For example, Stein claims that the conceptualization of disease in biomedicine in itself reflects cultural bias: "the mechanical-biological, pathogen-specific or organ-specific disease *is* the illness" (1977:15; italics in the original). Stein further points out such features as "single-factor" orientation, the isolation of variables rather than the demonstration of multiple determinants, or a heuristic rather than holistic mode of conceptualization as earmarks of the elements of "folk medicine" in Western medicine (1977:15–16). In addition, there is the question of the definition of science and of whether or not we recognize science in non-Western cultures. Thus, Leslie opposes the use of the term *scientific medicine* in referring to biomedicine and prefers the term *cosmopolitan medicine*. According to him, "By commonly recognized criteria, Chinese, Ayurvedic, and Arabic medicine are scientific in substantial degree" (Leslie 1976:7–8; see also Porkert 1974).

The problem of defining science is most significant and demands further deliberation that is beyond the scope of the present book. Of immediate relevance to my main theme, however, is a more pragmatic problem: the distinction between biomedicine as referred to in this book and so-called Western medicine. In my view, the two represent distinct, although somewhat overlapping, phenomena and thus must be clearly distinguished. Although biomedicine may, at least potentially, be viewed as culture-free, the way in which it is practiced is significantly influenced by the values and other cultural factors of a given Western society.

Gonzalez (1966) cogently argues that there is a need to distinguish between medicine and practice as healing techniques, and that it is in the philosophy behind the latter that we see the basic differences between what she refers to as Western modern medicine and non-Western medicines. She defines medicine as "any substance applied to or introduced into the body, which is believed by some specialist and/or the sick person to change the existing state of the body in the direction of better health" and medical practice as "any act undertaken by either the sick one or someone else, which may or may not directly involve the body, but which is believed to have an effect on the health" (Gonzalez 1966:124). However, there are many pharmaceutical products in American society that are not scientifically effective; pills are sugar-coated to ease the mind of the takers, just as suckers are thrust into the mouths of crying children to "pacify" them – a prevalent custom in American society. This fact suggests that Western medicine, as defined by Gonzalez, may indeed be culturally construed. In non-Western medical traditions, the meaning and functions assigned to herbs, decoctions, and other "medicines" are almost exclusively cultural products.

However, it is in medical practice that so-called Western modern medicine is most expressive of the cultural influence. Thus, a moral tradition of "moderation in all things, self-discipline, and a consciousness of our individual responsibility in keeping fit" lies behind the practice of much of Western medicine, as Gonzalez points out (1966:124). This Western moral tradition is not unlike the stress on balance and harmony that provides the philosophical basis of many humoral medicines in non-Western societies. Impersonal, technical, and often brief relationships between doctors and patients are also necessarily related to impersonal social relationships in highly mobile Western societies, making the introduction of biomedicine to another society difficult (Marriott 1955:263). Before simplistically equating biomedical categories and clinical processes as etic, we must first do ethnomedical studies of Western medicine so that we come to understand the "cultural transformations" involved (cf. Kleinman 1978b:29).

Within this framework of ethnomedicine as the study of illness as viewed by the people themselves, there are two major approaches. They reflect two basically different, but not necessarily contradictory, approaches in anthropology. At the risk of oversimplifying complex issues in theory and method, I label one approach *rationalist* and the other *empiricist*. Whereas rationalists are interested in the structure of ideas primarily in the unconscious and derive their data from the language and statements of informants, empiricists are interested in behavior and hence obtain their ethnographic data from observed transactions. The generalizations of the former relate to the sociocultural structure; those of the latter to the individual as an actor. In this book I take primarily the rationalist approach, although in Chapter 11 the empiricist approach is taken. Further discussion of the two approaches will be presented in Chapter 9.

Turning to the more specific problem of how to engage in an ethnomedical study with interests such as mine, an investigator first attempts to codify the domain of illness by asking the following questions: (1) What phenomena are seen as departures from the norm of health? (This question entails the delineation of the concepts of both illness and health.) (2) Is there a generic term for the entire domain of illness? (3) Is each illness identified by the same label? (4) Apart from the terminological system, what criteria are used to identify the phenomenon as an illness? (5) In regard to specific illnesses, what are the indicators – changes in the body and its functions, behavioral changes, sensory experiences, or feelings? (6) Do the people have explanations about the causes? (7) What do they prescribe, if anything, for the illness – materia medica, a ritual, or both?

In the balance of this chapter, I attempt to answer the first four questions for the Ainu case and delineate some of the important interrelationships among the concepts behind them.

The Ainu domain of illness

A brief look at the Ainu concept of health reveals not only their concept of illness but a basic tenet of their world view. The opposite of illness is described by them as *ramu pirika*, or "soul-beautiful." The term *ramu* means the soul as the metaphysical locus of feelings and thoughts, as well as the anatomical part of the body called the heart in English. *Pirika* is an important adjective in Ainu, denoting beautiful, sacred, big, and other qualities that are desirable. Thus, deities are *pirika* because they are sacred; a plant whose useful part is well developed is also *pirika*. The expression *ramu pirika*, that is, soul-beautiful, as an antonym of the state of ill health, reveals an essential unity of body and mind. If one's soul is in proper order through paying due respect to all the soul-bearing beings of the universe, then one's body too is in good condition.

Just as the maintenance of good health depends upon moral behavior, generalized cures of illnesses are religious in nature. Thus, the Ainu believe that dreaming about a wolf deity, such as about his howling, will cure any illness. Another all-purpose cure is help from the most important goddess in the Ainu pantheon – Grandmother Hearth. First, the plant called *nuhča*[1] and spruce branches[2] are burnt on the fire in the hearth, where this goddess is believed to reside. The smoke from the burning plants is then absorbed with wood shreddings on a ritual stick made from willow,[3] which are often used as offerings to deities and have a high ritual value. The entire body is wiped with the wood shreddings. The "polluted" ritual stick must later be placed on a bifurcated branch of a tree standing outside the patient's house in the direction of the sunset, which is considered to be the most profane of all directions (cf. Ohnuki-Tierney 1972).

In short, the Ainu notion of health reveals two basic themes in their world view: the fundamental unity of body and mind and the ubiquitous presence of their deities. Their notion of health and illness is deeply embedded in their world view.

With this basic notion, I now proceed to the more specific problem of delineating the domain of illness. In ethnosemantics, the standard technique for codifying a domain is to elicit a term that is both a generic designation of the domain and an identification of each subdivision – in the case of a medical domain, each illness. For illness, a few lexemes may be suitable as a label for the entire domain. A brief discussion of these terms may contribute to an understanding of the Ainu concepts of illness.

Araka is the term that most frequently appears as a part of illness labels. I attempted to determine if this may be the generic term for the entire domain of illness, and also to see if each departure from health may be referred to as *araka*. It soon became evident that most illnesses accompanied by pain, actual or potential, are readily identified as *araka*. Also, although not always accompanied by physical symptoms, all the illnesses caused by a spiritual being, referred to as *metaphysical illnesses* in this book, are clearly identified as *araka*. On the other hand, ordinary cuts and bruises, though accompanied by pain, are not considered illnesses unless they are serious or inflicted by a bear or other Ainu deities. In other words, the term *araka* is used to refer to either a pain in particular or an illness in general.

Another candidate as a lexeme for the domain of illness is *ikoni*, which also means either an illness or a pain. If contrasted to *araka*, this term means either a serious illness, as opposed to an ordinary illness, or a chronic pain, as opposed to a temporary pain. Likewise, another term, *tasum*, if contrasted to *araka*, means an acute pain rather than an ordinary pain.[4]

In other words, the term *araka* may be used at several different levels of contrast, each level having a different referent (see Table 3.1). In terms of the relationship between a concept and its linguistic expression, these different denotata in different contrast sets are important. It should be

Table 3.1. *The use of the term* araka

Illness (*araka*)
  Ordinary illness (*araka*)
  Serious illness (*ikoni*)
Pain (*araka*)
  Temporary pain (*araka*)
  Recurrent pain (*ikoni*)

  Mild pain (*araka*)
  Acute pain (*tasum*)

noted that both *araka* and *ikoni* mean either an illness or a pain, whereas a pain, although important and often present, is not a common denominator for all illnesses recognized by the Ainu.

Some illnesses are not usually identified as *araka*. When a phenomenon is categorized as an illness and yet is not habitually referred to as an *araka*, this may be due to several factors. First, the dual meaning of the term *araka*, illness in general or pain in particular, may create some difficulty unless the phenomenon is habitually referred to as *araka*. Second, in any culture there are many conditions that are not normal that are not consciously defined as illness or not-illness. For example, in American society, a headache or even a cold poses this problem: A person may not feel well, but is he or she sick? For that matter, does the individual have a disease, a sickness, or an illness? In cases of these ill-defined aberrant conditions, there is often considerable individual variation in classification; some Americans may consider a cold an illness, whereas others may not. Thus, although the Ainu clearly classify both headaches and colds as *araka*, there are other conditions of ambivalent status.

A strict terminological approach thus eludes the codification of the Ainu domain of illness. Furthermore, the presence of a culturally prescribed cure does not indicate that the phenomenon is considered an illness; some phenomena that are clearly classified as nonillnesses receive meticulous cure. Thus, cuts, burns, and bruises are regarded as departures from normal conditions, and the presence of disorder is recognized. Furthermore, there are several methods to treat these disorders. However, they are clearly not identified as illnesses.

In the Ainu case, any simplistic approach to the codification of illnesses is further complicated because on occasion these injuries may become illnesses – not habitual but metaphysical illnesses. Thus, when a burn is very severe, a metaphysical etiology is suspected, which in turn requires the performance of a shamanistic rite to seek its etiology and a special cure. Similarly, an injury inflicted by a bear, no matter how small, is considered a grave illness; the injured person must be placed in a special hut, called *kuča* in Ainu and made of tree bark. There the patient must be cared for by a postmenopausal woman. This treatment is necessary because a person injured by a bear temporarily becomes sacred through contact with a deity and should not be contaminated by the smell of menstrual blood or other polluting objects. Were the patient to remain at home, a menstruating woman might be present or might come to visit. Also, firewood contaminated by animal urine while lying outside unknowingly might be used in the hearth; in a hut only freshly cut firewood is used.

The primacy of culturally construed causes of illness therefore seems obvious. Ultimately, the Ainu illnesses are not independent biological entities. This basic nature of the Ainu conceptualization of illness illustrates that Ainu illness is fundamentally different from disease in biomedicine, in which biological symptoms and pathogens receive primary emphasis.

Within this domain of illness, there are two broad categories. The first is a group of illnesses for which the Ainu have both standardized diagnostic criteria and curing methods utilizing primarily materia medica, and in which no supernatural entity is directly involved. For lack of a better term, the expression *habitual illnesses* (Ackerknecht 1946:478) is used to refer to this group. The second is a group of illnesses in which a spiritual being such as a soul, deity, or demon is involved, either as a pathogen, as a source of curative power, or in the etiology. These illnesses are often referred to in anthropological literature as *supernatural illnesses*, expressing the involvement of a supernatural being. I use the term *metaphysical illnesses* simply to avoid the use of *supernatural*, obviously a misleading designation for Ainu deities, which consist of elements that in our perception constitute nature (e.g., bears, wolves, and the sun). There is no generic term in Ainu for the category of habitual illnesses or that of metaphysical illnesses.

A brief survey of the domain of Ainu illness immediately highlights several theoretical and methodological issues. First, it is uncertain whether the phenomena of illness are clearly separated from other phenomena. A number of illnesses are well demarcated as illnesses and labeled as such. But beyond this class of readily identifiable illnesses, there are intermediate states that are not really normal or healthy but are not necessarily illnesses, like our headaches and colds.

In regard to the question of a lexeme, *araka* may be viewed as a generic term for the domain of illness. However, because the term also stands for pain in particular, which is clearly not the common denominator for all illnesses, a one-to-one correlation may not be easily assumed between the conceptual form and its linguistic expression.

The presence of a lexeme for the entire domain, however, is an exception to the rule. The Ainu language characteristically lacks lexemes for the most inclusive domains, such as plants, animals, space, and time. This exception is especially intriguing because these unlabeled domains are in many ways better delineated than the domain of illness. These "unlabeled but real categories" (Berlin, Breedlove, and Raven 1968) will be considered further in a discussion of language and cognition in Chapter 10.

4

Habitual illnesses

General characteristics of habitual illnesses

Habitual illnesses are those that the Ainu diagnose on the basis of such symptoms as the nature of the pain or the appearance of the ailing part of the body. They usually employ standard treatments, using materia medica. Characteristically, though not in all cases, the label of an illness not only identifies a departure from health as a particular illness but also specifies the materia medica used for its treatment. If, for example, a person experiences a headache that simulates the sound of a dog gnawing on something hard, the illness is identified as *seta sapa araka*, that is, a dog headache – one of ten headaches that the Ainu recognize. This diagnosis, in turn, indicates that treatment requires the use of a dog – in this case, paste made from the powder ground from a dog's skull.

The diagnosis and treatment of habitual illnesses may be done by anyone, without the help of a shaman or accompanying rituals, although the choice of materia medica and the methods of application are said to have been originally revealed by shamans during rites in a distant past. In practice, adult women tend to get more involved in the diagnosis and healing of these illnesses as part of their domestic role. They assume the major responsibility of collecting and keeping a ready supply of materia medica.

The habitual illnesses may be grouped into four broad categories: (1) body-part illnesses; (2) bone illnesses; (3) skin abnormalities; and (4) others. The major characteristics of each category and its illnesses are presented here; the details of each illness and methods of cure within each category appear in Appendixes A and B (see also Ohnuki-Tierney 1977a and 1977b). In the following discussion, I use Frake's four diagnostic criteria (1961:125–230): pathogenic, etiological, symptomatic, and prodromal. Pathogenesis refers to "the agent or mechanism that produces or aggravates an illness," and etiology denotes "the circumstances that lead a particular patient to contract an illness." Symptoms are "the attributes of an illness currently perceptible to patient or observer," and prodrome refers to "a prior and diagnostically distinct condition."

39

Body-part illnesses. The illnesses in this category are identified by the Ainu primarily by the location of the ailment in a particular body part, including internal organs. Examples are nose illnesses (e.g., an infection in the nostril), head illnesses (e.g., headaches), and liver illnesses.

Only some of these body-part illnesses are further subdivided. The subdivision takes place in terms of the subsection of the body part where the ailment or other disorder occurs, as with an illness of the lower abdomen, instead of the abdomen in general; or it is differentiated into single illnesses on the basis of the nature of the disorder, as with the spruce branch abdomen illness, which is a stomachache characterized by a feeling as if spruce needles are prickling the lower abdomen.

I recorded twenty-six labels for body-part illnesses on a more general level of classification (e.g., *honi araka* = abdomen illnesses), with eighty-one specific names for single illnesses (e.g., *huhteh yamuhu honi araka* = spruce branch abdomen illness). (An analysis of the lexical construction of the illness labels is presented in Appendix A.)

The names of the body parts reflect the Ainu classification of the body, which differs from that of American English in the spatial divisions of the body. For example, ordinarily the Ainu do not express the English distinction between the hand and the arm or between the foot and the leg. Thus the term *teh* refers to the part that includes both the arm and the hand in English, and the term *parakita* is used only when the hand must be separately identified. In the case of the leg and the foot, only one term, *kema*, is used.

Further, by dividing the body into two parts at the lower end of the rib (*utohotuye* in Ainu), the Ainu assign greater importance and often a sacred quality to the upper half and an inferior and profane quality to the lower half. The assignment of contrasting values to each part of the bodily dyad is widely used in spatial perception of the universe, a river, a house, and so on. For example, the Ainu perceive the universe as dichotomized, with the mountains occupying the sacred upper half of the universe (cf. Ohnuki-Tierney 1972 for the details of Ainu spatial concepts). However, this division of the body and the respective values of each part are not significant features in the Ainu classification of body-part illnesses. Although the Ainu differentiate between the internal organs and the external surface, this distinction is not an important feature in their illness classification. Other possible differentiations of the body parts, such as proximal versus distal (cf. the Subanun distinction in Frake 1961), likewise are not meaningful in Ainu illness classification.

Bone illnesses. The term *poni tasum araka* (bone pain illnesses) is a general term for a category of illnesses in which the primary symptom is pain in the bones and joints. These illnesses are also called *poni čikoyki* *araka*, or simply *čikoyki araka;* the term *čikoyki* means to accuse or to nag. This category, as well as the category of skin abnormalities, cuts across the category of body-part illnesses in that bone or skin illnesses can also be referred to as body-part illnesses. Thus, *tuman araka* (hip illness) is an illness of the hip, but it is also a bone illness. On the other hand, a pain at the joints seems to be identified first as a bone illness, rather than as a body-part illness. Three of the most common bone illnesses are related to the joints: *kumsi araka* (kneecap illness), that is, pains at the knee; *sistoh araka* (elbow illness), that is, pains at the elbow; and *čirosi koyki* (wrist illness), that is, pains at the wrist.

Skin abnormalities. Some skin abnormalities are regarded as skin illnesses (*kami wen araka* = its-flesh-bad illnesses), whereas others are not. Because this category of illnesses illustrates the Ainu belief that external manifestations of symptoms are not the only criterion for identifying abnormalities as illnesses, my description here starts with skin abnormalities that are usually not classified as illnesses.

Abnormalities that are not considered illnesses include ordinary cuts, bruises, and burns, all caused by external agents. The Ainu definitions parallel English usage. *Mačiri* (cuts) refers to open skin, *ura* (bruises) are injuries from striking or pressing but without blood or open cuts, and *rimonke* (burns) are injuries caused by heat. Although they are not illnesses, the Ainu nonetheless meticulously prescribe cures for them. However, they may be considered illnesses if they are unusually serious, as in the case of a cut from an axe, or if an injury is inflicted by a deity. Thus, a cut inflicted by a bear, no matter how small, is a serious illness, requiring the performance of a shamanistic rite in order to decipher the precise etiology. Because the involvement of a spiritual being in the etiology and the requirement of a shamanistic performance are both characteristic of metaphysical illnesses (see Chapter 6), we see a curious phenomenon here. A small cut, which under ordinary circumstances does not constitute an illness, not only becomes an illness, but a metaphysical illness at that, if it is inflicted by a bear.

Boils, blisters, swellings, rashes, and other skin infections are skin abnormalities that fall under the category of *kami wen araka* (its-flesh-bad illnesses), a designation that also includes smallpox and measles, which are metaphysical illnesses (see Chapter 6). The skin infections that apparently receive the most attention are boils. The Ainu distinguish two types. The first one is *huhpe* (*huh* = to swell; *pe* = thing) – a large boil or swelling with a single locus of infection, perhaps corresponding to a furuncle. The second category of boils is small boils or blisters that are spread over a body part or the entire body. They are called *asispe*, which means a thing that erupts in multitudes (*asis* = to erupt in a large number; *pe* = thing). If the intensity of pain involved in a boil is to be emphasized, an alternate designation is *tasumpe* (*tasum* = to ache acutely; *pe* = thing). Although any of the *tasumpe* may be called *huhpe* or *asispe*, not all the *huhpe* or *asispe* are *tasumpe*.

Some boils are identified in reference to the afflicted body part. This seems to be the case with most *asispe* and some *huhpe*. Thus, *to: huhpe* (breast boil) is a closed swelling at the side of a woman's breast, and *etupuy araka* (nostril illness) denotes a growth in the nostril. Many other types of *huhpe*, however, are identified without reference to a body part. In these cases, the nature of a *huhpe*, such as its color, the presence or absence of fluid discharge, pain, and so on identifies it, for example, as a bat boil rather than a woodpecker boil. The bat, woodpecker, or other referents are analogies through which the Ainu express their perception of the particular nature of a boil. Thus the pain of a bat boil is thought to simulate the cry of a bat. Lexically, then, the term *keputenka* (bat) is added in front of *huhpe* to form the name of this boil, *keputenka huhpe*.

As mentioned earlier, any skin or bone illness, at least theoretically, may be considered a body-part illness. Although the social context or circumstances in which an individual identifies the illness may have some bearing upon the choice of the illness identification label, some illnesses are customarily identified as body-part illnesses rather than as skin or bone illnesses, or vice versa. For example, infections of the tongue are usually referred to as illnesses of the mouth rather than as skin illnesses, whereas skin infections on the arm would most often be identified as particular skin infections rather than as an illness of the arm. In other cases, the choice of the identification is a matter of free variation.

Others.   The illnesses in this category are not localized in terms of body parts. They are considered the most serious of all the habitual illnesses. Their treatments are standardized. The two most important illnesses, *kemasinke* and *hana*, are described here.

There are two types of *kemasinke* (*kem* = blood; *asinke* = to exit). The first kind, called *ihehpa araka*, is characterized by the spitting of a small amount of dark-colored blood, often mixed with phlegm. The cause is the "breakage" of the lungs. The blood is considered to be dead, and its color is referred to as *kurasno* (black) or *hu:re nuporo* (deep red). Diagnosis of this condition involves two prodromal symptoms. The blood spitting is preceded by a long period during which the patient becomes weak and pale, and by itching of the chest and throat. The second type of *kemasinke*, considered less serious, is called *urukay kemasinke* (short-blood-emission) and is caused by the lung "explosion." The blood is bright red and much more abundant than in the case of *ihehpa araka*.

The spitting of blood, however, does not automatically identify a case of *kemasinke*, because it could also be a case of sorcery. The presence in the blood of the following items verifies a sorcery case: if the victim is a man, an arrowhead and ritual shavings of the kind used by the Ainu as offerings to the deities; if a woman, a needle and ritual shavings. Because sorcerers are said to be nonexistent among the northwest coast Ainu, this happens only when sorcerers among the east coast Sakhalin Ainu or among the neighboring peoples (Gilyaks and Oroks) victimize the northwest coast Ainu. (For a further discussion of these sorcerers, see Chapter 6.)

A patient diagnosed as having *kemasinke* must immediately be removed to a temporary hut. This regulation is based upon a belief that "old blood" (*husko kem*), which consists of a variety of undesirable blood including menstrual and parturient blood, is offensive to the deities who reside in or visit the home. Once the patient is in a hut, numerous cures for this illness may be administered (see Appendix A). All of these treatments use plants, the majority of which are brewed as decoctions. If these treatments fail, the Ainu sometimes resort to a shamanistic rite in hopes of discovering a special cure. The rite must be performed at a house other than that of the patient – a house uncontaminated by the smell of blood. The Ainu are not optimistic about results, however, because the offensive smell of the patient's blood, which lingers even after washing, will ward off good spirits, without whose help the shaman cannot obtain the desired instructions from the deities.

Hana (a term whose meaning is not clear) is a condition that occurs when old blood is localized in a certain part of the body. Although it is dangerous anywhere in the body, if the blood goes from the throat and shoulder area to the area behind the ears, it will likely be fatal. Therefore, the patient should be treated before this happens, and one must always watch for any sign of darkening behind the ears. The symptoms of *hana* are quite complex, varying at times. Besides the darkening, *hana* may be identified by any one or a combination of the following symptoms: general fatigue, dizziness, nausea, headaches, and throbbing of the heart. A sudden death or paralysis is considered to be caused by *hana*.

The cure for *hana* utilizes the backbone of a shark, moistened by licking. The area where the old blood is presumably located is rubbed with the bone until it swells and bleeds slightly. When the old blood is let out, the illness is cured. If a shark bone is not available, one can use a Japanese coin or simply pinch the area with two fingers or, in the case of an infant, with the lips or teeth. It is claimed that this method is effective enough to revive a person who falls unconscious from an attack of *hana*. In addition, the use of this method enables *hana* to be distinguished from another illness called *čirayetehka araka*, which is also characterized by a partial or complete paralysis of the body. If blood, or old blood as the Ainu would specify, flows after rubbing, the patient is suffering from *hana;* otherwise, a diagnosis of *čirayetehka araka* is warranted.

There is a great deal of fear and concern about *hana,* because it can be lethal. It is said that everyone, including infants and elders, suffers from it at one time or another. Serious cases run in the family, although the illness is not contagious. Whenever she had a headache or felt heavy in the head, my key informant rubbed and "took out old blood" from the glabella area. She usually had a reddish line between the eyebrows as a result of her frequent bloodletting, although at times she chose the throat or the sides of the breast to work on. She also pinched the skin of her granddaughter's throat with her fingers whenever the child appeared to me to be suffering from a cold.

The decisiveness with which the Ainu diagnose this illness is quite remarkable, because to outsiders the symptoms are elusive. My own observation on this point is echoed in the observation by Chiri and Wada (1943:66-7); B. Wada was a medical doctor who worked extensively among the east coast Sakhalin Ainu. Although *hana* is very important to the Sakhalin Ainu regardless of the region, it is not recognized by the Hokkaido Ainu (Chiri and Wada 1943:66).

Healing of habitual illnesses

Just as the Ainu do not rely upon a deity and other spiritual beings in diagnosing habitual illnesses, their cure does not ordinarily involve a spiritual being or a ritual. Instead, materia medica alone usually suffices.

The materia medica for a particular illness seems to be chosen on the basis of analogy, ritual value, or practical efficacy. The large majority of cures are based on analogy. The most frequent analogy is the similarity between the nature or appearance of the abnormality and a materia medica, as noted at the beginning of this chapter. Thus, if the pain of a boil simulates the cry of a bat, then a tuft of hair from a bat is placed upon the boil or a paste made from powder ground from the dried meat of a bat is applied. For a crab headache, paste made from a ground crab shell is used, and for a crab eye illness, paste made from the ground eyeball of a crab is applied. In most of these cases, the name of the particular materia medica is present in the illness label itself. But even when no particular being is expressed lexically in an illness label, the choice of remedies for the illness often rests upon some analogy. In some cases, the analogy is made between the symptom and the cure. Thus, one of the treatments for *kemasinke* (blood-spitting illness) is to eat cranberries; the analogy is between the color of the blood that the patient coughs up and the color of the berry. In some cases, qualities of the affected body part are paralleled in the objects used to cure. For example, the remedies for *sampe araka* (heart illness), whose major diagnostic criterion is strong pulsation of the heart, include the use of a red heart-shaped pebble, a *sahpe sey*, or the blood, blood clots, or sinews from a dog's heart. Other examples are provided in Appendix A.

It is possible that, beyond an obvious analogy between some aspect of an illness and a particular materia medica chosen, the metaphysical value of these animals, plants, and objects is a factor in their choice. I have listed the number of times the name of a particular animal, plant, or object appears in illness labels (Table 5.1) or in prescribed treatments (Table B.1). By far the most frequently used item for a cure is some part of a dog. Fourteen different parts of the dog's body are used in cures, and the dog appears twice in the illness labels. Dogs are extremely important among the Ainu. Male dogs pull sleds, a crucial means of survival during the long cold winters; bitches are a welcome source of food; and puppies supply skins for garments. They are the Ainu's only domestic animal. Beyond these utilitarian values, dogs are also considered to be servants of bears – the supreme deities of the Ainu. However, the use of a dog in treatments seems to relate less to its symbolic value than to its availability. The Ainu often kill dogs for food or to sacrifice to bears (with later human consumption); this ensures that all parts of the dog's body are readily obtainable for medicinal use as well.

In addition, the Ainu supreme deities, the bears, appear in one illness label and the bear cage in another. Parts of the bear appear four times in cures and the bear cage once. However, there is no emphasis on the religious significance of the bears in the statements about the cause or treatment of these illnesses. Among the Ainu of the northwest coast, some land and sea animals and birds are deified, but fish and plants are not. Therefore, the reason for the choice of fish and plants as materia medica cannot be religious in nature.

In short, it is the analogy between the physical characteristics of these beings used in materia medica and the illness that provides the basis of their choice. The analogy, in turn, generates the power of what Frazer once called "sympathetic magic."

The second category of materia medica consists of a small number of items in the Ainu culture that are chosen as cures not through analogy but because they have a high ritual value. They are standard items of ritual paraphernalia but do not necessarily possess strong metaphysical power, such as that of a bear. The plants *nuhča* and *kito*[1] provide examples. During shamanistic rites, *nuhča* is used in the shaman's decoction and is one of the three plants burnt over embers to produce aromatic smoke. The Ainu brew tea using the leaves of this plant, and it is considered especially good to drink when one has a cold, trouble with the gallbladder, or any of the bone illnesses. Similarly, *kito* (leek) is burnt on embers during shamanistic rites for its aromatic effect. Its potent smell is believed to chase off evil spirits and demons, as well as bears and other deified animals. Thus, when the Ainu unexpectedly encounter a bear, they throw a few dried pieces of this plant (which they carry at all times) in its direction in hopes that it will ward off the bear. Because of medical ritual efficacy, its decoction is almost a cureall. Thus, a patient with various illnesses, including colds and cramps in the lower abdomen, would drink this decoction; it can also be applied to ailments of the uvula or penis. Leek is also an ever-present ingredient in many dishes that the Ainu consider not only as favorites but also as health foods.

The third category of materia medica is based on more practical efficacy. For example, resin (*ro:či* in Ainu) is used for wounds because the Ainu have observed that a wounded bear rubs its body against the resin on a tree trunk. Resin, however, is not used in any other context. Many of the materia medica in the first and second categories may also have a practical or biomedical efficacy. They may contain chemical substances that are effective in healing, but even in the absence of these substances they may be effective for the Ainu, who believe in their efficacy and thus are psychologically helped in the healing process. It would be interesting to see if there is any correlation between the presence or absence of biomedically effective substances in the materia medica and the symbolic value assigned to them. Although there are sources that specify the chemical components of some of the herbs (Batchelor and Miyabe 1893; Fukuyama and Nezu 1942; Mitsuhashi 1976; Miyabe 1939; Miyabe and Miyake 1915; B. Wada 1941:100–6), a systematic analysis of this field is beyond the scope of this book. The biomedical efficacy of the curing methods, however, must clearly be separated from the Ainu's perception of it. If a particular plant is seen as effective, it is not because of the chemical substance in the plant but because of the plant itself – the culturally defined meaning of it. Thus, from the Ainu point of view, the biomedical and symbolic values of a plant are one entity. Only a small number of materia medica in the third category possess purely practical efficacy even from the Ainu point of view, in the sense that they do not have symbolic values in other cultural contexts.

Last, it should be noted that the Ainu healing method is characterized by a multiplicity of available cures. Usually for each illness, there are a number of cures: cures for all illnesses (see Chapter 3); cures for all the illnesses in one category; and specialized cures for particular illnesses, of which there often are several (see Appendix A). For example, for the heart illness discussed previously, there are two other cures, both utilizing shellfish (*ikayuh sey* and *warawah sey* in Ainu; not identifiable). The remedies for this heart illness, then, include a land animal (dog), three kinds of shellfish, a plant, and an object (pebble), all of which may be tried one after another. The significance of multiple remedies is that they provide a mechanism for the infallibility of Ainu medicine. In this sense, Ainu medicine is a flexible system that allows room to fail and yet at the same time never lets the patient down, because for every failure there are still other alternatives.

I recorded 106 habitual illnesses, with 41 flora, fauna, and objects in their labels. For 6 of them, only symptomatic descriptions are available; for the remaining 100, there are 186 curative methods, with 121 flora, fauna, and objects recognized as suitable for treating these illnesses. For example, although only 6 species of plants appear in 6 illness labels (Table 5.4), 61 species appear 74 times in the treatment of the illnesses. In many cases, several parts of the same animal, plant, or object are used for the same illness; or different parts may be used for different illnesses, as in the case of a crab, whose eyeball is used for a crab eye illness and whose shell is used for a crab headache. Furthermore, the same part or the same substance may be used in different forms. There are at least ten different ways of preparing medicine, all of which are listed at the beginning of Appendix A. Appendix B and Table B.1 provide details of the Ainu healing methods.

Summary

The descriptions of the four categories of habitual illnesses indicate that those in the first three categories contrast in significant ways to those in the fourth category. The Ainu identify body-part, skin, and bone illnesses primarily through symptomatic criteria and prescribe standard treatments. In the case of these illnesses, causal explanations are rarely meaningful in their identification. A few exceptions are labor pains (*tuye ikoni*) and menstrual cramps (*čuhkes araka*), both of which are classified as illnesses of the abdomen together with what we would call ordinary stomachaches. There is always a possibility that they are linguistically referred to as *ikoni* and *araka* (both terms denoting either an illness or a pain) but are conceptually distinguished from other illnesses of the stomach. The rest of the illnesses in these three categories are diagnosed on the basis of symptoms alone. In contrast, the illnesses in the fourth category include pathogenic criteria as an essential part of their definition. Thus, *kemasinke* is not only defined in terms of hemoptysis but is also due to breakage of the lungs. Likewise, in the definition of *hana*, the presence of old blood is an integral part of the definition of the illness.

The types of pathogens chosen as the definitional criterion for the illnesses in the fourth category, however, distinguish them from the metaphysical illnesses discussed in Chapter 6. First, these pathogens are tangible body substances, that is, the lungs and blood, rather than the entities of soul, spirit, or wrath of the deities, which constitute the pathogens for metaphysical illnesses. Although shamanistic rites may be held for *kemasinke* when standardized treatments fail, none of the illnesses in the fourth category require the performance of shamanistic rites, which are a must for both the diagnosis and treatment of metaphysical illnesses.

In using symptoms as either the whole or a part of the definitional criterion, multiple symptoms usually constitute a syndrome. For example, in the case of the lamprey boil, the diagnostic symptoms include the presence of pus, an opening, the second stage in the development of a boil, a single locus of infection, tactile perception of the pain involved, and the unusual color and smell of the pus (see Chapter 5). Symptoms involved in defining the illnesses of the fourth category are even more numerous and complex. However, all of these illnesses are regarded as a single entity and hence receive a single label. Consequently, the cure for each illness aims at the elimination of the total complex involved. Headaches, however, pose a problem in that when the Ainu talk about the bear headache, dog headache, and so on, each constitutes a single illness. Yet a headache can be a part of the syndrome that characterizes other illnesses, such as *hana*. In the latter case, the headache in general, rather than a specific subcategory of headache, is seen as a symptom.

Even this cursory description of the habitual illnesses clearly indicates that the Ainu perception of illness is entirely different from biomedically defined disease. First, when an illness is defined through symptomatic criteria, the incubation period is not included in the illness. Even more complex are the illnesses of the fourth category. A simple equation of *kemasinke* with tuberculosis of the lung, a peptic ulcer, or both, cannot be established. All other stages of tuberculosis or ulcer are not included in Ainu *kemasinke*. On the other hand, some cases of these diseases are diagnosed not as *kemasinke* but as the result of sorcery. In the case of *hana*, certain stages of a number of diseases, such as high blood pressure, may be included. Yet, some cases of *hana* may not be regarded as a condition of disease. Similarly, among the Ainu, the materia medica are chosen because of the analogy and for other cultural/symbolic reasons rather than because of interaction between the chemical components and a microbe. However, their medical efficacy is just as real. To impose our notion of empiricism confuses the issue.

5

Classification of body-part and skin illnesses

In the previous chapter I illustrated, primarily through the lexical constructions of illness labels, that many habitual illnesses are further subclassified, although the degree of subclassification varies among illnesses. This chapter examines the principles involved in the classification of habitual illnesses. First, I examine the classification of headaches and boils, which show the highest degree of classificatory complexity. Second, some broader aspects of the classification of habitual illnesses are presented.

Taxonomy of headaches and boils

Table 5.1 presents a taxonomic classification of Ainu headaches. In three of the ten subtypes of headaches I recorded, the location of pain provides the specificity. Thus, when pain is located in the forehead, called *kistomoho* in Ainu, the headache is labeled *kistomoho araka*. The headache located in the part of the head next to the neck, called *kasuh* (spatula) in Ainu because of its resemblance to the kitchen utensil, is called *kasuh sapa araka*. The headache that attacks only one half, *ariki* in Ainu, of the head (migraine?) is referred to as *sapa ariki araka*.

The other seven subtypes of headaches are all located in the head in general, and their specificity derives from the particular nature of the pain. Thus, the bear headache is a headache that feels like the sound of a bear's heavy footsteps, whereas the musk deer headache resembles the light galloping sound of a musk deer. The dog headache simulates the noise a dog makes when it gnaws on a hard object, and the woodpecker headache sounds and feels like a woodpecker when it drills into a tree trunk.

Whereas these four headaches are not accompanied by a chill, the remaining three subtypes of headaches classified by the nature of the pain are. For these headaches, an aquatic animal rather than a land animal is used in the pain analogy. Thus, an octopus headache feels like the sucking motion of an octopus, the crab headache resembles the prickling feeling of a crab crawling over one's skin, and the lamprey headache feels as if a lamprey is digging into one's head (lampreys dig holes in rocks).

49

Table 5.1. *Taxonomic classification of Ainu headaches* (sapa araka)

Level I: headaches in the main part of the head (visual)		Level I: headaches in a specific part of the head (visual)
Level II: headaches of the terrestrial beings (auditory)	Level II: headaches of the aquatic beings (thermal/tactile)	
Level III		
Iso sapa araka (bear headaches)	*Ahkoype sapa araka* (octopus headaches)	*Kasuh sapa araka* (ladle headaches)
Seta sapa araka (dog headaches)	*Takahka sapa araka* (crab headaches)	*Kistomoho araka* (forehead aches)
Ni:na čikah sapa araka (woodpecker headaches)	*Ikurupe sapa araka* (lamprey headaches)	*Sapa ariki araka* (head-half aches)
Opokay sapa araka (musk deer headaches)		

Although the nature of these headaches is expressed through a single analogy, the diagnostic criteria involved in the analogy are multiple. They may even be viewed as constituting a syndrome, or a set of symptoms that occur together, although not in the ordinary sense of the term as it is used in biomedicine. Thus, symptoms relating to the specific nature of each headache include some or all of the following features: the degree of severity, the sound quality, continuous versus discontinuous pain (further specified in terms of its frequency or the interval between the attacks), the presence or absence of a chill, and possibly a few other features. Thus, in the case of the bear headache, specific symptoms involved are: (1) discontinuous pain, which comes at certain regular intervals and thus simulates the walking of a bear; (2) the sound quality, which is like the bear's heavy footsteps; and (3) the lack of a chill.

When the multiple features involved in the diagnosis of headaches are examined, a clear pattern emerges. All of the headaches with a land animal analogy in their labels are characterized by the absence of a chill and the presence of a sound quality (see Table 5.2). A particular sound feature reveals the nature of the headache: the heavy footsteps of a bear; the light galloping sound of a musk deer; the noise a dog makes when it gnaws on a hard object; or the sound of a woodpecker boring into a tree trunk. In contrast, in the descriptions of headaches with an aquatic animal in the label, the feeling of a chill is a thermo-tactile experience. Furthermore, additional diagnostic features are also of a tactile nature. Thus, the sucking motion of an octopus is certainly not as persistent as that of a lamprey, which, according to the Ainu, digs even into a hard rock. The crab, on the other hand, gives a feeling of the incessant prickling with multiple loci of pain when one is in contact with its legs.

Table 5.2. *Diagnosis of headaches: classification by pain*

	Pain		
Headache	Chill	Sound	Touch
Terrestrial headaches			
Bear headache	0^a	$+^a$	0
Dog headache	0	+	0
Woodpecker headache	0	+	0
Musk deer headache	0	+	0
Aquatic headaches			
Octopus headache	+	0	+
Crab headache	+	0	+
Lamprey headache	+	0	+

[a] Present = +; absent = 0.

What we see here is that the headaches are first experienced and diagnosed through multiple senses and then are translated into the Ainu perception of particular animals. Note that these animals are perceived in motion – a galloping musk deer and a crawling crab. Furthermore, we see an intriguing permutation between the classification of headaches through symptomatic criteria and the spatial classification of the universe. Thus, in terms of a diagnostic symptom, the presence or absence of a chill divides the headaches into two major categories: those with a chill and those without. These two categories, in turn, are expressed in terms of the spatial classification of the Ainu universe, in which land and water comprise the most basic dyad. The information on the headaches also indicates that the Ainu do more than perceive their universe cognitively. They also feel, touch, hear, and – as indicated in other ethnographic data – smell it. Therefore, a bear, a crab, and all other beings of their universe are not zoological and botanical species in Western scientific schema. They are the Ainu bear, Ainu crab, and so on, which are experienced through auditory, thermal, tactile, and olfactory senses, as well as through vision. Likewise, the Ainu space is not only seen but is perceived through other senses.

In terms of classification, headaches are divided into three taxonomic levels, as indicated in Table 5.1. At level I, the location of the pain is the classificatory principle. The seven headaches in the main part of the head are further subdivided, with the presence of a chill as the distinctive feature. The sensory receptor involved at level I is vision, whereas the audio-thermal-tactile receptors come into play at level II. In the distinctive feature analysis presented in Table 5.2, the presence or absence of three features – chill, sound, and touch – characterize the terrestrial headaches as one class and the aquatic headaches as another. However, because the presence or absence of a chill is the most widely used diagnostic feature, as we shall shortly see, we might conclude that it is the classificatory principle, and the two others are redundant.

It should be noted, however, that the presence of a chill may not really be a minimal distinctive feature because in level III of Table 5.2 none of the terrestrial and aquatic headaches are paired. Thus, if the bear headache and the octopus headache, for example, share all other diagnostic features except the presence of a chill in the octopus headache, then that feature may be considered a minimal distinctive feature. Nevertheless, the classification of the apparently minor ailment of headaches demonstrates regularity and consists of at least three taxonomic levels.

In order to demonstrate that the headache is not atypical of the Ainu perception and classification of habitual illnesses, I now turn to a description and analysis of boils. As noted in Chapter 4, the category of skin illnesses, or *kami wen araka* (skin-bad illnesses), consists of skin infections with a single locus of infection, *huhpe*, and those with multiple loci of infection, *asispe*. My attention is given to *huhpe* here.

I recorded nine types of *huhpe*, each identified on the basis of the nature of its infection. As in the case of the headaches, there are boils of the terrestrial beings and of the aquatic beings. The latter are characterized by the presence of fluid, that is, pus or blood. Of the land animal boils, the bat boil is described as causing a pain that simulates the cry of a bat. The pain of the woodpecker boil resembles the boring of the woodpecker. The fox boil is characterized by a reddish color like that of the fox. The beehive boil is a large boil with numerous small openings in it, resembling a beehive. Although there are a number of openings, this type of skin infection is classified as *huhpe*, rather than *asispe*, because the location of the openings is confined to a small area. The cormorant boil is characterized by a black ring that surrounds it. A very small amount of blood is discharged from the boil, distinguishing it from the lamprey boil (described later). I see no connection between the presence of a black ring and the appearance of cormorants, unless this name reflects a Japanese influence. The Japanese have a cormorant fishing ritual during which a rope is tied around the neck of the cormorant; thus the bird catches fish without being able to swallow them. Although the boils of the land animals are all characterized by a total absence of fluid, the diagnostic criterion of the cormorant boil is a small amount of blood discharge; the small amount, however, was emphasized in the description. This may have some relation to the choice of a water bird in the name for this type of boil; the cormorant's residence includes both land and water.

Of the aquatic animal boils, all of which are accompanied by the discharge of blood or pus, the lamprey boil is the largest and most dangerous. It erupts on any part of the body and is very painful, as if a lamprey is digging into the flesh. It is accompanied by a bad odor and a great deal of dark bloody pus, which is somewhat foamy. The crab boil has a bright red color like that of a crab, aches as if a crab is crawling on the skin, and is often itchy. The octopus boil is the color of an octopus, reddish but darker than a crab. It is accompanied by a large discharge of pus, and also by pain simulating the sucking motion of an octopus. The sea anemone boil is also reddish in color, like a sea anemone.[1] It is accompanied by much pus, a large swelling, and stinging pain, like that from a sea anemone.

On the basis of these descriptions, I have attempted to analyze the Ainu perceptual mechanisms involved in the diagnoses of these skin infections (see Table 5.3). As in the case of the headaches, I see the use of multiple senses and the permutation between the diagnosis of the infections and the spatial classification of the universe. Diagnostically, the single boils

Table 5.3. Classification of boils and diagnostic criteria

Diagnostic features of boils	Boils of the terrestrial beings					Boils of the aquatic beings			
	Keputenka huhpe (bat boil)	Ni:na čikah huhpe (woodpecker boil)	Sumari huhpe (fox boil)	Tomaka-či huhpe (beehive boil)	Uriri huhpe (cormorant boil)	Ikurupe huhpe (lamprey boil)	Takahka huhpe (crab boil)	Ahkoype huhpe (octopus boil)	Hewnay huhpe (sea anemone boil)
Pus[a]	0	0	0	0	0	+	+	+	+
Opening[a]	0	0	0	0	0	+	+	+	+
Stage[b]	0	0	0	0	0	+	+	+	+
Number of locus of infections	0	0	0	+	0	0	0	0	0
Pain									
Auditory perception	+	+							
Tactile perception						+	+	+	+
Appearance									
Color (of boil or pus)			+		+	+	+	+	+
Shape					+				+
Olfaction						+			

[a] Present = +; absent = 0.
[b] I = 0; II = +.

are classified most broadly into those that are accompanied by fluid and those that are not. It seems, then, that the boils of the land animals may represent the first stage of the development of boils; after they come to a head and start discharging fluid, they become the boils of the aquatic animals. For example, a fox boil becomes one of the reddish boils of the water animals depending upon which shade of red it assumes. It should be noted that these three diagnostic features (1–3 in Table 5.3) are redundant. From the Ainu point of view, the presence of fluid is the feature that distinguishes between the two types of boils; the presence or absence of an opening and the developmental stages are both corollaries.

Additional features identify each boil and distinguish it from other types of boils in the same category. The tactile perception of pain is involved in all water animal boils but not in any of the land animal boils. In contrast to the headache classification, however, auditory perception is involved in only two out of the five land animal boils. Noteworthy here is that bats are perceived through the auditory receptor; thus the analogy of the bat boil. Understandably, visual perception is frequently used for boils. Color perception is used for all of the aquatic animal boils and two of the land animal boils. Shape is used only for the ring surrounding the cormorant boil and the swelling involved in the sea anemone boil. Olfaction is involved only in the lamprey boil.

In terms of classificatory structure, a similarity between boils and headaches can be seen here. The presence of fluid is a minimal distinctive feature in that it distinguishes the terrestrial boils and the aquatic boils as a class, but none of the individual boils are paired so that each paired terrestrial and aquatic boil presents a set that shares all other features. In short, the binary opposition with the presence of fluid as a minimal distinctive feature is seen between the terrestrial boils and the aquatic boils as a class, but we do not have a situation comparable to, for example, American English consonants, which are composed of voiced and voiceless counterparts. As a taxonomic structure, the boils have only two levels, as opposed to the three levels in the headache classification.

A common feature in the classification of headaches and of boils is that both aquatic headaches and boils involve thermal and tactile features, whereas land headaches and boils do not. In addition, both aquatic headaches and boils are characterized by the absence of auditory features, which are present in all land headaches but in only two of the land boils.

In its relation to world view, the classification of boils is of particular importance in that not only Ainu space but also Ainu time is involved in the diagnosis. The two categories of boils represent two stages in the temporal progression of boils and are then translated into the basic dyad in the spatial classification of the Ainu universe.

Wet-dry opposition in the classification of other illnesses

The division of illnesses within a category into dry and wet is not confined to the headaches and boils. It is a principle used in the classification of many other illnesses for which the presence or absence of a chill or fluid is a diagnostic criterion. The symbolism of land versus water in the designation and the diagnosis of illness, however, is not always as systematic or evident as in the above examples. (For further details of the following illness, see Appendix A.) For example, of the eight eye illnesses, three are characterized by the discharge of fluid from the eye and receive their names from aquatic beings: *kaywantahpo* shellfish (unidentifiable) eye illness, crab eye illness, and lamprey eye illness. None of the dry eye illnesses, however, are named after dry beings. For example, a dry eye illness, in which the primary symptom is the reddening of the white part of the eye, is called *hu: saranpe araka* because of the similarity between the color of the eye and *hu: saranpe*, that is, a red garment imported from the Japanese. Tearing is not a symptom of this eye illness, and the red garment is not associated with water. Although the remaining four eye illnesses are also dry, they are not named after a dry being, perhaps because they are characterized by a growth and other symptoms not comparable to those of the wet eye illnesses. Similarly, two of the seven throat illnesses recorded are characterized by an excess amount of saliva; their labels bear the term *ota*, or sandy beach, which may be covered by water during high tide. Of the rest of the dry throat illnesses, one is called a *bear cage throat illness* and thus is associated with a land animal, and the other is associated with a dry plant, but the remaining three have little to do with dry animals or plants.

A slightly different picture exists with the illnesses of the mouth. Reflecting the ever-present liquid or saliva, six of the seven mouth illnesses bear the names of beings associated with water; the meaning of the seventh label is not clear. Thus, the four are named after fish (sturgeon, shark, cod, and smelt), and one is called *snail mouth illness* (snails are wet with slime). The sixth is named after a *parakinači* plant.[2] Although the resemblance between the tongue in this illness and this plant is offered as the primary reason for the name, the plant, as the Ainu are well aware, always grows near water. Likewise, among the *asispe*, that is, skin infections with multiple loci, an illness characterized by blisters covering the entire hand and the joints of the fingers is called *imukina tasumpe* (*imukina* = an impatient plant; *tasumpe* = a thing that aches).[3] Again the primary explanation for this designation is the resemblance in appearance between the skin infection and the plant, but this plant too grows on wet land and its association with blisters, which hold water, seems obvious.

In drawing an analogy, there is a choice, then, among land mammals, birds, dry plants, and dry objects for an illness characterized by the absence of a chill or fluid. Likewise, for a wet illness, an analogy can be drawn from fish, shellfish, other marine animals, wet plants, or wet objects. I tried to find a pattern explaining the relationship between a particular kind of illness and the specific choice of a being or object for the analogy. For example, is there any definite reason why a particular wet illness is analogous to a shellfish rather than a wet plant?

The reason for the choice of fish is simple; it is confined to illnesses of the mouth, which is always wet, like the sea in which fish live. The shellfish labels may predominate because most of these creatures live near shore and hence are more readily available to women, who have the major responsibility of curing and for whom it is taboo to go fishing in deep water. It may also be that they are familiar beings of the universe and yet conceptually distinguishable from food. Although they are abundant in the area, the Ainu eat mainly mammals and fish, and do not use shellfish, octopi, crabs, and other marine creatures extensively. Food is to be internally consumed, and many of these medicines are only externally applied, although there are a few medicinal foods that may be taken internally either as a decoction or as cooked food. Also, the manner in which the shellfish spits out water provides a most appropriate analogy to the condition in which pus or water spurts out of skin infections. As to the choice of a wet plant over shellfish, for example, the only pattern seems to be that the condition of a particular illness is most analogous to the appearance of a particular wet plant.

Regarding the illness labels (see Table 5.4), out of thirteen objects and plants (which appear fourteen times in the illness labels), five items or species (with six occurrences) are chosen because of their positive or negative association with water. This means that out of 106 (100%) illness labels, shellfish appear in 6 (5.7%), fish appear in 9 (8.5%), other water creatures appear in 11 (10.4%), and plants and objects associated with water appear in 6 (5.7%). Therefore, 30.3% of 106 illness labels are associated with water. In contrast, of 106 illness labels, land mammals appear in 10 (9.4%), birds in 5 (4.7%), and objects and plants in 8 (7.5%). The total is 21.6%. Thus, over half (51.9%) of the illness labels are chosen on the basis of this criterion.

In order to determine the significance of this diagnostic criterion, one can attempt an etic/emic correlation by examining all 106 illnesses to see for which ones the presence or absence of fluid/chill can be considered important from the biomedical point of view; the results can then be compared with illnesses for which the Ainu regard the diagnostic criterion to be important. Not only is this task difficult, because occurrences of each illness must be observed, but it judges Ainu medicine on the basis of biomedicine. The fact that more than half of the illness labels emphasize

Table 5.4. *Frequency of appearances of beings and other terms in illness labels*[a]

Beings and other terms	No. of species and items[b]	Frequency of appearance	
Terrestrial beings			
Land mammals	7 (17.1%)	10 (9.4%)	14.1%
Birds	3 (7.3%)	5 (4.7%)	
Aquatic beings			
Shellfish	6 (14.6%)	6 (5.7%)	
Fish	6 (14.6%)	9 (8.5%)	24.6%
Other water creatures	6 (14.6%)	11 (10.5%)	
Plants	6 (14.6%)	6 (5.7%)	5.7%
Objects	7 (17.1%)	8 (7.5%)	7.5%
Body parts in the label	n.a.	34 (32.1%)	32.1%
Others[c]	n.a.	17 (16.0%)	16.0%
Total	41 (100%)	106 (100%)	

[a] The above categories of the beings of the Ainu universe are those utilized by the Ainu. I also followed the Ainu schema in identifying each being in the categories.
[b] The percentage is calculated on the basis of the total number, 41, from which "body part" labels and "others" are excluded.
[c] "Others" includes such labels as *kemasinke* (blood exit), which involves a lexeme for a major symptom, and several names, such as *hana*, whose meaning is not clear.

the presence or absence of a chill or fluid seems enough to indicate that this criterion is significant in Ainu diagnosis.

A crucial question here is why the criterion is so significant in the diagnosis. Although land and water are the basic spatial dyad of the universe, it is too hasty to conclude that this dichotomy is the blueprint for the illness classification. As noted in my 1972 publication, it is the human body that provides the prototype for the image of space. Thus, the universe is seen as a human body lying with its head in the mountains and its legs stretched toward the sea. Likewise, a house is pictured as a body lying prostrate on its back with its head toward the mountains (our east), its legs toward the sea (our west), and its right hand toward the Ainu border (our north). It seems then that the image of the human body is translated into the image of the Ainu universe and phenomena within it, but the quality of the spatial division – that is, dryness and wetness of the land and the sea, respectively – is translated into the illnesses that afflict the human body. One important point, however, is that although the dyad in the spatial classification is based upon the binary opposition between the sacred and the profane, this particular symbolic contrast is not carried over to the division into dry/land and wet/aquatic illnesses.

For the remaining 48.1% of the 106 illnesses, the presence or absence of fluid and chill is not a relevant diagnostic criterion. Among these illnesses, 32.1% simply have a lexeme for the affected body part. As for the rest ("Others" column in Table 5.4), some labels themselves express symptoms, as in the case of *kemasinke* (blood exit), and the meanings of other labels are not clear, as in the case of *hana*.

In the section on the taxonomy of headaches and boils, I emphasized that the presence of a chill or fluid is a classificatory principle but not, strictly speaking, a minimal distinctive feature. The examples at the beginning of this section related to the eye, mouth, and throat illnesses indicate that this diagnostic feature, as it applies to these illnesses, may not even be a classificatory principle. In other words, although this feature characterizes all the wet illnesses within the same category, the dry illnesses often do not have a comparable set of symptoms and hence do not even receive names of dry beings. It may be best understood that whereas the presence of chill/fluid is a classificatory principle for a few illnesses, such as headaches and boils, for many others it operates as a common denominator. In fact, these illnesses, regardless of their classification as a body-part or skin illness, are collectively called *sey araka* or shellfish illnesses (*sey* = shellfish), although octopi, crabs, and lampreys are not called *sey* under other circumstances.

The use of the chill/nonchill factor as a diagnostic criterion suggests that there is some element of humoral medicine in the Ainu concepts of illness. As with other humoral medicines (cf. Molony 1975), the feature of chill comes from its association with water. Theoretically, the absence of chill can mean either the nonpresence of chill, which is its neutrality, or the presence of fever or heat, which is its polar opposite. The Ainu data suggest the former, because there is no mention of *se:seh* (fever) in the description of the illnesses without chill. Also, the chill/nonchill opposition in symptoms is equated with the tactile/auditory opposition in the perception of aquatic versus land animal illnesses; the auditory receptor does not register temperature. The Ainu medical concepts differ from other humoral medicines in that the chill/nonchill opposition is used only in the classification of habitual illnesses; it does not extend to the classification of medicinal objects, food, and others. Furthermore, humoral medicine in other societies is often related to the cosmological emphasis on harmony and balance; this feature is also not particularly emphasized in Ainu medicine.

The nature of pain as a classificatory principle

In addition to the wet/dry feature, pain is of paramount importance in the diagnosis, as reflected in the choice of analogous illness terms. On the basis of the type of pain involved, there is an implicit category of crab illnesses, including the crab headache, crab boil, and crab eye illness, or lamprey illnesses, including the lamprey headache and lamprey boil. Although crab or lamprey illnesses are not explicit categories in Ainu medicine, *nius araka* is. This category includes all the illnesses whose primary symptom is sharp pains at multiple loci, as if wooden skewers were suddenly driven into the ailing part. The term *nius* means wooden skewers stuck in abundance; *ni* means wooden skewers, which the Ainu use in smoking trout, and *us* is an intransitive verb used when a number of things, such as needles or skewers, pierce a surface simultaneously. The label *nius*, then, describes the nature and degree of pain as well as the manner of occurrence (sudden assault), all in one analogy. One example is *nius takuh araka*, characterized by the pain striking the shoulder (*takuh*). For any of the illnesses in this category, a cure is to simulate the motion of pounding a wooden skewer, nail, or drill into the ailing part.

It is tempting to suggest that illnesses can be classified based on the nature of the pain. For example, if the pain has multiple loci but is fairly mild and the illness is wet, then it is one of the crab illnesses; if dry, however, it is a spruce branch illness, like the spruce branch abdomen illness, characterized by a prickling feeling of pain in the lower abdomen (see Chapter 4). If, however, the pain has multiple loci but is acute, without a chill or fluid, then it is one of the wooden skewer illnesses (*nius araka*) just discussed. A second category would be the illnesses characterized by pain that has a single locus and penetrates deep. If it is dry, then it is one of the woodpecker illnesses, such as the woodpecker headache or woodpecker boil. But if it is wet, then it is a lamprey illness, such as the lamprey boil or lamprey headache.

For these few cases of illness, a flow chart using the presence of a chill or fluid as a minimal distinctive feature is possible. However, beyond these cases, the other descriptions of pain do not lend themselves to systematic typology.

Illness classification and grammatical structure

In this last section, a possible correlation between the classificatory structures of illness and linguistic structures is briefly discussed. The illness classification discussed so far indicates that the single versus multiple loci is a frequently used criterion. Thus, boils are first divided into *asispe*, with multiple loci of infection, and *huhpe*, with a single locus. Likewise,

the wooden skewer, crab, and spruce branch illnesses are all characterized by multiple loci of affliction, whereas woodpecker, octopus, and
lamprey illnesses involve only a single locus. Just as the number of loci of
pain is the definitional criterion of these habitual illnesses, three out of
eight aspects of Ainu verbs (Chiri 1942:93-5; Kindaichi 1960:162-7) relate
to the number of occurrences of sound, motion, and behavior. The
momentane aspect [sic], characterized by a suffix of *-kosanu* (pl. *-ko-
sampa*), is used when the motion occurs only once, briefly. For example, *humkosanu* is used when a sound is emitted only once, as with the
single honking of a car horn. The successive aspect [sic] involves a suffix of
-rototo (or *-rototke*) and is used when the motion is repeated; it also
implies intensity of motion. Thus, *humrototke* is used when a loud, intense sound is emitted repeatedly, as when a car horn honks loudly
several times. The multitudious aspect [sic], accompanied by the suffix
-atki (pl. *-atkipa*), is chosen when intense multiple loci of movement are
involved. For example, it is used when a number of car horns honk
simultaneously and loudly. Although many of the examples given by Kindaichi involve sound, these distinctions are also applicable to other types
of motions and movements. For example, the momentane aspect is used
when a person falls or gets up, and when these motions occur only once
and suddenly. The multitudious aspect may be used when a person
shakes vigorously and repeatedly from the cold. Other aspects of the Ainu
verb specify the nature of the motion. As noted in Chapter 10, the Whorfian hypothesis, which emphasizes the relation of grammatical categories
to world view, has been more or less discarded by many anthropologists.
Yet, this partial concordance between the illness categories and the aspects of Ainu verbs seems worth noting.

Also of relevance here in regard to illness classification and the Ainu
language is that the classification of boils by stage of development is
paralleled in the classification of many important animals and plants by
their stage of growth. A young *Petasites japonicus*, used for *okuy eskari*
abdomen ache (see Appendix A), emerging from the snow in early spring
is called *etetara*, whereas an adult plant receives several lexemes, each
denoting a different part of it. Similarly, important animals such as salmon, bears, and seals receive different lexemes depending upon their
stage of growth.

Whereas time seems to be one of the features used in the classification
of several domains, it is important to note that the Ainu scheme does not
denote quantitative time. Thus, it is not the amount of time that marks
the division between a land animal boil and a sea animal boil; regardless of
the measurable time involved, a boil becomes a marine animal boil when
it opens and emits fluid. Likewise, different growth stages of plants and
animals are perceived as qualitative rather than quantitative distinctions.

The qualitative perception of time as reflected in these classification systems is consonant with the classification and perception of time itself, as revealed in other ethnographic data (see Ohnuki-Tierney 1969b, 1973c). Returning to Ainu grammatical structures, it is noteworthy that Ainu verbs have no tenses but distinguish many aspects (Chiri 1942:77, 91–2), as noted earlier, making fine distinctions with regard to the nature of the action or behavior but expressing neither measurable time periods nor temporal sequence.

Summary

Several conclusions may be drawn about the classificatory structure of habitual illnesses. First, some of these apparently minor illnesses, such as headaches and boils, are meticulously classified into a taxonomic structure consisting of several levels. Second, not all the habitual illnesses receive equal attention in classification. Thus, although the presence or absence of chill and fluid is a widely applicable classificatory principle for many illnesses, it is simply the most important diagnostic feature for many others. The nature of the pain may also serve to classify several illnesses. However, except for a small number of meticulously classified illnesses, a diagnostic feature such as a chill, fluid, or pain simply serves as a common denominator for a number of illnesses to be grouped together. Third, the diagnostic feature of the presence or absence of chill and fluid is closely aligned with a basic perceptual structure such as the spatiotemporal arrangements of the universe. The Ainu illness classification is therefore intimately linked with the basic structure of the world view. Fourth, the above analysis of habitual illnesses clearly demonstrates that the Ainu perceive their universe with various senses. Thus, they not only see but also hear and feel their universe. This sense-rich universe is mirrored in their perception of these minor illnesses. Fifth and last, there seems to be some concordance between the principles of illness classification and those of the grammatical and lexical structures of the Ainu language.

6

Metaphysical illnesses and their healing rituals

In contrast to the previous two chapters, this and the following chapter focus on afflictions that are often referred to as *supernatural illnesses* in anthropological literature. The term is misleading in the case of the Ainu, whose deities, such as the sun and bears, are beings of *nature* as we define the term. For lack of a better term, I refer to Ainu souls, spirits, deities, and demons as *metaphysical beings*. The metaphysical illnesses are all characterized by the involvement of metaphysical beings, either in the etiology, as a pathogen, or as a source of curing power, and all of the illnesses require the performance of shamanistic curing rites. This chapter is devoted to descriptions of metaphysical illnesses and their healing rituals. It begins with a discussion of smallpox and influenza epidemics, that is, illnesses accompanied by physical symptoms that afflict a great number of people. It then describes illnesses that involve physical symptoms but that afflict only individuals. Next, illnesses characterized by mental conditions that the Ainu recognize as abnormal are presented. The chapter ends with a detailed description of shamanistic healing rites, the spirits and deities involved in them, and sorcery. Chapter 7 presents a symbolic interpretation of metaphysical illnesses.

Epidemics

Smallpox and influenza epidemics have threatened the Ainu several times in the past, causing a drastic reduction in population and leaving a fearful imprint in the Ainu mind.[1] Referred to as evil illnesses (*wen araka*), epidemics are thought to be spread by demons.[2]

The major effort of the Ainu in relation to epidemics is directed to their prevention. With news of an approaching epidemic, a respected male elder recites *hawki* (epic poems), which constitute the most sacred genre of the Ainu oral tradition and which only male elders can recite (cf. Ohnuki-Tierney 1969a:3). In the Ainu scheme, the beneficial power of the deities is not directly involved in eliminating or retaliating against demons or other evil elements of the universe. The deities, however, can assist the Ainu by providing instructions as to how to combat evil. The *hawki* epics relate what occurred at the beginning of the world, when the demons threatened the existence of the Ainu. With aid from the deities, the Ainu were able to slay the demons or otherwise eliminate their threats. By reciting these epic poems, the performer and the audience psychologically reenact the drama of a successful combat against the demons and feel reassured of the favorable attitude of the deities toward them; thus the recitation of the epic poems provides the Ainu with extra fortitude against the threat of an epidemic.

The preventive measure of the epic poem recital is followed by the construction of a series of elaborate charms rich in cultural meaning. *Inaw* ritual sticks and wooden swords are placed at the entryway to each home. The ritual sticks, which are ordinarily offered to the deities, will hopefully ward off the demons with their positive power, and the wooden swords will be activated to combat the demons. The Ainu also hang a plant called *sikataro kina* (unidentifiable)[3] at the upper corner of their doorways. The plant's strong smell is believed to expel demons.

Next, the men of the settlement, often under the direction of its religious and/or political leader, collaborate in making and erecting various charms along the sides of a path that connects the Ainu settlement to the shore, because demons who live offshore use the path to come up to the settlement, just as the Ainu do when they are finished with their fishing. One kind of charm, *oken*, is a large statue of a man carrying a sword. The Ainu construct a number of these statues, using three kinds of trees: alder, elder, and white birch. Aromatic juniper branches are placed on the *oken* statues and are also hung from the right and left sides of the entrance to each home, both inside and outside. In addition, large bundles of sedge grass fastened on wooden sticks are placed along the path, and puppies are killed so that their skulls can be stuck on wooden sticks erected on the sides of the path.[4]

When the demons come up the path, the wooden statues come alive, swinging their swords right and left to kill them. The sedge bundles sway their bodies from side to side, and the puppy skulls return to life and bark at the demons, trying to chase them away. In other words, the charms thus become animated to perform an exorcism rite. (For details of this exorcism rite described as a part of a tale, see Ohnuki-Tierney 1969a: 67–72.)

A brief description of the cultural meaning of the plants used in demon exorcism is in order here. As noted, the *oken* statues are made from alder, elder, and white birch. The bark of alder soaked in water for a few days produces a red solution for dying that is also believed to be a blood substitute; a woman drinks this at the time of excessive hemorrhaging during menstruation or parturition. Because menstrual and parturient blood are offensive to both deities and demons and thus have the power to expel them, alder is effective in exorcism. This tree, used for *oken* statues, is also employed to make various charms for daily use. Consequently, it is strictly taboo to use alder for anything related to deities.

Elder is called *osokoni,* or a tree with excrement,[5] and its smell is considered to drive off not only humans but also demons. Elder is hence used also to make various charms.[6] Conversely, elder is the only tree that is taboo for use for firewood; when burnt, its smoke darkens everything in the house, including treasures. Because treasures signify offerings to the deities as an expression of respect and goodwill, the Ainu cannot afford to tarnish them, lest they risk offending the deities. White birch too is used to make charms. It is the tree chosen to make ritual sticks for the Goddess of Hearth and other female deities.[7]

Juniper, whose strong smell is considered good, purifies people and objects contaminated with death and sickness. A few branches of this tree are always hung in the upper corners of the doorway to keep out evil spirits. When there is a sick or mentally ill person in the house, juniper is burnt in the hearth. Its smoke purifies not only the afflicted person but also the entire atmosphere as it emerges from the chimney. When one becomes ill, one must, upon returning home, be purified at the doorway with freshly cut branches of juniper or with smoke from a burning branch. In addition, a solution made from boiling juniper branches, preferably with berries, in water is a good medicine for a number of illnesses.[8]

Once one is stricken, the most powerful antidote against smallpox is menstrual blood, which is smeared on the affected parts of the victim's body; its offensive smell expels the demons that spread the disease. A substitute medicine for a smallpox victim is red bog moss,[9] whose color resembles menstrual blood. Fresh in summer or dried in winter, the grass is boiled and pressed over the victim's body. In addition, the victim is urged to drink as much water as possible, because the high fevers accompanying smallpox will burn out the victim's stomach.[10]

In order to avoid contagion, some Ainu move away from their settlement, leaving the victim behind. Among the Hokkaido Ainu, this was done regularly; it is reported that some even left behind immediate family members who had already been stricken (Kubodera and Chiri 1940:126). The northwest coast Ainu did not resort to such drastic measures, although pregnant women were sometimes moved to a more isolated place, as in the case of my informant's mother.[11]

Somatic illnesses afflicting individuals

The following five types of illnesses are somatic illnesses, but unlike epidemics, they afflict only individuals. They are similar to habitual illnesses described earlier, but their cause involves a metaphysical being.

Unlike epidemics, which are caused by demons, these illnesses are caused either by souls or spirits, which are in themselves powerless, or by deities, which ordinarily exercise beneficial power. These benign or beneficial beings, however, cause illnesses when the humans break taboos, or mistreat or show disrespect to these metaphysical beings.

The *aymawko ahun* is identified by a sudden attack of sharp pain localized in a part of the body such as the stomach, chest, or sides of the torso. The reason for the name is that when one experiences this illness, one feels as if the spirit (*maw*) of an arrow (*ay*) has been shot (*ahun* = enter) into the body. This illness is caused by one person's harsh words against another. The victim is often not the violator of the code or the one verbally attacked, and there may not necessarily be any kinship tie between the victim and the two individuals involved. It is said that if one person verbally assaults another, someone in the community will suffer from this illness.[12]

A common cure for this illness is to grind a stone arrowhead or spearhead into powder, which is placed on the affected body part. An arrowhead or spearhead wrapped in ritual shavings may also be placed on the affected part instead. In addition, a shamanistic rite must be performed in order to determine the specific etiological factor, unless the etiology is immediately apparent. Also, rubbing the patient's body with wooden shreddings (called *ro:či* in Ainu), which have a high ritual value, is considered efficacious. Some administer a decoction to the patient.[13]

The *mokoro esaman kohka* (sleeping punishment by an otter; *mokoro* = sleep; *esaman* = otter; *kohka* = to punish) is another category of illness caused by a breach of a taboo. The only diagnostic symptom is excessive sleeping, which indicates to the Ainu that a relative of the victim has taken home an uninjured dead otter, either to eat it or to use its fur. In the Ainu code of behavior, an uninjured otter must be left alone; without a hole in the body, the otter's soul has not been able to leave its body to rest peacefully in the world of the dead. It therefore wanders around, inflicting this illness upon a relative of the offender. Although there is little treatment that assures a complete cure, usually a piece of an otter's fur or hide is wrapped in cloth and placed under the patient's pillow.[14]

When an estranged soul of a dead human causes an illness, it is referred to as a case of *isam aynu ramatuh iko ahun* (the entrance of a dead human's soul). When a human corpse does not receive a proper funeral, its soul cannot rest in peace in the world of the dead. Therefore, the soul afflicts someone with this illness as a reminder for the neglectful behavior of the survivors. Again, there is usually no necessary connection between the estranged soul, the offender of the Ainu code in the treatment of the dead body, and the patient, who often is an innocent victim.

When offended, the deities, who are the most powerful group of beings of the Ainu universe, cause an illness called *kamuy iramohkari* (punishment by the wrath of a deity). As in the case of possession by an estranged human soul, this illness is not identified by a standard set of symptoms, although there is always a feeling of total exhaustion without localized pain. But unlike possession by an estranged soul, when an illness is caused by the wrath of a deity, it is not altogether clear whether or not it entails entry into the body and subsequent possession. Only a shaman can identify an illness as *kamuy iramohkari*, which strikes when an Ainu engages in some form of disrespectful behavior toward a deity. For example, one case was diagnosed when the victim unknowingly built a house where bear bones were once enshrined; the structure had long since decayed and disappeared. Nevertheless, the bear deities were offended by the presence of the humans, especially the women with their polluting menstrual blood. Again, there may be no relation between the victim of the illness and the offender of the code. If a shaman reveals that an illness is a result of an offense toward bears, which are the most powerful deities of the Ainu pantheon, then an elaborate rite must be performed in order to apologize to them. All men who are closely related to the patient must participate in making the *inaw* ritual sticks, which are favored by the deities and hence are effective in appeasing them. They must then sacrifice a carefully chosen dog (dogs are considered to be messenger-servants of the bears), which is brought to the bone pile and cooked. After the consumption of the animal, its bones are enshrined at this location.

Whereas the illnesses described above are characterized by physical symptoms, the symptomatic criterion of *iramahsahkare* (the loss of one's soul) is a sudden loss of the sense of direction. When this occurs, one cannot recognize where one is, even when one is next to one's house. The illness, as the Ainu define the phenomenon, is caused by soul loss due to fox bewitchment. Thus, the eyes of a victim sometimes change to look like those of a fox. The foxes, deities of the Ainu, are assigned both a positive power of foretelling future events and a negative power of bewitching people. When fox bewitchment is suspected, one can resort to cursing (*topahse* in Ainu), which is a common measure used in an emergency. If one sees a ball of light, one can spit and curse in that direction, because the soul of any deity, including foxes, is said to fly like a ball of fire. Another measure considered efficacious for fox bewitchment is to offer prayers to the deity to which one feels closest, asking for help. Some, however, may not be able to pull themselves together to resort to these measures and may get lost in the woods or mountains. If they manage to return home, however, a shamanistic rite must be performed for a cure. Fox bewitchment is not very common among the northwest coast Ainu. The fox plays a much more prominent role among the Ainu of the east coast of Sakhalin (cf. Pilsudski 1912).

In three of the illnesses described above, the soul plays an important role. The *mokoro esaman kohka* is caused by an otter's soul, *isam aynu ramatuh iko ahun* is caused by the soul of a dead Ainu, and *iramahsahkare* is caused by soul loss. In order to fully understand the Ainu concepts of these illnesses, a brief discussion of the Ainu notion of the soul is in order. The common denominator of most beings of the universe is ownership of a soul; those without a soul are of little significance to the Ainu. Every Ainu, a newborn baby, a plant, and an animal, has a soul. So do most of the material objects made by the Ainu, including tools, kitchen utensils, and even grass mats. When inside a being, the soul is invisible. In the case of humans, it is located somewhere either in the head or in the heart. Its presence in the human body is seen in the expression of emotions; the soul is the seat of anger, joy, sorrow, and other strong emotions.

An important capacity of the soul is its ability to leave the body and act independently of it. Its presence becomes even more clearly demonstrable when it is outside the body than when it is inside. When people dream, their soul frees itself from its sleeping owner's body and travels to places distant in time and space. This is why in our dreams we visit places where we have never been. By the same token, a deceased person may appear in our dreams, because the soul can travel from the world of the dead to visit us during our dreams. Likewise, during a shamanistic performance, a shaman's soul travels to the world of the dead in order to snatch back the soul of the client who is "already dead," thereby reviving the dead. The departure of a soul is also an explanation for such phenomena as fainting and "temporary deaths" during which the person sleeps or is unconscious for an unusually long time while his or her soul visits the world of the dead Ainu.

Whereas these phenomena are due to a temporary parting of a soul from the body, death is explained as being caused by a permanent departure of the soul. A smooth transfer of the soul of the deceased to the world of the dead and a successful afterlife are guaranteed only when a proper funeral is given. Otherwise a restless soul may trouble the living in order to remind them of the proper treatment that is still required. A funeral for nonhuman beings means a proper treatment of their remains, whether the bones of fish or animals after human consumption or broken pieces of tools. Thus the Ainu must place the bones of animals and fish at their proper bone piles, called *keyohniusi* in Ainu; each species has its own bone pile at an appropriate place – for example, in the mountains for bears and close to the shore for sea mammals. In the case of large animals, the skull is placed on a ritual stick with its bifurcated tips piercing the eyeholes.

Thus, the soul and the dead body are intimately linked and yet can move about independently. A similar relation is also seen between words and their spirits, as in the belief that the illness is caused by the spirits of words. Further, as expressed in the notion that illness is caused by the wrath of a deity, emotions, whether of humans or nonhuman beings, have the power to move about and engage in acts of serious consequence. Without a thorough understanding of the Ainu beliefs concerning the soul, spirits, and emotions, one cannot comprehend Ainu metaphysical illnesses. Above all, the Ainu concepts of the soul, spirits, and emotions indicate the inappropriateness of applying the Western dichotomy between mental and physical diseases. The illnesses described above are characterized primarily by physical symptoms; yet their cause lies in nonphysical entities. These illnesses are therefore neither purely somatic nor spiritual or mental, but both, precisely because the body and the soul of human and nonhuman beings are closely related to each other.

Mental illnesses

Whereas the illnesses described in the previous section are caused by metaphysical beings but are characterized by physical symptoms, there is another category of illnesses that affect the mind and correspond approximately to the Western concept of mental illnesses. Just as mental illnesses are relatively ill-defined in Western societies, Ainu mental illnesses are also not well articulated and elude systematic classification. The identification of pathogens or of the etiology of an illness may differ from time to time even when made by the same individual. In what follows, I describe only one of the better-articulated types and briefly discuss others as best I can.

The best-articulated illness has the most severe symptoms, including delusions, lack of touch with reality, and physical violence against oneself as well as others. For example, a middle-age woman harmed herself until her body was bloody, and she insisted on eating her children. Thinking that water offered to her was the urine of a fox and that other food was animal excrement, she refused to drink or eat at all. Another older woman started to beat people and set fire to various places following the death of her son. Because of these violent actions toward others, the afflicted are often confined. The Ainu may build a wooden structure outside the house that is similar to a bear cage, with an opening to insert food for the confined. Or, as with the woman who lost her son, the afflicted may be confined to a storage house, which is an elevated structure outside the house. In the woman's case, with the approach of winter, her family built a semisubterranean pit house at a short distance from the house, because the storage house would have been too cold.

Although this illness can be caused by the estranged soul of a dead human, it is most often said to be caused by possession by demons. Thus, the labels for this type of insanity often include the term *oyasi* (demon), as in the case of *wen oyasi karape* (*wen* = evil; *oyasi* = demon; *kara* = possessed; *pe* = person), or *wen oyasi astepe* (the meaning of *aste* is not clear). Two types of demon exorcism rites are performed in an attempt to cure individuals suffering from this type of insanity.

The most frequently used method involves the following. First, a shamanistic rite is performed in order to secure a diagnosis. If successful, the spirit that enters the shaman's body will tell him or her what has possessed the patient. The curing process begins by rolling the patient, wrapped in a mat, down a hill. At the foot of the hill, male and female elders wait for the arrival of the bundle to perform a rite called *yohaykoyki*. This consists of the ritual swinging of swords, long ones for males and short ones for females, over the patient. The male elders then cut open the mat. In a severe case of insanity, the rite may have to be performed repeatedly until the patient becomes normal. At that time, a male elder purifies the patient by waving fir branches over the now presumably recovered individual and rubbing the body with wormwood – a favorite plant food of the Ainu.[15] After being brought home, the patient is again purified by the elders, who light a piece of cloth, wrap it over the head, and wave a fir branch over the individual. As a finale, a shamanistic rite is performed and the patient's relatives make offerings to the deity who has provided the diagnosis and etiology of the illness.

The *yohaykoyki*, or the rite of swinging swords, is a common demon exorcism rite. The Ainu believe that by cutting a demon to pieces and feeding its meat to the beings of the universe, they prevent a demon from being reborn, just as the proper treatment of corpses of beneficial beings of the universe will insure their rebirth. Thus, Ainu tales often end with a passage in which a hero cuts a demon to pieces and feeds its meat to trees, grasses, the ground, and all other beings of the universe to prevent its rebirth. The rite of *yohaykoyki* thus not only chases off a demon possessing the patient but also symbolically eliminates the demon from the Ainu universe.

A less frequently performed demon exorcism rite is *imos rimseka*. It is used in a settlement without a hill to perform the above-mentioned rite. The term *imos* refers to a large fir tree stump on which facial features are carved. The Ainu use fir for objects in events related to sickness and death. The patient is placed in the center of a circle made by shamans, who move around (*rimse* = to dance), each in turn lifting and dropping the tree trunk; this movement is synchronized with loud, rhythmic shouting. For additional purification, the patient's body is passed through a wreath made of fir branches.

The Ainu are sympathetic to the victims of this affliction, just as their penal code is aimed at rehabilitation rather than punishment of the offender. (For details of the Ainu legal code, see Ohnuki-Tierney 1974a:76–7.) They do not demonstrate an unusual fear of the insane, and they do not ostracize them. For example, the woman who lost her mind following her son's death was a shaman. Therefore, her family built a hearth in the center of the pit house and provided her with all the necessary paraphernalia for shamanistic performances. One day she was found unconscious, with her mouth full of spruce leaves given to her for her rituals. The family brought her back home, where she started to recover. If the period of confinement in an outdoor structure stretches into winter, however, the patients have little chance of surviving in the subarctic climate.

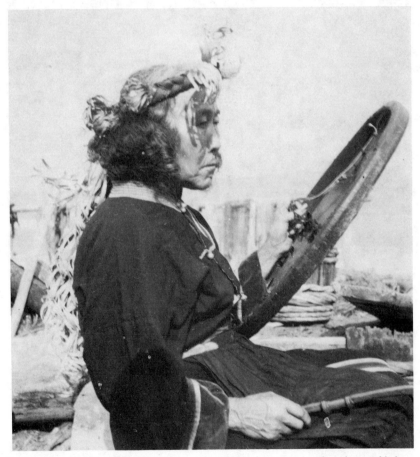

Kasuga Fumi, a shaman from the Ni:toy settlement on the east coast of southern Sakhalin. (Courtesy of T. Yamamoto.)

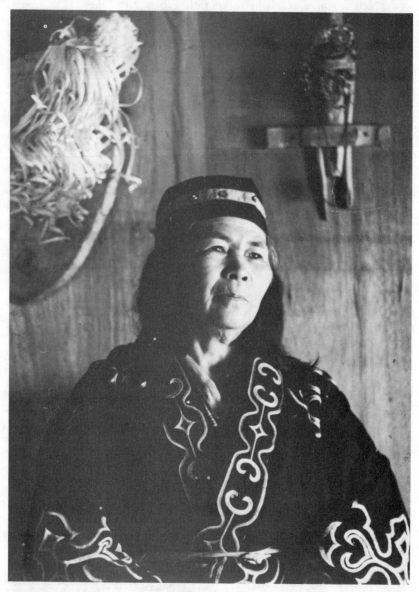

Husko, a shaman from the Rayčiska settlement on the northwest coast of southern Sakhalin. Her drum and ritual shavings for shamanistic rites are on the wall to the left, and her amulet and ritual shavings are on the wall to the right. (Taken in the 1950s; courtesy of Husko.)

Besides insanity involving violence, there are some minor types of mental aberration not necessarily considered illnesses by the Ainu. These are less articulated phenomena, and the data defy a systematic description. For example, those who feel sorry for themselves and cry excessively are said to suffer from *yayrampoki wen yayramsahka* (to feel sorry and lose one's soul). Another state of psychological aberration is a type of soul loss called *ramuču uhpe*. Its onset is marked by sudden withdrawal; a normal person suddenly becomes very quiet, as often occurs at the death of a spouse. It is perceived as a state in which the soul has already traveled to the world of the dead Ainu; thus these people are said to die shortly after experiencing this condition.

There are several types of mental aberration that afflict only shamans. A shaman may begin performing a rite involuntarily, even during the daytime, and continue this activity for several days. Only neophytes perform rites involuntarily when they are overcome by an urge; for experienced shamans who perform the rites only at the request of clients, it is strictly taboo to perform during the day. Apart from this behavioral aberration, these individuals act normally and carry out their daily responsibilities. Although the causes of this condition seem to vary from time to time and are not altogether well defined, some believe that it is caused by possession by a small animal such as a mouse or a crow. This condition is also called *ramuču uhpe* (soul loss).

Another mental aberration that befalls only shamans is the desertion of a shaman by his or her spirits. This occurs when a shaman violates a religious taboo and angers the spirits. The shaman will become like a fool, or a person without a soul, and will no longer be able to perform rites.

Shamanistic healing rites

As noted earlier, the performance of a shamanistic rite is a must for all of these metaphysical illnesses. The Ainu term *tusu* refers to these rites, as well as to everything involved in being a shaman. Shamanism is an age-old practice of the Ainu; it appears even in their oral tradition, where it is called *kinra* (Chiri 1954:143–4; Kindaichi 1914:36, 109, 159–60). In this section, I describe the shamanistic healing rites, the identity of shamans' spirits, and the deities involved; a discussion of shamans as social persona will be found in Chapter 11. Although both men and women have access to the profession, in the recent past most shamans have been women; the shamans I have personally known are all women. Therefore, in the following description, I refer to shamans as women.

There are strict rules for the performance of a shamanistic rite. Most importantly, it may take place only after sunset. Although a rite may be performed at any time of the year, in actual practice more rites are held during winter, when the Ainu are less busy, than during the summer fishing season. A menstruating woman may never be present, either as a shaman or as a member of the audience. The rite is always performed inside the house beside the hearth, where glowing embers provide the only light. The Ainu hearth is centrally located and square in shape. It is regarded as a miniature universe (cf. Chiri 1944:44) and is where the Goddess of Hearth resides. Two ritual sticks, male and female, are stuck at the northwestern corner of the hearth for her. She is called *Unči Ahči*, or Grandmother Hearth, and mediates between the Ainu and their deities at all times, including all the rituals.

Although there is no official announcement of the performance, when the shaman signals its beginning by beating a drum, people in the settlement start to gather at her house. To produce smoke, an assistant to the shaman places three aromatic plants on the embers (listed in order of their closeness to the embers): a branch or two of Yesso spruce or, if the shaman is a woman, of larch, a plant called *nuhča*, and minced dried leek.[16]

Throughout the rite, the shaman drinks sea water from a bowl in which the following items have been soaked: a twig of Yesso spruce, some *nuhča*, and dried tangle.[17] During the winter, when the sea is frozen, plain water from a river is used as the drink but becomes quite salty from the tangle. Though the Ainu consider the solution too salty for human consumption, a shaman often consumes two or three bowls of it during a rite, because it is supposedly the spirit, not she, who drinks it. The solution is also used at the beginning and end of the performance, when the shaman exorcises evil spirits by spraying it from her mouth.

The shaman commences the rite by asking the Goddess of Hearth and other deities for help. She then presents the specific case for which the rite is being performed, describing the symptoms of her client's illness. In contrast to the prayers recited in fixed forms during group rituals, the shaman's invocations are always impromptu, geared to the specific purpose of the rite.

Amidst the smoke from the plants, the sound of drumming, and the crowd of people packed into the small one-room Ainu house, the shaman becomes possessed by a spirit. The salty drink the shaman swallows may also help the process of possession because the *nuhča* plant is mildly narcotic (Miyabe and Miyake 1915:308-9). The Ainu discern two stages in the process of spirit possession. The first is *kamuy maw koro*, which means "to acquire the power of a deity" (a spirit is commonly referred to as a deity). This stage of spirit possession is easily identifiable by observers, because the shaman's facial expression and voice are replaced by those of the spirit that has possessed her. If a rough spirit possesses her, her behavior becomes rough; if it is an animal spirit that hops, such as a grasshopper, she hops around the hearth. Although the behavior of a shaman during this period is determined by the spirit, a shaman often has a small repertoire that she usually employs. It may include, for example, certain movements of the body, whistles, groans, and rapid oral utterances like "ya, ya, ya." The second stage is the climax; it is referred to in Ainu as *kamuy ko ahun* (the deity, that is, the spirit, enters). It is during this stage that the information eagerly sought from the deities is released by the spirit through the shaman. Although some shamans say that they remember what they have said during the trance, the majority seem to experience amnesia.

The drum, called *kačo* or more politely *senisteh* (a term used for charms in general), is an important element in Sakhalin Ainu shamanistic rites. In addition to being an effective inducer of a trance, the drum functions both as a means of summoning the spirits and calling the attention of the deities and as a charm against the evil spirits that always try to interfere and prevent a successful performance of the rite. The drum is composed of one oblong membrane made of a musk deer skin fastened to a wooden frame made of larch or a plant called *raramani*[18] using fish glue. The drum stick is wrapped in a dog's skin. Shamans do not wear special garments for the performance, and their paraphernalia includes only a special headdress, a headband to which various charms are attached, a necklace, and ritual sticks with shavings called *inaw*.

In addition to the shaman, the presence of two or three other individuals is necessary in order to conduct the rite properly. One, an assistant to the shaman, is called *kamuy ču:tehpe* (literally, a servant of a deity). The assistant prepares the necessary items for the performance, adds herbs to keep the smoke going, and makes offerings to various deities at appropriate times. No special qualifications are required, nor is the assistant always the same person. Usually a shaman chooses a family member or a close relative who is available at the time.

Because the shaman's trance is usually followed by amnesia, the second requisite person is the one who interprets to the audience the information received from the deities and related by the spirit through the shaman. This assistant is called *inu: aynu* (the person who listens) and is usually an older person who is well versed in both the language of the deities and the language of the elders, because a shaman's message involves an extensive use of these two sets of lexical and grammatical forms. The language of the deities, *kamuy itah*, is used exclusively by male elders in their communication with the deities, such as the prayers offered during group rituals. The language of the elders, *onne itah*, is used among elders, both male and female, during their conversation. Because the language of the deities is involved, a male elder is best suited for this role. However, many female elders have a basic understanding of the language, which they do not necessarily display and are forbidden to use.

The presence of a third person, who must be a shaman, male or female, is required when a rite is performed for a sick person. It is this person's duty to remove the ritual stick, or *inaw*, which is used in purifying the patient, and to deposit it outside the house toward the west, the direction associated with death. Because of the pollution incurred by handling the ritual stick, this person must stay outside the house for a period after the performance.

Although in most cases shamans are consulted about the diagnosis and treatment of illnesses, they can also obtain other types of information from deities or perform "miracles." (For details of the Ainu shaman's power, see Chapter 11.)

An additional ethnographic fact is that the Ainu perform shamanistic rites for sick bears. As noted in Chapter 2, the Ainu raise a bear cub for a year and a half in order to send it off in an elaborate ritual. If the cub becomes very sick during this period, the men in the settlement take it out of its cage and bring it into the house through the ordinary entrance that the humans use. Although a slain bear during the bear ceremony must be brought into the house through the "sacred window," through which no human can enter, this window is not for a living bear. The bear is placed beside the hearth on a layer of freshly made ritual shavings and spruce branches. Male shamans perform rites throughout the night, taking turns, so that the performances themselves cure the illness. Unlike a human sickness, no diagnosis or cure is sought; there is no medicine for the illnesses of a bear. While male shamans perform the rites, older women of the house or in the settlement apply cold water in which ritual shavings have been soaked to the forehead of the sick bear, or force its mouth open and drop cold water into it. When the bear is returned to the cage, freshly made ritual shavings are liberally placed inside. The great amount of ritual shavings throughout the treatment period is thought to cause recovery through the potent healing power they possess.

Spirits and deities involved in shamanistic rites

A number of spiritual beings are involved in shamanistic rites. Major deities, as noted above, are the ultimate source of information sought during the rites. The Goddess of Hearth, a major deity in the Ainu pantheon, plays a critical role. As a mediator, she only delivers messages from the Ainu to deities if she is favorably inclined to the humans, but she is also thought to inject her opinions about the matter in question.

Shamans' spirits, *kosimpuh* in Ainu,[19] are difficult to identify, although I repeatedly attempted to do so throughout my three fieldwork sessions. My key informant, Husko, for example, who is otherwise always eager to teach me the Ainu way, was vague and often peculiarly possessive about her knowledge in this area. She had to be in the right mood and the right physical condition to discuss the subject; otherwise her mental and physical well-being might have been endangered. Even under the right circumstances, she claimed that such deep knowledge cannot be expressed in words and that the only way for me to understand was to become a shaman myself. Although my key informant did have the knowledge, because she did not totally lose consciousness during her performances especially during the recent past, other shamans claimed that they themselves had little knowledge because of amnesia. Pilsudski (1961) and Chiri and Wada (1943), authors of the only detailed reports on Sakhalin Ainu shamanism available today, do not elaborate sufficiently on the shamans' spirits to provide any additional information or insight. The following descriptions represent my piecing together of information about the spirits given on different occasions.

The animals that are most commonly thought to become spirits are grasshoppers, crows, ravens, cranes, ducks,[20] demon birds called *kawawe:*, and the worms called *ruroyaw*. I have not been able to identify the last two. The *kawawe:* are female birds, the males being called *hu:ni*. The onomatopoeia of their cry, after which the birds are named, is the only identifying feature, because they cry only at night when they are not visible. Their cry may foretell a death or may cause either insanity or death. (For further details on this belief, see Ohnuki-Tierney 1968:269–70.) The *ruroyaw*, according to the Ainu, are sea worms that look like snakes (*oyaw*) but have many legs. It is taboo to step on them, as they instantly break into many pieces. The Ainu abhor snakes, but they neither deify them nor consider them to be spirits.

There are other spirits that are not identifiable in terms of actual species of animals. For example, *suruku e kamuy* is a spirit that causes a shaman to eat the root of aconite (*suruku*). Although the root is poisonous, a shaman possessed by this spirit during a rite may eat it without being poisoned; it is the spirit that consumes the root and not the shaman, who is consequently not harmed.

Although shamans' spirits are respectfully called *tusu kamuy* (*tusu* = shamanism; *kamuy* = deity), the Ainu do not assign them the status of deities. Unlike other Ainu, who are said to deify a multitude of beings in nature,[21] the northwest coast Ainu include only a restricted number of land and sea mammals and some birds in their pantheon. Conversely, they maintain that none of the major deities, such as the bears, seals, the God of the Sea, the Goddess of Sun and Moon, and the dragon deities become shamans' spirits.

The Ainu consider certain spirits as either male or female or sometimes undifferentiated in terms of sex. There is no connection between the sex of a shaman and that of his or her spirit. Nor is there any rule explaining why a shaman receives a male or a female spirit. Some spirits specialize in certain types of work. For example, the aforementioned worm spirit and the spirit that consumes the aconite root are both considered especially efficacious in curing illnesses.

No permanent relationship is established between a shaman and a particular spirit because possession by a spirit is more or less haphazard. The Ainu emphasize the helplessness of the shamans, who have no control over which spirits possess them at a certain time. Usually a shaman seems to have a pool of spirits, one of whom possesses her during a particular performance. Some shamans have evil spirits in their pool and may occasionally become possessed by one of them, as in sorcery (discussed in the following section). The audience can easily determine which spirit has possessed the shaman by the way the shaman starts to act, as noted earlier.

Another group of spiritual beings involved in Ainu shamanism is referred to in Ainu as *seremaka* or *turenpe* – guardian deities. Again, the precise nature of these deities is difficult to determine. These Ainu terms are also used to refer to personal guardian deities, to guardians of all the Ainu of a particular settlement, or to guardians of all the Ainu. Moreover, because shamans' spirits help the Ainu in getting information from the major deities during the shamanistic rites, the deities may be referred to as *seremaka* or *turenpe* in this context. Direct questioning on the relationships between these various groups of metaphysical beings elicited no satisfactory information. However, taken together, various statements made on different occasions seem to indicate that a number of deities and spirits who are favorably inclined to the shaman collaborate more or less indirectly to achieve a successful result in a particular rite. Often these are spirits and deities who have in the past aided the older relatives and ancestors of the shaman. Even the deified ancestors of the shaman can render help during the rites. It would seem, therefore, that all these varied spirits and deities must be included among the guardians or *seremaka*.

Sorcery

The power of the sorcerer is the polar opposite to that of the shaman, the healer. Instead of healing illnesses, sorcery causes them. Shamans' spirits that harm people are called *sipes oyasi* (cannibalistic demons). As the designation indicates, these spirits are conceived to be demons who kill people to drink their blood and eat their flesh. The northwest coast Ainu claim that there were only a few such shamans among them in the past and that there are none at present. They assert, however, that among the east coast Ainu, and among the Gilyaks and Oroks, evil shamans abound, and that from time to time some of the northwest coast Ainu are victimized by them; in other words, these peoples are their enemies.[22]

More common among the northwest coast Ainu are shamans who occasionally become possessed by evil spirits. The Ainu emphasize that it is not the shamans who are wicked, because they have no control over the spirits that possess them and do not realize that they are evil until after the harm has been accomplished. Evil spirits are called *wen tusu kamuy* (evil spirits) or *semun ranne kamuy* (delinquent deities). Despite my repeated attempts, their identity, except for the quality of their behavior, remains unknown.

There are definite indications that a person has become the victim of an evil shaman. As noted earlier, if the victim is a man, he will vomit blood in which one can find an arrow point and wooden shavings of the kind used by the Ainu as offerings to the deities. If the victim is a female, she too will vomit blood, but it will contain wooden shavings and a needle. The relatives of the victim may take revenge by offering the shavings and the arrow tip or the needle to their own spirits, if they themselves are shamans, or to the spirits of the shamans they consult. The spirits that are ordinarily good then return these objects to the evil shaman, who, it is believed, will consequently die.

Evil spirits are thought to disguise themselves as birds in traveling to the place where their possible victim is located. Sagacious elders are consequently always on the alert and shoot these birds whenever they spot them. According to the Ainu description, the bird in question looks like a kite.[23] It has long claws and large eyes like those of a cat, and is reddish brown with a tinge of gold. Although kites are common in Sakhalin, the Ainu neither use them in any way nor attach any metaphysical power to them.

Because the pool of spirits of some shamans includes both good and evil spirits, a battle between the two sometimes takes place within the shaman. If an evil spirit wins, the shaman falls on the floor. It is the duty of people in the audience to help the good spirits to win such a battle. When they observe a battle taking place, the men will swing their daggers to the right and left and shout – a common method by which men exorcise evil spirits. The women participate by swinging branches of fir or ritual sticks made of willow to purify the shaman. When the rite is over, the fir branches or ritual sticks are carried outside and placed in the crotch of a tree that stands west of the house.

The Ainu do not see the involvement of kinship ties between sorcerers and their victims. This is a restatement that there is no sorcerer among them because most of the inhabitants of the northwest coast settlements are somehow related to one another.[24]

Summary

The illnesses described in this chapter are perceived by the Ainu to involve a metaphysical or nonmaterial agent in the etiology, as a pathogen, or both. The Ainu descriptions of these illnesses indicate that the worst cases of human misfortune – epidemics and severe cases of mental illness – can be attributed to the demons, the innate evil in the universe. Epidemics can wipe out the entire population or at least cripple Ainu society. The mental illness attributed to the workings of demons not only causes one to lose one's mind but is also responsible for violent antisocial acts – behavior essentially identical to the workings of demons, whose business is to destroy human beings. Neither case offers much hope of recovery. By ascribing their causes to demons, the Ainu avoid blaming their fellow members for the worst and most hopeless misfortunes. Likewise, sorcerers are said to exist only among others. This aspect of their illness perception is in accord with other aspects of Ainu culture, such as a lack of emphasis on punishment in their legal codes and a strong emphasis on sharing among members of the society.

In contrast, somatic illnesses that afflict individuals or milder cases of mental illness are caused by a being of the Ainu universe who is either beneficial or powerless in ordinary circumstances but who can cause illnesses when mistreated. The power of the deities is demonstrated to the Ainu not only through their beneficial power in providing abundant food and general welfare but also through their power to punish by causing an illness if offended. A soul is usually benign; however, if a body is mistreated by humans, then the soul may exercise its power by causing an illness. Likewise, words, when misused as an antisocial weapon, can physically harm people by causing an illness. In other words, the ultimate cause of these illnesses lies with humans, who can please these beings so that they remain beneficial or benign or break a taboo and bring about their own misfortune. Thus, an illness is incurred by breaking moral codes against deities or other soul-bearing beings of the universe, or by breaking social codes against fellow Ainu with the use of offensive remarks. Because illnesses are seen as expressions of disharmonious relations between the Ainu and nonhuman beings of the Ainu universe, they also serve to enforce both religious and social control – a point I shall return to in Chapter 11. The control of individual behavior through illness affliction as it works in Ainu society is again nonpunitive in nature because the Ainu do not stipulate a particular relation between the violator of the code and the victim of illness.

If the locus of negative power is seen in illness pathogens and etiologies, then the source of positive power may be seen in the Ainu rituals for illness healing and prevention. In regard to epidemics and in the worst cases of mental disorder, male elders play an important role. The physical power of combat by young men is also symbolically expressed in the prevention rites of an epidemic. Above all, however, it is the shamans who play the crucial role in healing the afflicted. Women too play an important role here. Shamans are usually women, and the female deity, that is, the Goddess of Hearth, is the most important deity in the ritual.

A characteristic of the Ainu is their notion that the shamans are helpless victims of spirits who possess the shamans at will – contrary to Eliade's description of shamanism (1972:6). Ainu shamanism involves both the impersonation of spirits and amnesia experienced by most shamans following the performance; these two features are defining characteristics of what Bourguignon calls "possession trance" (1973a:12–13). Like shamanistic practices in many other societies (cf. Eliade 1972:508–9), Ainu shamanism is antidemonic and defends life and health, but it does not deal with fertility and sex.

7

A symbolic interpretation of metaphysical illnesses and healing rituals

This chapter focuses on the interpretation of negative and positive symbolic powers as expressed in the Ainu concepts of metaphysical illnesses and their treatments. The description in Chapter 6 of Ainu metaphysical illnesses and their preventive and healing rites illustrates that these illnesses are concrete manifestations of the interrelationships among deities, demons, spirits, and souls in the Ainu universe. But in order to locate negative symbolic power in the Ainu symbolic structure, as expressed in illness pathogens and etiologies, and the positive symbolic power of healing, we must examine what these beings of the universe represent in the basic symbolic structure.

I begin with an interpretation of deities and humans in Ainu symbolic classification and proceed to an interpretation of demons. Next, the symbolic nature of illness and health is analyzed to determine its relation to the basic structure. This is followed by a detailed discussion of symbols that appear in the Ainu medical rituals of exorcism, purification, and healing. To further determine the nature of the mediation symbols involved in medical rituals, the power of transcendence held by these symbols and the source of this power are explored. The relationship between demonic anomaly and marginal symbols of mediation is determined in the following section; both share features other than normal, but demonic anomaly destroys the structure whereas marginal symbols restore it. After the importance of the use of senses in Ainu symbolic perception is discussed, the symbolic emphasis of cooking and women in shamanistic rites is examined with reference to the /nature:culture/ opposition. Next, shamanism is contrasted to Ainu group rituals in order to explore the possibility of the presence of more than one set of symbolic systems. Anthropological concepts underlying the discussions in this chapter are reexamined in Chapter 8 from theoretical and cross-cultural points of view with reference to interpretations by other scholars.

Deities and humans in Ainu symbolic classification

The Ainu term *mosiri* (universe, world) in its most inclusive sense means the total sphere of Ainu physical and mental activities and phenomena. It is the land of the Ainu, living and dead, their deities, demons, and numerous other beings, including nondeified animals, plants, and fish. It is, in our view, southern Sakhalin, the adjacent sea, and the sky above. As noted in Chapter 2, the Ainu have been in contact with other peoples possibly since the first millennium A.D. (Stephan 1971:19–29; see also Hora 1956) and were active participants in the Santan trade. However, when they talk about their *mosiri* and their way of life, all other lands and peoples disappear and the *aynu*, that is, the Ainu, become the only humans. The most meaningful unit of social organization for the Ainu is the society of the universe, in which they interact intimately with their deities and demons.

The Ainu believe their deities are more powerful than humans, but this power is not necessarily physical; it is perceived at a symbolic or metaphysical level and is beneficial toward the Ainu unless the deities are offended. For example, although bears are physically more powerful than humans and have the remarkable capacity to survive the winters simply by licking the salt on their paws (as the Ainu believe),[1] the power of the bears as perceived by the Ainu is, above all, their capacity to reign as the supreme deities who determine the welfare of the Ainu. If pleased, they provide abundant food and protect the Ainu from the demons, but if offended, they can punish the humans by harming them. Similarly, the Goddess of Hearth has the physical capacity to provide warmth for survival and fire for cooking in this subarctic region; however, she is revered, above all, as a mediator between the Ainu and the deities. If pleased, she will speak positively on behalf of the Ainu, but if angered, she will refuse to deliver their messages. Therefore, even though physical capacities of the deities transcend human capacities, it is their metaphysical power that is more real and more important for the Ainu.

Although these deities are seen as super-Ainu, they are not altogether different from the Ainu. The Goddess of Hearth is called *Unči Ahči*, or Grandmother Hearth, the bear deities are addressed in prayers as grandfathers, and the bear cub the Ainu raise for the bear ceremony is referred to as their grandchild. If the bear slain during the bear ceremony is a female, she is adorned with necklaces and other ornaments just as a human woman would be, and a ritual stick dedicated to the Goddess of Sun and Moon is carved to symbolize her earrings. Further illustrations of the fact that the deities are perceived much the same as humans are found in folktales. For example, in one tale a human who is married to a bear deity takes along elders from her settlement to the country of the deities; the elders find the deities to be in human form, living with their families in houses just like those of the Ainu (Ohnuki-Tierney 1969a:167–70). In fact, one of the marks of *nupuru aynu* (holy men), who have the extraordinary power of communicating with the deities, is their ability to see a bear or other deities in this human form rather than in their animal forms, as ordinary people see them. Along this line, Chiri (1944:27–8; 1954:359–61; Chiri and Oda 1956:235–6) presents an interpretation that, in the Ainu view, all animal deities are actually human in appearance and live as humans do when in their own country. Only when they visit the Ainu country do they disguise themselves in the forms of animals by wearing special fur or leather garments. The purpose of this disguise is to bring a present when visiting as an expression of goodwill.[2] Although the northwest coast Ainu do not explicitly entertain this concept, there is sufficient ethnographic evidence, such as the above-cited tale, to support Chiri's interpretation.

In terms of symbolic classification, the anthropomorphic nature of Ainu deities leads to the belief that in the Ainu perception of the society of the universe, both deities and humans belong to the same general category of beings. Deities are distinguished from humans only in that they are super-Ainu, that is, sacred. We may say, therefore, that deities and humans are in binary opposition, with the sacred quality as the minimal distinctive feature characterizing the deities (see Table 7.1).

If we go down a level in the taxonomic structure of the beings of the universe, the domain of analysis is the human society. In this very small society, there is no such elaborate social organization as moities. The Ainu kinship organization is basically bilateral, with some emphasis on patriliny in certain areas, and a basic flexibility in the exercise of rules. The most meaningful division of the Ainu society is that of men versus women – a division rigidly observed by a strict allocation of sex roles. The Ainu explain that men engage in activities that deal directly with the deities. All religious rituals except shamanistic rites are officiated by men, especially male elders, and the male head represents the family before the deities in family rituals. Because some of the animals hunted are deified and fishing takes place at the residence of a sea deity and involves the products of this deity, both hunting and fishing are viewed as activities dealing with deities.

From the point of view of sociopolitical structure, these activities lie in the public domain, that is, they take place beyond the localized family unit. (For a discussion of the public and domestic domains, see Chapter 8.) Because an important qualification for political leaders in the community is their ability to communicate with the deities, which is manifested in their hunting and fishing skills, the political arena becomes an exclusive territory for men. This intricate triad of men, hunting, and political structure is nowhere more expressive than in the bear ceremony. A high cultural value is placed upon capturing a newborn cub, raising it for a year and a half, and sending it off in an elaborate ceremony that lasts for days. The host, who distributes the bear meat along with other ceremonial dishes to all the guests, receives admiration for his generosity. An added bonus here is that the host can get rid of his excess food and other items of property in the process, because the bear ceremony is held just before the migration to the Ainu winter settlement. Although bear meat is considered by far the greatest food by the Ainu, it is not a dependable food source (it is eaten only several times a year), nor is bear fur particularly valuable, because it collects snow. The high value placed upon the bear does not derive from its food or other economic values but from its political role in the distribution of goods. Among the scholars who point to the political importance of the distribution of goods in noncapitalistic economic systems (e.g., Forde and Douglas 1967:22; Gluckman 1965:esp. Ch. 2), Sahlins (1960:411) expresses the situation most succinctly: "It is not, however, the possession nor consumption of goods that gives chiefly power, but their dispensation; hence generosity is the *sine qua non* of chieftainship." In short, the host of the bear ceremony, who is often a political leader of the community, converts his excess food into generosity, which in turn provides him with political power. When we realize that guests are invited to the bear ceremony even from distant settlements, whereas all other Ainu rituals are held only on a family or individual basis, then the political significance of the event looms large.

An opposite picture holds for women and their economic activities. Thus, the plant food gathered by women does not receive high ritual value, despite its well-recognized food value, because it is not distributed publicly, as the bear meat is. The Ainu again explain the situation from the ideological viewpoint; the smell of menstrual and parturient blood, too potent to disappear even after washing, is offensive to the deities. Hence the taboo against women's participation in the economic and political activities. Consequently, women gather plants, cook, sew, and bear and raise children – all in the domestic domain. (For a detailed discussion of the political dimension of the economic roles of Ainu men and women, see Ohnuki-Tierney 1980b.)

The degree to which sex determines social position in Ainu society is, however, mitigated by the effects of another ascribed status – age. The Ainu believe that one gets closer to the deities as one becomes older. The elderly, both male and female, therefore, are sacred and thus superior in status to the young. They alone use the previously mentioned language of the aged (*onne itah*), which consists of a special set of vocabulary and grammatical usages. When the age and sex criteria conflict, as in the case of young men versus older women, there usually are situational rules. For example, during the bear ceremony young men take a superior or more sacred role than older women as a group in that young men can actively participate in the ceremony, whereas all women, regardless of age, must follow certain rules that restrict their behavior. Although the older woman of the host's family receives a special privilege during the cere-

Table 7.1. *Basic dyads of the society of the Ainu universe*

	Dyad	
Domain	Sacred	Profane
Society of the universe	Deities	Humans
Human society	Men	Women
	Aged	Young

mony by heading the ritual process, she too must follow the same rules (see Chapter 2).

The combined factors of sex and age bring the elderly males closest to the deities. They alone have the right to officiate in group rituals, during which formulaic prayers are dedicated to the deities. Another special language mentioned earlier, the language of the deities (*kamuy itah*), is used in these prayers because knowledge of it is a prerogative of male elders; it provides the basis for their exclusive access to the role of officiants in the rituals. Although some of these male elders are no longer capable of hunting and fishing, they remain productive members of society by transmitting their accumulated wisdom regarding hunting and fishing, by acting as managers in social affairs and, most importantly from the Ainu point of view, by communicating with the deities through prayers and dedication of rituals to ensure abundant food and the general welfare of the Ainu. The superior position of male elders is expressed daily in the seating arrangement in their houses (for details, see Ohnuki-Tierney 1972). They sit at the most sacred side, where offerings to the deities are placed and where the slain bear is seated during the bear ceremony.

This discussion of the symbolic classification of the beings of the universe is summarized in Table 7.1. It consists of two taxonomic levels, with the /sacred:profane/ opposition acting as a classificatory principle. When the domain is the most inclusive universe, deities are contrasted to humans and are the sacred half of the dyad. When the domain is human society, men and the aged are the sacred half of the dyad, contrasting to women and the young, respectively, who comprise the profane half. Because the contrast in these two levels represents a complementary opposition that does not signify the possession of a specific property or properties, it can operate on more than one level, as I discuss in detail later in this chapter. Although details are not directly relevant for the theme of this section and therefore are not presented, it should be pointed out that the deities and other beings of the universe are further classified, just as time and space and various other phenomena are meticulously classified (Ohnuki-Tierney 1969b, 1972, 1973c).

Demons in Ainu symbolic classification

Against the background of a meticulously classified universe, we can now examine the structural identity of demons, some of which are vividly described in Ainu folktales. Most of these tales take place at the beginning of the world, when both demons and deities were more numerous than now, and demons often threatened the survival of the Ainu. The most dreaded demons then were a male and female pair who lived in caves in two adjacent mountains. They are depicted as having one eye like a full moon, impenetrable skin, an upper jaw that touched the sky, and a lower jaw that dug into the ground (for details, see Ohnuki-Tierney 1969a:10–52). Morphologically, they are anomalous; they have one eye instead of two and unusual skin. In addition, their bodies are depicted as traversing more than one spatial category, that is, the sky and the earth. As described in my 1972 publication, in the Ainu spatial classification the vertical sphere is divided into the sacred sky and the profane earth or ground.

More often, demons in Ainu tales are those beings of the universe who ordinarily are benign but who temporarily turn evil as a result of human misconduct. For example, two of the demon stories are based on the Ainu code that when one moves away from a settlement and has to leave behind a musical instrument, a loom, or any other soul-bearing object, it must be broken apart so that its soul can leave the "dead body" to rest in peace in the world of the dead. This treatment is comparable to a funeral for humans or the bear ceremony, whose function is to send off the soul through a proper ritual so that it may be reborn in the world of dead humans or the deities.

In one story (Ohnuki-Tierney 1969a:53–66), a pair of *tonkori* musical instruments that were left behind intact by their owner turned into cannibalistic demon brothers who went to Ainu settlements asking who they (demons) were. When the Ainu could not determine their identity, they engaged in a wholesale assault on the settlement. When they came to the settlement of the culture hero, however, he had been instructed by his guardian deity through a dream and was thus able to tell them that they were the children of musical instruments. The demon brothers instantly disappeared, and all that remained were two musical instruments lying on the upper side of the hearth; the culture hero took them out of the house and broke them apart with an axe. This story contains symbolic representations of two types of anomaly: first, the anomaly of being out of place – the souls of the instruments could not belong to the world of the dead; second, the anomaly of lack of identity – in Ainu society, in which kinship is of paramount importance, a child who does not know its parents is a person without social identity.

In another story (Ohnuki-Tierney 1969a:130–7), a loom left intact by the owner turned into a cannibalistic demon in the shape of an old woman who resided in an empty house in a deserted settlement. Travelers unknowingly seeking shelter were cooked and eaten by the demon, who, like the musical instrument demons, represents the anomaly of being out of place; its soul is out of its proper place, which is the world of the dead.

Other Ainu demons (see Ohnuki-Tierney 1969a) are characterized by invisibility, extraordinary size, or other anomalies. Therefore, although demons constitute a class of beings at a surface level of Ainu classification, they personify symbolic anomaly. The demons in Ainu tales are the antithesis of order, that is, the classified world of the Ainu, and threaten the Ainu conceptual framework. The male and female demons who lived in caves in the beginning of the world represent a permanent disorder and innate evil in the universe, whereas the demons in the other two stories represent temporary anomaly and disorder. (Theoretical discussions of the notion of anomaly in symbolic classification are presented in Chapter 8.)

Illness and health in Ainu symbolic classification

In myths, both intrinsic and temporary demons are said to take human lives; intrinsic demons exterminate whole settlements, and temporary demons kill individuals. Although the method of killing is not specified in these myths, it was noted in Chapter 6 that the cause of illnesses with little hope for recovery (epidemics and the severest cases of insanity) are ascribed to intrinsic demons, whereas other illnesses are ascribed to temporary causes, including the estranged soul. There is a close concordance, then, between the demons described in myths and those that appear in the description of illness pathogens and etiologies. It follows that in the Ainu scheme of things, real threats to human lives and society, such as death and illness, are personified as demons, which, from the viewpoint of symbolic structure, are either permanent or temporary anomalies.

The structure that the demonic pathogens and etiologies threaten is the classified universe of the Ainu (see Table 7.2, A), described in the previous section. But as we saw in Chapter 6, apart from demons, causes of illness include disharmony in the social network between the deities and humans or among humans themselves (see Table 7.2, B); these too may be seen as anomalies in the social relations among the beings of the universe, although not all of them are personified as demons.

The maintenance of individual health may therefore be seen to correlate symbolically with the cherished world of the Ainu in which the deities, humans, and other beings are classified in a hierarchical but

Table 7.2. *The Ainu symbolic structure of health and illness*

	Structure – order	Antistructure – anomaly
A. Beings of the universe	Deities, humans, and other classified beings	Demons
B. Social relations within the dyad	Harmony	Disarticulation
C. State of human life	Health Normal time	Illness Liminal period
D. State of the individual	Complete social persona	Incomplete social persona
E. Value	Cleanliness Good	Pollution Evil

orderly fashion and maintain harmonious relations (see Table 7.2, C). Illness, on the other hand, is equated with anomaly in the Ainu cognitive structure as well as anomaly in social relations. In terms of temporal categories, it is a liminal period hovering between life and death and requires medical rites of passage to exorcise the demons, purify not only the patient but also the defiled structure, and then restore the patient's health and the classified world of the Ainu.

In terms of the state of the individual, the sick person departs from the norm in two ways (Table 7.2, D). First, he or she is no longer a whole social persona, because the sick cannot perform some or all of their roles. A woman may no longer be able to perform her economic roles, such as plant gathering, although she may continue to carry out her kinship roles as a mother or wife until the illness becomes too serious for her to function at all. Second, causes of illness such as an arrow intrusion, spirit possession, and soul loss threaten the identity of the sick as an individual. The person is no longer "I" with a clear boundary around the ego, because either a part of the body, such as the soul, is elsewhere, or a foreign entity, such as the spirit of an arrow, has entered. (Cf. Kapferer 1979, who presents an interesting application of Meadian social phenomenology to an interpretation of the demonic illness in Sri Lanka during which the subjective "I" and the objective "me" merged.)

In terms of values (Table 7.2, E), the need to perform purification rites for the sick most succinctly expresses the belief that illness is dirty and polluting, whereas health is clean. Thus the function of the purification rites is to cleanse and free the patient from pollution inflicted by the pathogenic demons. Because demons are evil by definition, we can further translate the elements listed in the right-hand column in Table 7.2 to stand for evil, whereas those in the left-hand column stand for good

(Table 7.2, E). Here an insightful remark by Vansina about the Bushong poison ordeal is pertinent. He points out that the poison ordeal is not simply a judicial procedure; it is a meeting of the supernatural with the human, with "its ambitious aim to eliminate evil and death" (Vansina 1969:245). Similarly, Ainu medical rituals claim to remove the basic evil from the universe.

Symbols in medical rituals

Before interpreting each medical symbol, I summarize the nature and purpose of three types of medical rituals:

Medical rituals	Place of action	Ultimate purpose
Exorcism rites Purification rites	At the interface between the structure and anti-structure	Fortification of the structure from without
Shamanistic rites	Categorical boundaries within the structure	Fortification of the structure from within through mediation

An important first step in the healing process is to identify an illness – the act that corresponds to placing even an anomaly into an ordered scheme by naming and identifying it. Actual healing takes place, however, only with the restoration of the structure of the cherished categories that have been threatened either by demons from outside the structure or by social disharmony within the structure. In contrast to the rituals of purification and exorcism, which take place at the boundary between structure and antistructure (anomaly), the act of mediation in the healing rites of shamanism takes place within the structure, that is, between the deities and humans – the most important part of the classified world of the Ainu. The healing of a patient as a result of successful mediation, therefore, is a testimony of the renewed dyad, that is, the reinforced relationship between the sacred and the profane. The restoration of this dyad further symbolizes the victory of the classified world of the Ainu over the threat of disorder. Thus, whereas the role of the purification and exorcism rites is to fortify the endangered structure from without, the role of mediation is to invoke the deities on behalf of the humans, with the ultimate purpose of fortifying the entire classified world of the Ainu from within (see also Figure 7 in Ohnuki-Tierney 1980a).

As described in Chapter 6, in the exorcism rites performed to ward off epidemics, a male elder recites epic poems and offers ritual sticks to the deities in an effort to solicit their help on behalf of the settlement in preventing the spread of an epidemic. This ritual act suggests that although the Ainu believe the sacred has the power to help them to counterattack the anomaly, it is the humans, or the profane, who have the power to oppose the anomaly directly. Further, symbols of combat are displayed – wooden swords at the entrance, *oken* statues representing men with swords, and bundles of sedge grass representing "combat soldiers" – showing that in the Ainu belief system one of the sources of power to counterattack the demons is *human* physical force.

Two other properties that the Ainu believe have the power to retaliate effectively against an attack by demons are human excrement and menstrual blood. Human excrement is symbolized by the use of elder and *sikataro kina* of the *Allium* family; their smell resembles that of human excrement. The third plant, alder, is chosen to make *oken* statues because its color resembles that of menstrual blood. The only antidote for smallpox victims is menstrual blood itself or red bog moss, which simulates the color of the blood.

The ritual for insanity cases involves two types of medical rites. First, the exorcism of demons is carried out by the swinging of swords and other physical behavior, which, as in the case of the demon exorcism in the epidemic prevention, can be interpreted to symbolize human physical force. Second, the purification rite uses fir and wormwood. Sometimes referred to as *mahteku ni:* (female tree), fir symbolizes women, and wormwood, a favorite plant to eat, symbolizes human food; thus both women and food are associated with the power to cleanse the defilement caused by demons. (For the nearly universal association of wormwood with women, see Lévi-Strauss 1966:46–8.)

The symbols involved in shamanistic rites seem to cluster around two themes: cooking and mediation, both of which involve women. Shamanistic healing rites are always held beside the hearth, where the Ainu do all cooking. The sea water, tangle, and spruce branch in the shaman's drink are all essential ingredients in Ainu cooking. The Ainu, who do not extract salt, use sea water for their cooking. Before the turn of the century, when they moved to their winter settlement farther inland at the onset of the cold season, they used river water with dried tangle, which is thickly coated with salt and has a good flavor. Spruce is also a favorite herb extensively used in cooking meat and fish. The three plants placed on embers – spruce or larch, *nuhča* plant, and dried minced leek – are all closely related to Ainu dietary practice. The leek is perhaps the most favored plant ingredient and flavor for the Ainu; an important activity during the summer is to collect and dry enough leeks for the winter supply. Although not an ingredient in cooking, the *nuhča* plant is the most commonly used plant for brewing tea (two other kinds of plants are used when *nuhča* is not available). The embers themselves symbolize the completion of cooking, because wood was the only fuel used by the Ainu until the introduction of coal by the Russians and Japanese. Smoke in this context is also a symbol of cooking.

The second set of symbols represents the act of mediation. In the Ainu symbolic system, the female sex, deity or human, is often assigned the role of mediator. Thus, Grandmother Hearth, whose residence – the hearth – provides the site for the performance of rites, mediates between humans and deities; prayers offered by human male elders would not reach the deities without her mediation. Her role corresponds to the mediating role of human women, who in folktales marry deities and who, among humans who practice patrilocal residence, become a bridge between otherwise unrelated settlements whose core members consist of patrilineally related men. As additional evidence for assigning a mediating role to women, let me point out that the Goddess of Sun and Moon, although not featured in the medical system, also mediates between humans and deities. During the waning moon, when the goddess is ill-disposed, no human prayers will reach the deities. This provides the basis for the religious rule that all rituals must be performed during the first half of the lunar month.

Besides Grandmother Hearth, both shamans and their spirits are assigned the role of mediation; they fetch information from the deities for human benefit. The predominance of birds and such flying insects as grasshoppers as spirits is probably due to their ability to traverse different spatial categories of the universe; they can travel to the world of the dead or to the world of the deities in order to bring back a diagnosis or method of healing an illness. Likewise, the water in the shaman's drink travels between two separate spatial categories; water in rivers travels from the mountains to the sea. Another symbol of mediation, smoke from the embers, also travels from the land to the sky. (For a further discussion of smoke as a marginal symbol, see Ohnuki-Tierney 1976b.)

To recapitulate, the majority of symbols involved in the Ainu medical rituals represent the most profane aspects of human life: human physical force (combat), procreation (menstrual blood and other symbols of women), and consumption (various foods, cooking, and excrement). In the Ainu symbolic scheme, then, it is the profane, or the Ainu way of life, rather than the sacred that is called upon to fortify or restore the Ainu symbolic structure under the threat or attack of anomaly. These symbols are not symbols of the sacred. Thus the analysis of symbols in medical rituals bears out one of the basic beliefs in the Ainu world view: The deities do not counterattack the demons directly, but they help humans to do so.

The power of anomalous symbols

Among the medical symbols of the Ainu, there are two types of anomalous symbols – first, menstrual blood and excrement, used in the demon exorcism rites, and second, mediation symbols, used in the shamanistic healing rites. Because bodily dirt is considered both polluting and powerful in almost every culture (as we shall see in Chapter 8), the use of menstrual blood and excrement as medical symbols requires interpretation not only in the context of medical rituals but also against the background of Ainu uses of other types of bodily dirt.

A hunter carries at all times a piece of his mother's or wife's *činki*, the front part of a women's skirtlike undergarment. Its smell is believed to protect him when he unexpectedly encounters a deity, such as a bear, or a demon. *Činki* is also used to make shoes and garments for a sickly infant to ward off demons. When a fire starts, someone must wave a woman's undergarment toward it; this is believed to be effective in extinguishing the fire. As seen earlier, the very reason given for the exclusion of women from all activities dealing with the deities, that is, hunting, sea fishing, and group rituals, is the potent smell of their menstrual blood. The belief in the polluting nature of blood at childbirth requires that parturient women be placed in a separate house from the regular one where hunters must live. Not only is it taboo for a husband to engage in sexual inter-course with his wife after childbirth, but he too is contaminated by associa-tion and hence may not go hunting for about a week after the birth of the child. The Ainu cite examples of the violation of this taboo that resulted in the killing of a hunter by a deity. The incompatibility of "old blood" and the sacred is nowhere expressed more clearly than in the Ainu belief that at the beginning of the world, men menstruated through the knee. How-ever, because it was inconvenient for men, who must hunt, the deity in charge of human births switched the function to women. The blood, then, is above all seen to be incompatible with the sacred, because it is pollut-ing and offensive to the deities. At the same time it is powerful in expel-ling not only the demons but also the deities when an encounter with the latter is not welcome.

Excrement is used not only in the demon exorcism rite but in other ways to expel demons. When an infant sneezes, which signals the ap-proach of a demon, the adults present sing a song in which the infant is described as being covered with excrement; the song is believed to deter a demon from approaching the infant. Urine too is believed to have power. When passing by a snow bank, a traveler should urinate; the smell, referred to as *aynu hura* (human smell), will prevent the snow from falling on the person. (It is uncertain whether a demon or an evil spirit is believed to be involved in the snow bank.) Nasal mucus is used only to insult another person, and other bodily dirt, including semen, receives little attention by the Ainu.

Menstrual and parturient blood are seen to be anomalous by the Ainu, who refer to them as old blood (*husko kem*) instead of new blood (*asiri kem*), that is, blood in the body. The Ainu believe that during menstruation the old blood leaves the body as new blood is formed in the body from the water women drink at this time. Likewise, excrement is something rejected by the body as food enters it. In other words, they are both characterized by being out of place – one of the five types of anomaly that I discuss in detail in Chapter 8. It is the anomalous quality of these matters that makes them some of the most frequently used and most powerful symbols of the Ainu. Although they are structurally anomalous, these symbols represent the essence of that which is human – procreation and consumption; so again, it is the human or profane quality that can expel both demons and deities.

In terms of classificatory identity, the beings chosen to mediate may also be seen to possess characteristics that make them anomalous members of the category to which they belong. Grandmother Hearth represents women; however, she is an old, postmenopausal woman and therefore may be seen as a peripheral member of the female sex, whose most important function in the Ainu view is procreation. The shaman's spirits also have characteristics that distinguish them from ordinary birds and insects. Ducks are birds that swim like fish and yet walk more extensively than other birds. Crows, ravens, and cranes are all characterized by eating habits that are unusual for birds; crows and ravens scavenge for carrion, and cranes occasionally eat frogs and snakes, the two most abhorred animals of the Ainu. *Kawawe:* birds are characterized by a lack of visual identity; they also cry only at night, when most other birds are asleep. Grasshoppers are recognized as insects, but their peculiar habit of hopping marks them as odd. The worm (centipede?), is thought to break into pieces when someone steps on it – it becomes amorphous; similarly, smoke and fire are characterized by formlessness. In other words, all of these beings and phenomena are characterized by an anomaly of one type or another (see Chapter 8).

I think the source of the power of these symbols to mediate derives from the very characteristics that render them anomalous. Being anomalous, they can transcend the boundaries imposed by the classificatory scheme in order to mediate. Because of their peculiar behavioral characteristics, ducks are able to move between three spatial categories – air, land, and water – rather than being confined to air and the tops of trees, as most birds are. Birds are usually active only during the day, yet the *kawawe:* bird is active at night. In the Ainu temporal classification (Ohnuki-Tierney 1969b, 1973c), the day is divided into the light half (day) and the dark half (night); thus the *kawawe:* bird demonstrates an ability to transcend the temporal category assigned to it. Similarly, the formlessness of water and smoke enables them to traverse land and sea, or land and air, respectively.

The power of the mediation symbols to override classificatory confinements is most succinctly expressed in the Ainu notion of the power held by shamans, who often traverse both spatial and temporal categories during their healing rites. Spatially, they travel back and forth between the world of the living Ainu and other worlds. In order to receive instructions about the diagnosis and cure of an illness, for example, they go to the world of the deities. The Ainu belief that shamans are able to see the deities in this world as they are in their own world – namely, in human forms – also expresses the capacity of shamans to transcend spatial categories. Shamans also visit the world of the dead Ainu when they perform a rite to revive a person who is "almost dead." In Ainu belief, a person dies when his or her soul travels to the world of the dead; hence, the job of a shaman entails a trip to the world of the dead to retrieve the client's soul quickly before it permanently settles there.

Shamans also transcend temporal categories during their performances. In diagnosing certain illnesses, shamans may find a pathogen or an etiological factor in misconducts of the patient's ancestors that took place long ago. Similarly, a shaman's drum summons the souls of the shaman's ancestors or their spirits, if the ancestors themselves were shamans, to aid the shaman. Thus past and present merge into one during a shamanistic performance. Because of their ability to transcend temporal boundaries, shamans are given credit for all that the Ainu know about the beginning and end of the world; the knowledge was revealed to some shamans during their rites. The Ainu belief that shamans have a special vision that allows them to see things at a distance, in both time and space, expresses their ability to transcend both space and time.

Just as the power of the symbols of mediation derives from their anomalous quality, the transcendental power of shamans too seems to derive from their anomalous status as members of Ainu society in that they are often women, who, as we saw earlier, are peripheral members of the society. Men who become shamans are often those who cannot pursue the regular route to power and fame through an ability to hunt and fish, as in the case of a noted blind shaman of the Rayčiska settlement. (For details of shamans as social personae, see Chapter 11.)[3] Like demons, they each constitute a category of people (women, shamans) at a surface level, but they symbolize anomaly or structural inversions.

To recapitulate, in terms of symbolic structure, the power of transcendence derives from the structural anomaly of the mediation symbols and the marginal status of shamans in the society. To be somewhat off center is to have freedom from the restrictions imposed by the existing classificatory structure. This freedom and consequent power for transcendence are used by these anomalous symbols and persons to solicit favors from the deities with the ultimate purpose of restoring the existing system of the Ainu, which has been threatened by a liminal state of illness in the individual's life and by anomaly in the symbolic system.

Anarchic anomaly and creative anomaly: demons and other anomalous symbols

We saw in the previous discussion that there are two types of anomalous symbols: excrement and menstrual blood in the control of epidemics, and the mediation symbols in shamanism. Both sets of symbols have positive functions, the former to counterattack the demons and the latter to fetch information from the deities. In terms of the symbolic structure, both work to fortify it. However, how does one reconcile the anomaly of these symbols, on the one hand, and the anomaly of demons, on the other? Demons threaten to destroy the classified world of the Ainu. Both demons and the other symbols are characterized by anomalies, and yet their respective roles in relation to the structure constitute polar opposites: destruction versus fortification. Demons are anarchic anomalies, whereas the other symbols are creative anomalies.

Here I view symbols of creative anomaly as located within the classificatory structure; they are anomalous but still belong to a class. Thus, ducks are definitely birds and grasshoppers are definitely insects. But they are peripheral rather than representative members of those categories because they have peculiar habits. In contrast, demonic anomaly is a total juxtaposition of categories and therefore is not within the structure; anarchy lies outside of an orderly world. As an additional feature that distinguishes the two, I suggest that symbols of creative anomaly are either ordinary fauna or flora or other natural phenomena (e.g., water and smoke) in the external world, which may be perceived through sensory organs. By contrast, a demon, whether a one-eyed monster or the restless soul of a musical instrument, is a metaphysical construct, although it is as real to the Ainu as a duck.

As the Ainu draw no hard and fast line between these "real" and "metaphysical" phenomena, the respective roles that they assign to the two types of symbols are not altogether fixed. Although they are both symbols of mediation in shamanism, a stray crane can be a demon as a result of human misconduct (Ohnuki-Tierney 1969a:73–85), and the *kawawe:* bird may cause insanity. Similarly, fire can cause extensive damage and water can bring about floods or drownings. The anomalous nature of these natural symbols not only enables them to traverse the categories within the structure but also endows them with the power to cross over to the antistructural side. Conversely, demons are often benign; we recall the Ainu refer to them as deities in the hope that flattery will keep them benign. Various types of anomaly and the power assigned to anomalous symbols are further discussed from cross-cultural perspectives in Chapter 8.

The use of senses in Ainu symbolic perception

Chapters 4 and 5 show that the identification of habitual illnesses rests heavily upon the use of the senses. The Ainu use auditory, visual, and tactile senses in perceiving and identifying headaches, boils, and many other ailments. As described in Chapter 6, metaphysical illnesses are also perceived through various senses. Extensive use of the senses applies to the choice of objects and beings used in medical rituals as well. For instance, both alder and red bog moss are chosen to symbolize menstrual blood because they have a red color similar to that of blood; thus, vision is used in the choice of these plants.

Vision, however, does not generally play a significant role in the Ainu perception of the universe. Instead, the olfactory sense is far more important. Thus, to the Ainu the essence of menstrual blood is not color but smell. It is the smell that is offensive to the deities and provides the basis for the permanent exclusion of women from hunting, fishing, and group rituals; the smell also expels demons. Similarly, elder wood is used to make *oken* statues for the demon exorcism rite because it smells like human excrement. Another plant with the same smell, *sikataro kina*, which belongs to the *Allium* family, is placed in doorways to ward off demons. On the other hand, wormwood is used in rubbing and purifying the sick during shamanistic rites because its smell is refreshing to the Ainu. Spruce branches, leeks, and *nuhča* plants are placed on embers during shamanistic rites to produce not only smoke but also a particular aroma. The olfactory sense is especially important during shamanistic rites, because they are performed in a house after sunset with embers as the only source of light. We recall that the efficacy of the leek as a medicine is based upon its potent smell.

The auditory sense also plays an important role in illness definition, prevention, and healing. For example, illness can be caused by harsh words against a fellow Ainu, and recitation of epic poems is believed to help prevent epidemics. Spoken words, therefore, have an enormous power. The crucial role of the drum in shamanistic rites is another example. As its sound echoes in the Ainu universe, it signals an invitation to good spirits and deities while repelling evil spirits and demons. In addition, it may play a crucial role in inducing a trance in the shaman. (In the absence of laboratory tests to show that the amount of *nuhča* plant consumed and the method used are sufficient to induce mental alteration, I can only propose the possibility that the beating of the drum plays a role in inducing the trance. Kats and de Rios emphasize "the crucial role that music plays in structuring the area of culturally determined subjective experience arising from drug-induced states" [1971: 320].)

Through powerful appeals to multiple senses, the Ainu symbols evoke the strongest emotions. These sensory-emotive dimensions of symbol perception are even more important for the efficacy of symbols.

/Sacred:profane::nature:culture/

In previous discussions, I briefly equated the sacred with nature and the profane with culture. In this section, I further elaborate this equation, primarily by reexamining symbols of cooking and of women that appear in the shamanistic healing rites.

Cooking represents culture and thus the profane half of the dyad. Because the Ainu abhor raw food, especially raw meat, cooking is the only means to sustain life. Cooked food signifies life and represents the Ainu way of life, that is, culture, as opposed to raw nature, which represents death. The use of uncooked food is limited to ritual consumption by men of the blood and brain of a bear during the bear ceremony,[4] and to occasional raw fish in brine with leek (the latter, I suspect, is the result of Japanese influence). The Ainu cook food, and they cook it for a long time.

The plants used in the healing rites also symbolize life and culture. For instance, *nuhča* and leek serve not only as a tea and an herb for the Ainu but also as medicine – a means to restore life when threatened by illness and death. *Nuhča* is used for several kinds of illness, including bone aches, common colds, and stomachaches. Leek is considered one of the most potent medicines. It is used not only for bone aches but is considered especially efficacious when used either after childbirth or for illnesses of the sexual organs. Thus, the symbolic association of leek with reproduction and consequently with life itself is obvious.

In addition, in Ainu folklore the smoke from cooking is a recurrent symbol of both culture and life as opposed to nature, that is, the deities. It is said that the smell of smoke from an Ainu house (referred to as *unči hura yuhke*) is too potent for the deities to approach; thus as long as smoke is coming from a house, the deities will not come close. When an Ainu traveler sees an Ainu house, he or she determines whether smoke is coming out of the skylight; if it is, the traveler is usually relieved, because it means hospitality by the host. Smoke, then, represents the presence of life in the Ainu house as well as a guarantee of life for the traveler.

The Ainu emphasis on cooking has another dimension. For the Ainu, cooked food distinguishes their way of life from that of the neighboring Oroks and Japanese, who eat raw meat and raw fish, respectively. Because of their eating habits, the Ainu feel justified in considering their life to be civilized and in looking down upon their neighbors as barbarians with disdainful customs.[5] In fact, in one tale (Ohnuki-Tierney 1969a:173–6) a war between the Ainu of the Rayčiska settlement on the northwest coast and the Oroks is said to have started when the Oroks mistook a placenta, which the Ainu placed on a crotch of a tree, as is their custom, for animal intestines and ate it. Upon discovering what they had done, the Oroks were angered and set out to take revenge. Similar stories are found elsewhere in Sakhalin.[6] Thus, cooking not only distinguishes the Ainu, that is, the humans, from the animals, that is, nature, but on another plane of consciousness where the Ainu recognize other human populations, cooking serves to distinguish them from their barbarian neighbors. It is a vital element in their ethnicity.

Cooking thus is a dominant symbol in Ainu culture. The Ainu cooking method clearly specifies that the meat of land animals may never be cooked in the same pan with fish; in fact different pans must be used for each. Above all, there is a special pan for bear meat that cannot be used for anything else. In general, the Ainu prefer to cook different species of animals, whether meat or fish, separately, rather than together in the same pan. This meticulous separation of animal species contrasts to the way they mash vegetable foods and mix them together. Because culture may be equated with the classified world at the most abstract level, we may say that for the Ainu, cooking symbolizes not only the conversion of nature to culture but culture, the classified world, itself.

Apart from symbols of cooking, there are several symbols in the healing rituals that represent women. In addition to having the major responsibility for cooking, Ainu women are also in charge of making clothes for everyone. Needless to say, clothing is vital for survival in this subarctic climate. Women thus transform raw hides of sea mammals, dogs, foxes, and other animals into warm garments; make fish skin garments, bags, and shoes from trout and salmon (cf. Ohnuki-Tierney 1974a:40–8); and weave garments from nettle fiber and elm bark. It is they who convert nature, that is, animals and plants, into culture, that is, clothing. They are nurturers of the Ainu way of life, that is, culture, through their cooking and sewing roles.

The third role of women in relation to the cultural process is reproduction. Although the Ainu do not equate menstruation with the reproductive process, they do emphasize the woman's role in reproduction and pay little attention to the man's role. In fact, the crucial measure of the importance of women is said to be their reproductive capacity; without women there would be no Ainu. The Ainu equate a large population with the prosperity of the settlement. In tales, this prosperity is usually expressed as follows: "There were so many people in the settlement that the sleeves of their garments became worn out as the result of people rubbing each other as they walked" (cf. Ohnuki-Tierney 1969a:172).

People wish to have as many children as possible so that some of them will survive and be willing to take care of them in their old age when they can no longer actively engage in hunting, fishing, and plant gathering. Twins are welcome and are considered special gifts from the deities. This emphasis on population increase, rather than control, may be due to the ecological-demographic factor of any small nonsedentary foraging population: The more people there are, the better the chance of their group survival. Whatever the etic reason may be, the emic rationale justifies an interpretation that women's reproductive capacity is seen as a vital means to sustain the Ainu way of life, that is, culture.

Just as the activities expressed through symbols of cooking and of women represent culture, the healing process for which these rituals are performed is itself a cultural process. It is the process of re-creating health from the shattered state of illness.

It is in this context of the structural meaning of culture that my most cherished symbol – the shaman's drum – takes on a profound significance. As noted earlier, in the Ainu perception the drum functions to chase off evil spirits and summon good spirits. Cognitively, it wards off antistructural threats and fortifies the structure by summoning the aid of the sacred. This is done, through music – patterned regularity, that is, the epitome of culture (cf. Lévi-Strauss 1969b). As the shaman's drum creates music, it sings of the triumph of the cherished world of the Ainu over threats to its cognitive integrity. It is noteworthy that the symbolism of the drum is not simply related to the cognitive structure, which remains unconscious for the most part. It also has a powerful appeal to the emotions and senses of those who listen to its beat, especially in a dark, crowded, one-room house.

Finally, let me emphasize that the dominant symbols of culture in medical rituals indicate that culture is not a static state but a process of creation – creating food from raw materials in nature, creating a human being from the body, re-creating a healthy body from a sick one, and creating music from the animal and plant material used to make a drum – which contrasts to both untamed nature and the uncivilized ways of life of other peoples. In short, the notion of culture involves a syntagmatic chain or melody, rather than a paradigmatic association of harmony (cf. Leach 1976:15–16, 25–7).

Multiplicity of belief systems

In the previous section, we saw a systematic symbolic equation of women with the healing process, and I stressed the equation of women with culture. Some readers may have already wondered whether men do not have an equal claim to be associated with the cultural process, symbolically and otherwise, because it is they who get the raw meat, hides, and even elm bark from which the women make cultural products.

I suggest that the Ainu symbolic system validates both types of equation - /nature:culture = men:women/ and their inversion - the former expressed, as we have seen, in individual rituals and the latter in the group rituals. In order to illustrate this point, let me first briefly outline the contrasts between individual rituals of shamanistic rites and group rituals, which include the bear ceremony, the fox ceremony, and the ash renewal ceremony for Grandmother Hearth.

In terms of time, shamanistic rites are held only at night, whereas all group rituals are held during the day. The Ainu consider daytime to be the Ainu portion of the day, during which humans engage in their activities, whereas nighttime belongs to both deities and demons. Furthermore, group rituals have fixed dates in the sense that each ceremony is performed at approximately the same time of the year and month. Also, they must all take place during the first half of the month when the Goddess of Sun and Moon is believed to be cheerful, so that she can mediate between the humans and the deities. Shamanistic rites, on the other hand, may be performed at any time of the year or month.

Spatially, shamanistic rites are the only rituals of the Ainu that are held inside the house. All other rituals are held at the sacred altar located outside but near the house and facing in the sacred direction, that is, the mountains. In Ainu spatial classification, the shore belongs to humans and the house symbolizes this human part of the universe. In contrast, the mountains and sea belong to the deities. The high mountains in the interior, in particular, are believed to be the most sacred part of the Ainu universe, and the altar represents the interior mountains. In terms of time and space, then, shamanistic rituals take place during the nonhuman portion of the day and in the human part of the universe, structurally opposing the group rituals, which are held during the human portion of the day and in the nonhuman part of the universe.

The contrast between shamanistic rites and group rituals is also seen in the types of metaphysical beings involved in the respective rituals. In group rituals the major deities, such as bears, foxes, Grandmother Hearth, and the Sun-Moon Goddess, are the direct recipients of prayers and nonverbal forms of worship by the Ainu. In contrast, during shamanistic rites, those directly involved are the shaman's spirits, which are not bona fide deities. Major deities are important - Grandmother Hearth as the mediator and other deities as the ultimate sources of power. But humans are using them, as it were, rather than worshipping them, as they do during group rituals.

Another distinction between group rituals and shamanistic rites lies in the nature of the communication that takes place. Communication between the deities and the Ainu during group rituals is one-way. Offerings are made and the Ainu convey their respect and ask for general welfare, such as an abundance of food, from the deities concerned. But these behaviors represent only a long-range presentation; the deities are asked to repay only at some unspecified time in the future. In contrast, during shamanistic rites, communication is two-way and at close range. Offerings demand immediate repayment in the form of specific help from spirits and, ultimately, from the deities. Spirit possession in particular represents an intense and intimate contact between a shaman, that is, a human, and spirits and deities.

Most important of all, especially for the purpose of our discussion here, is that all group rituals celebrate the death and subsequent rebirth of a deity – the death of a bear, in the case of a bear ceremony, for example, so that it can bring meat and fur for the Ainu, and rebirth so that it can again visit the Ainu with these gifts. In addition, this process of death and rebirth is dramatically ritualized to emphasize the fact that the entire process lies in the hands of men; only men can officiate at these rituals, and women must stay at the periphery. In fact, the spatial arrangement of participants during group rituals mirrors the hierarchy in Ainu society at large, with male elders in the center closest to the altar, followed by young men, older women, and younger women. It is noteworthy that in the case of the bear ceremony, the most important group ritual of the Ainu, the men not only dominate the ceremony in general but also cook the meat of the slain bear, which has been ritually shot by a chosen marksman early in the ceremony. In other words, the bear ceremony vividly enacts the conversion of raw material in nature into human purposes – the cultural process – by man the hunter.

We have then a situation in Ainu culture whereby two sets of ideology and symbolic representation co-exist side by side, one expressed through group rituals and the other through shamanistic rites. The set expressed through group rituals is the official or formalized version that Ainu men and women have been taught and therefore can articulate more or less systematically. The other set is a less conscious one, but is systematically expressed through the symbols involved in shamanistic rituals. This covert ideology is quite intriguing in that its content shows systematic inversion of the formalized ideology. Thus, in the formalized version humans are powerless against the deities, whereas in shamanism humans are assigned strong power. Although officially proclaiming that shamans are at the mercy of spirits that decide to possess or not possess them, shamans in fact manipulate the spirits and ultimately the deities to achieve the desired results. Shamans symbolize humans who are formally powerless against the deities and yet unofficially possess power to manipulate them. Likewise, women, who are at the bottom of the social hierarchy, and are seen as such during group rituals, receive a strong symbolic assertion in the language of shamanism. It is in this context that the double nature of menstrual blood is best explained. In official ideology and the cultural activities based upon it, the sacred (deities and men) prevails, and menstrual blood, symbolizing the most profane of all human activities, is taboo, because its presence implies mixing of the sacred and the profane. It has a positive power, however, in a nonformalized context, that is, individual rituals and emergency situations.

Summary

This chapter has examined the relationship between symbols used in the Ainu medical system and the basic Ainu symbolic structure. Ainu definitions of illness indicate that, symbolically, illness constitutes an anti-structural threat to the classified world of the Ainu, which corresponds to health in an individual's life. Pathogenic demons represent an intrinsic and permanent juxtaposition of categories, whereas disjunctions in the social network of the universe also are seen to cause illnesses and are temporary anomalies caused primarily by human misbehavior.

In healing endeavors, the Ainu solicit favors from deities. This is seen in the recitation of epic poems at the time of epidemics and through symbols of mediation in shamanistic healing rites. Analyses of Ainu symbols in exorcism, purification, and healing rites indicate, however, that above all it is the symbolic power associated with the profane, or the Ainu way of life, that counterattacks demonic/pathogenic anomalies. Some of these medical symbols may be seen as anomalous; they are menstrual blood, excrement, and mediation symbols. The power to expel demons, in the case of the former, and the capacity to transcend classificatory boundaries and thereby mediate between the sacred and the profane, in the case of the latter, are seen to derive from the very nature of their anomaly.

The creative power of these anomalous symbols to fortify the Ainu symbolic structure is contrasted to the destructive power of demonic anomalies. Symbols of creative anomaly are close to the boundary but still within the limits of a category; that is, they are more peripheral than anomalous; demonic anomaly, in contrast, is a total juxtaposition of categories. In addition, symbols of creative anomaly are flora, fauna, or other natural phenomena, whereas demons are metaphysical constructs that are not sensorily perceived. It is noteworthy, however, that the difference between the two types of symbols and their respective power is not always clear. Beings chosen as symbols of creative anomaly may also exercise negative power at times.

Systematic representation of women through their roles of cooking, sewing, and childbearing and rearing in the symbols of shamanism is interpreted to equate women with the cultural process. This equation is examined further in a comparison of the rituals and belief systems in shamanism with those in group rituals. My finding is that the two types of rituals involve two sets of belief systems, one being the inversion of the other. Thus, in group rituals the equation of men with culture is symbolically expressed.

In short, healing in the Ainu medical system involves not only the sick individual but also the symbolic structure, which has been threatened by anomalies. A most ambitious aim of healing is achieved through the use of powerful symbols in the Ainu medical rituals, which appeal to the cognitive, emotive, and sensory dimensions of Ainu perception.

8

Theories in symbolic studies and the Ainu data

In the previous two chapters, I interpreted symbols involved in the perception of Ainu metaphysical illnesses and their healing rituals. I did so without explaining my method, and I used anthropological terms and concepts without much reference to similar terms and concepts used by other scholars. In fact, my use of these terms and concepts is very different from the way they are used by other scholars. In this chapter, I attempt to relate my findings on the Ainu symbolic system, as revealed in their notion of metaphysical illnesses and their healing rituals, to various theories and findings based upon data from other societies.

This chapter begins with a clarification of my method in the interpretation of Ainu symbols. In subsequent sections, I focus on the Ainu /sacred:profane/ dyad in relation to the use of these terms in anthropological literature, the /nature:culture/ opposition, another frequently discussed opposition in anthropology, and, in relation to both of these, the /men:women/ opposition. I then deal with the problem of anomalies. Different types of anomalies and various kinds of power assigned to anomalous symbols are examined. Last, I explore the possibility of the presence of more than one ideological or symbolic system in a culture and seek mechanisms that explain the simultaneous presence of symbolic oppositions and their inversions, as well as the presence of often contradictory referents of a single symbol. The purpose of this chapter, then, is to elucidate further the Ainu symbolic system and to evaluate critically existing theories in symbolic anthropology in the light of Ainu data.

Interpretation of symbols

A major problem in the interpretation of symbols is how to arrive at their meaning. First, what is the source of information upon which an interpretation is based? Turner proposes three levels of meaning for a symbol: the exegetical, the operational, and the positional (Turner 1967:50–2). The exegetical meaning is obtained from informants in response to the investigator's questioning. Although the Ndembu in Turner's studies are most articulate about the meaning of symbols, I found that even the best Ainu

105

informants offered little explanation of symbolic referents, especially when direct questions were asked. Although I would not categorically disqualify native explanations and conscious models as inaccurate, as Lévi-Strauss does (1967:273–5; 1969b:295), I think symbolic referents at the structural level are rarely articulated in the minds of the people (cf. Hallowell 1964:50; Lévi-Strauss 1967:19, 21, 273–4). Therefore, as sources of information for my interpretation of symbols, I relied on the operational meaning, that is, the meaning in the use of symbols, and the positional meaning, that is, the meaning in relationship to other symbols in a totality (Turner 1967:51). Thus the referent of a symbol was determined on the basis of the referents of other symbols in the same context, and with the aid of knowledge of its use in other rituals, its appearance in oral tradition, daily life, and various other ethnographic contexts. This involved a thorough examination of ethnographic data, piecing together various contexts in which a symbol occurred. The task demanded a close scrutiny of each case, because dominant symbols often have various, even contradictory, symbolic meanings, as I discuss shortly.

In interpreting symbols, Lévi-Strauss and Turner again differ. The former seeks the basic structural meaning expressed in a variety of symbolic forms, whereas the latter emphasizes the multivocality of dominant symbols. In interpretation of Ainu symbols, I found both approaches to be useful. Operationally, I began by distinguishing a particular meaning for each symbol in a context, such as in the shamanistic rites, from other possible meanings of the same symbol. When all the symbols within a context are interpreted, there emerges a configuration of meanings expressed by all the symbols. For example, the dominant themes of cooking and women emerged only after a certain referent of each symbol in the shamanistic ritual was carefully chosen from among various other meanings that each of the symbols could express. Taken together, the picture of shamanism reflected in these symbols becomes more than the sum total of cooking and women. These two themes jointly express another concept at the highest level of abstraction, that is, the primary process of converting nature into culture, in which the Ainu way of life is triumphantly asserted.

The choice of a particular referent of a multivocal symbol, however, is not always easy. Southall's criticism (1972:104) that Turner's treatment of multivocal symbols lacks "discernable rules" for "contextual distinction" is pertinent here. Only when we specify the reason why one referent is symbolized over the others in a particular context can an interpretation of a symbol of an alien culture become convincing to the reader, who may otherwise criticize this approach as simply arbitrary and subjective, as many have done already.

Although Turner (1967:50–2) finds a consistent relation between the exegetical, operational, and positional meanings of the Ndembu multi-

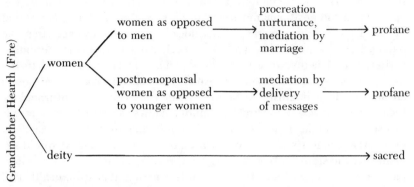

Figure 8.1. Choice of referents of a multivocal symbol. (From Ohnuki-Tierney, 1980a, *American Ethnologist* 7 (1):145.)

vocal symbols, I find that Ainu multivocal symbols have contradictory meanings even at the structural level. For example, as shown in Figure 8.1, the choice of the immediate referent for Grandmother Hearth can be either women or deity. When interpreted as women, its structural referent is the profane, but when interpreted as deity, its structural affiliation is the sacred, as discussed in Chapter 7. The choice is crucial in determining what type of power is solicited in counterattacking the demonic anomalies. In interpreting the symbolic meaning of Grandmother Hearth in shamanistic healing rites, the place of shamanism in Ainu religion as the domestic and individual ritual (cf. Chapter 7), and the presence of numerous other symbols that represent women and their roles of cooking and mediation are the factors I find to be crucial in choosing the referent of the female sex rather than a deity. Put another way, the symbolic referent is only the sacred, and not women, in a context in which Grandmother Hearth as a deity is contrasted to humans.

Another major concern in the interpretation of symbols is the problem of the extent to which a given meaning is public (Geertz 1973:12) or a "*collective* representation," rather than a personal meaning peculiar to a particular informant or a projection of the investigator's own thought. For that matter, if the meaning is solicited from an informant, it could even represent a meaning that the informant more or less concocted. If an investigator not only relies on the exegetical meaning but also systematically examines the operational and positional meanings, then some of these problems are eliminated. In interpreting Ainu symbols, the exegetical meaning was rarely available and the examination of the operational and positional meanings often yielded an amazing consistency in terms of the symbolic referent, especially at a deeper level. As noted earlier, rich ethnographic information on the Sakhalin Ainu obtained by Chiri, Pilsudski, Wada, and Yamamoto has been very helpful in ascertaining the operational and positional meanings of these symbols and in assuring that my data are not idiosyncratic. This does not mean, however, that the perception of a particular symbol by each Ainu is identical. As noted earlier, the structure of a symbolic system is rarely articulated in the minds of the people concerned; it usually remains unconscious. Although an analogy to a linguistic structure is not fashionable in anthropology today, the best way to illustrate the public nature of symbolic structure is to use an example from the composition of stops in American English. Other than linguists, no native speaker of American English would explain that the stops /p, b, t, d, k, g/ are the voiced and voiceless counterparts in binary opposition. However, it is precisely that structure that all English speakers use in order to communicate with each other; the structure is public, although unconscious.

/Sacred:profane/ opposition

In Chapter 7 I used the term *profane* to denote the Ainu way of life. It is equated with the way of life of humans (the Ainu) vis-à-vis deities, because in the Ainu world view the Ainu are the only humans. In contrast, the term *sacred* is used to refer to the way of life of the Ainu deities, who, in the Ainu view, possess power over them. The Ainu dualism of the sacred and the profane, however, corresponds only in a limited sense to the sacred/profane dualism used by many other scholars (e.g., Durkheim 1965:52 et passim; Eliade 1961:10 et passim; Smith 1972; van Gennep 1961:1 et passim). Leach (1967b:97) summarizes the anthropological use of these terms, stating that *sacred* refers to the abnormal, special, other-worldly, royal, taboo, and sick, whereas *profane* refers to the normal, everyday, worldly, plebeian, permitted, and healthy. However, the Ainu sacred does not involve the abnormal, taboo, and sick; as we saw, in the Ainu symbolic structure these characteristics belong to anomaly, which is neither profane nor sacred. Hertz (1960:94–5), a most influential scholar in the early development of symbolic classification, equates the profane with the impure, stressing that the profane is an active and contagious nothingness in that it is "the antagonistic element which by its very contact degrades, diminishes, and changes the essence of things that are sacred." In contrast, the Ainu regard themselves as powerless and are at the mercy of the wishes of the deities, whose moods determine human fate. The Ainu profane, therefore, is not as powerful as Hertz defines.

The sacred in the Ainu dyad is characterized by power that is beyond human control, and in this sense the Ainu sacred is similar to the sacred in the world view of other peoples. It departs significantly, however, from the sacred or holy as defined by such scholars as Smith, Durkheim,

Leach, and Douglas, whose reference is often the Judeo-Christian concept of God. According to Douglas, God in the Old Testament creates
order, with binary opposition, we might say, as his tool of classification. In
Genesis, therefore, God creates heaven and earth, light and darkness,
day and night, evening and morning, waters and firmament, above and
below, and so on. In marked contrast, Ainu deities are much more humble. They are not above the universe creating order in the human world
below; they are simply part of the order. The presence of order in the
Ainu universe precedes the deities, not necessarily in a temporal sense
but in logic. Thus, in the beginning, the gods and humans were already
there (Ohnuki-Tierney 1973b:285–6). There is a conspicuous absence of a
creation myth in the Ainu oral tradition.

   This fundamental difference between the sacred by the aforementioned
scholars and the sacred of the Ainu stems in part from the fact that Smith,
Durkheim, and many others considered the dualism of sacred and profane
or holy and mundane within the context of established, or what they
called advanced, religions such as Judaism and Christianity. Furthermore, these scholars excluded what they called magic from their
treatment. Of the contemporary scholars, neither Douglas nor Leach
makes evolutionary distinctions between religion and magic. However,
their notion of the sacred seems to rely heavily on the Judeo-Christian
tradition. Although the understanding of the pangolin cult of the Lele
created Douglas's lifelong interest in anomaly, the principal theme in her
1966 work that God represents order and thus disorder represents defilement is based more on the interpretation of the Old Testament than on
that of the Lele religion. This is also true of her later work (1975). Leach
also discusses the Old Testament extensively in his recent works, although his discussion of anomaly (e.g., 1963, 1968) is more general. I do
not make a sharp distinction between religion and magic or between
established religion and tribal religions. However, there is a basic and
significant difference between God in established religions and the deities
in such religions as that of the Ainu. In most established religions, God is
clearly distinguished from nature so that God, nature, and humans constitute a triad, whereas in many tribal religions, especially those of
hunting-gathering societies, nature and the deities are one and the same.
As Redfield observes, "The radical achievement of the Hebrews in put-
ting God entirely outside of the physical universe and attaching all value
to God is recognized as an immense and unique achievement" (1959:102).
This basic difference between the two types of religion, as I see it, is
schematically illustrated in Figure 8.2. In the world view of the Old
Testament, God created the dyad in which the world of humans is opposed to the world of nature and its creatures, whereas in the Ainu world
view, deities and nature form one half of the dyad and humans form the

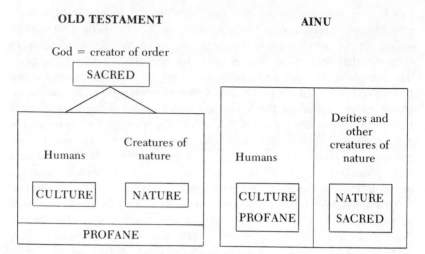

Figure 8.2. God in the Old Testament and Ainu deities.

other half. In the Ainu world view, nature is sacred and culture is profane by definition.

/Sacred:profane::nature:culture/

Beginning with Rousseau, many scholars in different fields have pointed out the cognitive necessity for humans to distinguish themselves from nonhuman animals. Douglas (1975:210) relates this "boundary between us and animal creation" to the boundary between spirit and matter and points out that "every great revolution of thought has touched that boundary." In anthropology, Lévi-Strauss made a significant contribution on the subject through his discussion of the /nature:culture/ opposition. These scholars have discussed the matter as a universal phenomenon in human cognition. From the point of view of formal analysis, the /nature:culture/ opposition is a pan-human mode of thought. However, there must be various types of the /nature:culture/ opposition across human cultures. I postulate that the variations depend on the nature of the sacred, that is, religion as discussed above. Thus, the type of opposition between nature and culture depends on whether or not the nature part of the dyad includes the sacred, that is, god or deities. In religions in which animals are deified as sacred beings who possess positive and beneficial powers over humans, the metamorphosis of humans into animals or vice versa is not uncommon and is in fact often highly welcome, because it certainly does not signify any degradation on the part of humans. In marked contrast, in religions in which animals are considered lowly creatures, humans must differentiate themselves from the "beasts." More-over, if the religion dictates, as does the Old Testament as interpreted by Douglas, that the opposition between nature and culture is an important part of the order created by God, it then becomes imperative to make a sharp distinction between humans and animals in order to please God. Conversely, lack of order, or anomaly, is not simply antistructural but a major sin against God. Therefore, pollutants are blasphemous. It follows, then, that there is a greater need for those peoples to observe the well-marked boundary between the two categories so that there is no uncer-tainty about their identities. I think this is the kind of society that Douglas discusses; her examples of hunting-gathering societies are confined to occasional mention of the !Kung San (Bushmen), Hadza, and a few others.

Lévi-Strauss, on the other hand, draws his examples heavily from horti-cultural populations of South America, although he also refers to some North American natives. His argument (1969b) generally follows the equation /sacred:profane = nature:culture/. His placement of raw food midway between nature and culture, however, seems to correlate with the fact that the peoples he studied are horticulturalists, whose raw food would be domesticated plants and animals, that is, things of tamed na-ture, in contrast to the raw food of foraging populations, which comes from wild nature.

Although I noted above that Douglas seldom discusses hunter-gatherers and Lévi-Strauss draws his examples from South American hor-ticulturalists, the mode of subsistence by no means imposes a rigid struc-ture upon the mode of thought. Consider, for example, various peoples in Asia. The Ainu, hunter-gatherers of northern Japan, deify animals, but so do the Indians of south Asia, who are agriculturalists. Another agricultural group in Asia, the Japanese, deify beings of nature such as the sun but consider animals as lowly cousins of humans, as expressed in the Japanese definition of monkeys – humans minus three pieces of hair. Perceptively pointing out the difference between the Western and Japanese views of the relationship among humans, deities, and animals, Umesao (1960:esp. 262-7) suggests that the evolutionary theory would have been too natural to be conceived as scientific theory by the Japanese, because they have always viewed animals as related to humans but of lower status.

Clearly, then, the mode of thought is not a functional byproduct of praxis: "[The nature] rules only on the question of existence, not on specific form" (Sahlins 1976a:209).

/Nature:culture::men:women/, or its inversion?

Another opposition, or transformation, as Lévi-Strauss would call it, that has received attention in anthropological literature, especially in the recent past, is the /men:women/ opposition as it relates to the /nature:culture/ opposition. The propositions advanced by Ortner and Lévi-Strauss deserve critical evaluation.

Using a tripartite approach, Ortner (1974) explains that we see the equation /nature:culture::women:men/ in all cultures. The first part of her argument rests on woman's physiology. Here she relies heavily on de Beauvoir (1974), who interprets woman's body as serving no apparent function for the health and stability of the individual. Instead, the woman is adapted to the needs of the egg rather than to her own requirements; hence her bodily functions are only sources of discomfort, pain, and danger (Ortner 1974:74). Following de Beauvoir, Ortner thus points out that men assert creativity externally, artificially, through the media of technology and symbols:

> It is not the killing that is the relevant and valued aspect of hunting and warfare; rather it is the transcendental (social, cultural) nature of these activities, as opposed to the naturalness of the process of birth. Thus, if male is, as I am suggesting, *everywhere* (unconsciously) associated with culture . . . female seems closer to nature. (Ortner 1974:75; italics mine)

This statement is an anthropological extension of de Beauvoir (1974:72), who stated, "it is not in giving life but in risking life that man is raised above the animal; that is why superiority has been accorded in humanity not to the sex that brings forth but to that which kills."

Ortner's second point is that woman's social roles are seen as closer to nature. Here her argument has two parts. First, woman's roles as childbearer and rearer place her closer to nature because infants are universally considered to represent nature until they go through initiation rites, which transform them into socialized beings. Ortner's second step combines the concept of the public/domestic opposition developed by Rosaldo (1974) and the concept of exogamy developed by Lévi-Strauss (1969a). According to Lévi-Strauss, the universal prohibition of incest and the rule of exogamy ensure that a biological group, which is reproductively a closed system, becomes a social group bound to other social groups. According to Ortner, then, the sex roles confine women to a domestic group, that is, a biological group representing nature, whereas men's activities are in' the public domain, that is, a social group, symbolizing culture.

Ortner's main argument, however, does not stress the equation of /nature:culture::women:men/ so much as the ambivalent position of women between nature and culture. Thus, it is women who are in charge of both socialization and cooking – the two primary processes seen by Lévi-Strauss to represent culture – but they somehow do not receive full credit for their roles. Ortner explains this ambivalent position by stating that in most societies the socialization of boys is transferred at some point to men and that cooking becomes a male role when it becomes part of the public domain; professional chefs are males.

The third part of Ortner's thesis is that the woman's psyche is seen as closer to nature (1974:81). However, because my concern here is the symbolic alignment of women and men with culture and nature or vice versa, which does not directly deal with the psychology of women and men, I will not pursue her argument here.

Although the /nature:culture/ opposition became prominent in anthropology because of Lévi-Strauss's exposition of this theme, and because many scholars who have discussed the relation of this opposition to the symbolic opposition between men and women credit their ideas to Lévi-Strauss, his own position on the transformation between these two oppositions is not clear. The ambiguity in his presentation stems primarily from the fact that he is concerned basically with the /nature:culture/ opposition; his references to the other opposition are therefore unsystematic. For his idea of culture, three concepts are perhaps most important: exogamy, socialization, and cooking. We have already noted that Lévi-Strauss sees the incest taboo and the rule of exchange of women as the cornerstones in the formation of human society. On the last point, he is clear about who gets the credit: "In human society it is the men who exchange the women, and not *vice versa*" (1967:45). According to him, the exchange of a marriage partner is up to the men, on empirical rather than logical grounds. Because this particular cultural role – to transform a biological group into a social group – is assigned to men, and because this process is considered essential to the formation of human culture, the inference is obvious that men should symbolically be equated with culture. Lévi-Strauss also sees a close analogy between cooking, which transforms raw food in nature to edible food in culture, and socialization, during which a human infant in the natural state, as it were, becomes transformed into a socialized being. However, he is not directly concerned with the allocation of these roles to a particular sex.

On the other hand, Lévi-Strauss is fairly articulate in equating women with nature on the basis of physiology. Thus, interpreting the vaginal odor, which receives much emphasis among his Brazilian Indians, as representing nature, he leaps to his favorite universality: "And woman is everywhere synonymous with nature, even among the matrilineal and matrilocal Bororo, where the men's house, strictly out of bounds to the opposite sex, acts as a sanctuary for the religious life, at the same time as it offers the living a reflection of the kingdom of souls" (Lévi-Strauss 1969b:270). Here the argument is that these Brazilian Indians explicitly equate the vaginal odor with rotten fruit, nuts, and so on. In his scheme, the rottenness symbolizes nature in contrast to the cooked state, which symbolizes culture.

Elsewhere, Lévi-Strauss presents a slightly different argument. He contrasts parturient women and pubescent girls, on the one hand, to unmarried women, on the other; the former are equated with culture and the latter with nature. He writes about "cooked" women:

Individuals who are "cooked" are those deeply involved in a physiological process: the newborn child, the woman who has just given birth, or the pubescent girl. The conjunction of a member of the social group with nature must be mediatized through the intervention of cooking fire, whose normal function is to mediatize the conjunction of the raw product and the human consumer, and whose operation thus has the effect of making sure that a natural creature is at one and the same time *cooked and socialized.* (Lévi-Strauss 1969b:336)

An unmarried woman, on the other hand, is "a person who, still unmarried, has remained imprisoned in nature and rawness, and perhaps even destined to decay" (Lévi-Strauss 1969b:338). He thus concludes that the parturient and pubescent girls are "burned" (overcooked), whereas unmarried women are "rotten" (too fresh). I infer from these statements that Lévi-Strauss sees women as a group to be universally equated with nature when they are compared with men, but when the domain of analysis is women, pubescent girls and parturient women represent an exaggerated culture, whereas unmarried women represent an exaggerated nature.

In using women's physiology as the basis for the cultural equation of women with nature, La Fontaine (1972) advances a slightly different proposition. She sees a correlation between an ideological system and a social system. She explains the ritual significance placed upon defloration by the Gisu of Uganda as follows:

While defloration is one step in the chain of physical events that result in the maturation of a child into a fertile woman, it is also the one step that can be controlled by the society. First menstruation and first childbirth can be ritualized into social significance, but no human act can determine when they will occur. (1972:178)

We can say, in Lévi-Straussian idiom, that men's powers are part of culture, women's of nature . . . Defloration is the point at which nature and culture meet. (1972:179)

La Fontaine's interpretation of the Gisu defloration rests heavily upon their kinship organization; defloration symbolizes the act of control of women by men in this strongly patrilineal and male-centered society.

The point La Fontaine does not develop in this article and yet is implicit is another transformation – /nature:culture::uncontrolled:controlled/. Douglas (1975:213–14) offers an insight:

To domesticate an animal means to teach it to bring organic process under control. To socialize a child means the same thing... Living organisms shed their own used products. Excretion, urination, vomitting, spitting, nail-paring, hair-losing, these are the processes which rank lowest. Other physiological processes which are not part of discourse *should* be controlled: sneezing, hiccups... The more important the social event, the greater the demand for bodily control, and the lower the threshold of tolerance of bodily processes.

Although Douglas does not mention here the symbolic value of menstruation, it is one physiological function that cannot be under human control. It is therefore an apt symbol of nature. In some societies, in which women are equated with uncontrolled nature, menstruation may further represent uncontrollable sexuality symbolically assigned to women. Two conditions are necessary, however, before menstruation becomes a symbol of nature. First, a given culture must see the transformation of /nature:culture::uncontrolled:controlled/. Second, there must be an underlying symbolic equation of women with nature. Again, I propose that this equation of [nature = uncontrolled = women] is likely to take place in cultures in which the deities are not a part of nature.

In short, whereas de Beauvoir, Ortner, Lévi-Strauss, and La Fontaine propose the [nature = women] equation and their argument may be convincing as far as their respective cultures are concerned, a leap from these cultures (the nineteenth-century Western European cultures for de Beauvoir and Ortner, Brazilian Indians for Lévi-Strauss, and the Gisu for La Fontaine) to human culture seems to negate their own contention that these symbolic valuations of men and women are a result of cultural patterning. It is equally plausible to find the opposite equation of men with nature. For that matter, both types of equation are likely to be present within one culture, as I have shown with Ainu data in Chapter 7.

Sex roles too are subject to cultural interpretations. There are two possible fallacies in the argument for the [men = culture] equation, which is based upon the rule of exogamy proposed by Lévi-Strauss. First, even though the assertion that men are in charge of the exchange of marriage partners is ethnographically correct, a cultural interpretation can just as well equate women with culture, because it is women who facilitate this transformation from a biological to a social group; women are "valuables *par excellence* from both the biological and the social points of view," as Lévi-Strauss himself notes (1969a:481). Another weakness of this argument is that scholars have been increasingly critical of the universality of the rule of exogamy as Lévi-Strauss has depicted it. For example, Leach, who is often sympathetic to Lévi-Strauss, points out (1970:esp. 110, 113) that Lévi-Strauss's concept of exogamy is based on a unilineal descent system, which is not widespread enough to form a universal model of human kinship; Keesing (1975:91) estimates that at least one-third of tribal societies were without unilineal descent systems (see also Murdock 1960:2). Lévi-Strauss's assumption of the universal presence of an incest taboo, which provides the basis of the universality of exogamy in his scheme, has also been criticized because of ethnographic evidence that "normal" incest taboos are absent in many societies, past and present (Leach 1970:110). It seems, then, that an inference about the universality of the [women = nature] symbolic equation on the basis of the custom of exogamy falls short of ethnographic facts. Also, even when it is present, it can be interpreted to the contrary – to link women with culture, provided there is such ethnographic evidence.

The role of cooking is likewise subject to alternative interpretations. Ortner's point that professional chefs are males indicates that when any activity is transferred to the public domain, whether sewing (tailoring) or cooking (chefs), it is held by men, because women are barred from engaging in public activities. However, this point does not illustrate the /nature:culture::women:men/ equation, except when the domestic is already equated with nature and the public with culture. Assuming that cooking is relegated to women in most societies, there are still two alternative interpretations. First, because cooking is done by women and is the process of converting nature into edible food, that is, culture, women should be equated symbolically with culture. Second, one can argue that because men obtain raw meat, without which cooking cannot take place, men should be equated with culture. This second point needs further deliberation because women too gather raw food. Not only among agriculturalists, where women often do as much farming as men, but even among foraging populations it has recently been pointed out that plant food gathered by women is a significant part of the diet. The most frequently cited finding is Lee's work on !Kung Bushmen, 60%–80% of whose total diet by weight consists of vegetable foods collected by women (Lee 1968:33). Martin and Voorhies calculate that among ninety foraging societies listed by Murdock (1967), plant gathering done by women is the primary mode of subsistence in fifty-two (1975:181). Therefore, we cannot assume that it is men who always get the raw food from nature. A further complication, however, is that even though women may obtain a major portion of the food, this does not always mean that their society views them as the breadwinners. The credit for food getting often goes to the sex that brings in culturally valued food, which is often not the staple food. There is increasing evidence that even the foragers do not simply go after food to fill their stomachs; they place high value on nonstaple foods, which are often harder to obtain. The Ainu rely heavily upon plant food, which women gather, and fish, which men catch, but their highest esteem goes to bear meat, which they eat only several times a year; there is also more risk involved in bear hunting than in other food-getting activities. Siskind (1973, 1974) points out that, among the Sharanahua, it is not readily available food but the meat of animals caught during the special hunt that receives the highest valuation, although people can easily live without it. The men go infrequently and only unwillingly, when forced by the women, because the hunt in the jungle is very dangerous. In a number of his publications, Turner also states that the social importance of hunting among the Ndembu does not derive from the objective contribution to the food supply by the hunt but from the high ritual status of the hunter and also from the Ndembu association of hunting with masculinity. Turner, however, turns the tables and finds that it is the status of men, and not the meat they obtain, that renders hunting among the Ndembu socially significant. In short, inferences from the cultural activity of cooking are many. Should men be equated with culture because they obtain raw meat or culturally valued meat, or should women be equated with culture because they cook and may obtain much of the food supply themselves?

A discussion of cultural perceptions of food getting inevitably leads to a discussion of the cultural view of hunting. We saw above that both de Beauvoir and Ortner stress the transcendental nature of hunting and warfare and use this cultural notion as ethnographic evidence to equate men with culture. We also saw that both scholars expand this equation, making it universal. However, Rosaldo and Atkinson (1975) provide a convincing emic view of the equation of hunting with killing. Of the Ilongot, a group of hunters and swidden agriculturalists in Northern Luzon, Rosaldo and Atkinson (1975:58) state, "An examination of the similes used in magic suggests that hunting is equated with headhunting, that killing of animals is like killing of men, which is a focal cultural theme." With ample ethnographic evidence, they demonstrate that among the Ilongot the men, who engage in hunting and headhunting, are symbolically equated with life taking, whereas the women, who engage in agriculture and childbirth, are equated with life giving. Turner also convincingly demonstrates that among the Ndembu, women are associated with the life-giving force; they are nourishers as symbolized in the *mudyi* "milk tree" (1967:e.g., 57) and healers (1969:38). Ndembu men, on the other hand, are hunters, whose business, as seen by the Ndembu, is to kill (1969:e.g., 18). In a slightly different vein, the Stratherns (1968:198) find that among the Mbowamb of New Guinea, women, with their impure fertility, are symbolically equated with the domestic domain, whereas men, with their nonmenstrual powers of growth, are equated with the wild.

In interpreting symbolic associations of men and women among the Bakweri of Cameroon, Ardener (1972) focuses not on the economic roles of men and women per se but on where these activities take place. The Bakweri men live inside the fence with their livestock, whereas the women go outside the fence for firewood collecting and farming. Thus, the men stay within the fence, that is, the cultural domain, and the women spend their day outside the fence, that is, in nature (Ardener 1972:145):

> The women are all day in the forest outside the fence, returning at evening with their back-breaking loads of wood and cocoyams... screaming with fatigue at their husbands... It is no wonder that the women seem to be forest creatures, who might vanish one day for ever.

Ardener's interpretation is far more complex than a simple equation of the spatial dyad and the /man:woman/ dyad. Thus, the basis for the equation of women with the wild rests upon the symbolic equation of women's reproductive powers with nature; reproductive powers, which are central to women, do not fall under male control. As told in a Bakweri myth, "although the men bound off 'mankind' from nature, the women persist in overlapping into nature again" (Ardener 1975:143).

Two other sex roles are childbearing and nurturing, or socialization. Although childbearing is the only biologically based sex role for women, the conception of childbearing varies from culture to culture. First, men are not always credited with a role in conception, as in the case of the Ainu. Second, as with the Ainu and the Ilongot, childbearing may be regarded either as the life-giving process sui generis or as a natural biological process antithetical to the cultural process. The subsequent stage of nursing may similarly be interpreted either way. It may be regarded as the only way to sustain life, or simply as a biological and hence natural function. It should be noted here that for foraging populations, among whom there are no milk substitutes such as cereal grain or animal milk, the nurturing role during this early stage becomes at the same time a biologically based role and yet is even more vital than among agriculturalists or pastoralists, who have substitutes. In regard to the socialization process, Ortner, as noted earlier, points out that the socialization of boys in many societies is transferred to men at some point. This is the case with many societies but especially the hunters and gatherers, among whom hunting is done exclusively by men, who therefore must teach the boys. Until then, however, both male and female children are socialized primarily by their mothers. Therefore, the responsibility for transforming an infant into a socialized being again can be assigned to either sex.

In short, no matter what aspect of the physiological or sex roles may be chosen, that feature can be interpreted in various ways. Only through a systematic analysis of the emic view can one arrive at a particular transformation between the /nature:culture/ opposition and the /men:women/ opposition. In fact, both the /nature:culture::men:women/ equation and its inversion may be found within a culture, as I have demonstrated with the Ainu in Chapter 7. Although I think that both the formalized and non-formalized symbolic systems of the Ainu are held by both men and women, Ardener (1972) points to a possibility that men and women may hold separate ideologies and suggests as an example that menstruation may be viewed as marginal in men's world view and as central in women's (1972:143–4). It is high time anthropologists systematically investigated the multiplicity of symbolic systems and focused on the discovery of mechanisms that facilitate "the organization of diversity," to use Wallace's terminology (1970:23–38).

Anomaly: problem of definitions

The problem of determining how people classify their universe must necessarily include the problem of what they do with symbolic expressions of the unclassifiable. Having used the term *anomaly* with only a brief definition, I begin this section by defining it more fully. Anomaly refers to symbolic expression of some type of structural inversion. By *structural inversion*, I mean a state opposite to a classified world. That is, it is a state in which a culturally defined classificatory structure is inverted, reversed, contradicted, abrogated, nullified, or, in general, not in accord with the given structural principles. Babcock's definition of *symbolic inversion* (Babcock 1978:14) and Needham's (1979:38–47) concept of *transformations* both are akin to my notion of structural inversions. Thus, my concept of anomaly is characterized by the notion of the unclassifiable, although being a symbolic expression, anomaly is not synonymous with the unclassifiable. Some taxonomical unclassifiables may never receive symbolic meaning or power in a given culture, as will be discussed shortly. Likewise, as expressions of inverted structure, symbols that represent structural inversions at a particular symbolic level of abstraction may be classified beings at a lower level. Such is of demons and shamans, which were discussed earlier.

Anthropological awareness of the problem of anomaly has a long history, although it has long been part of only such interests as taboo and pollution. The major credit in drawing attention to this problem should go to van Gennep, whose classical treatment of rites of passage (1961, first published in 1908) is saluted by many; these rites function culturally to facilitate the passage of liminal periods. Robertson Smith (1972, first published in 1889) has also made an invaluable contribution to the anthropological understanding of this problem. Among contemporary anthropologists, major credit for emphasizing the theoretical import of the concept of anomaly and its power goes to Douglas, whose seminal work (1966) is devoted to the subject. The contributions of Steiner, Leach,

Turner, Tambiah, Bulmer, and Beidelman, to name only a few, are also indispensable.

In discussing anomaly, the two major issues are the concept of anomaly in relation to the concept of the sacred, discussed in this section, and the symbolic power ascribed to anomalous beings, discussed in the next section. In defining the concept of anomaly, some scholars see it as synonymous with the concept of the sacred. Leach uses the terms *ambiguous* (1968:39–40), and also *dirt* and *abnormal* (1967b:96–7), and defines the notion:

... the ambiguous categories that attract the maximum interest and the most intense feelings of taboo. The general theory is that taboo applies to categories which are anomalous with respect to clear-cut category oppositions. (1968:39)

Whatever taboo is sacred, valuable, important, powerful, dangerous, untouchable, filthy, unmentionable. (1968:37–8)

Likewise, Turner equates his *liminal* with the sacred (1969:106).

Douglas has pursued the problem of pollution and anomaly in relation to holiness. As noted earlier, the theme in her 1966 publication is basically that God created order and therefore God and order are holy, whereas confusion or a lack of classification is unholy, polluting, taboo. The definition of anomaly, however, is better articulated in her 1975 publication (e.g., 266, 282). She defines anomaly as follows:

For the purpose in hand, it is enough to speak of creatures which in their morphology show criteria of more than one major class, or not enough criteria to enable them to be assigned to any one class, and of creatures which in themselves belong clearly enough to a recognized class but which have either the habits or which stray into the habitat of another class. (Douglas 1975:282)

She thus discerns four types of anomalous creatures (1975:282): (1) creatures that show criteria of more than one major class in their morphology, for example, the pangolin of the Lele – the favorite symbol of Douglas; (2) creatures that do not have enough criteria to be assigned to any one class, for example, the cassowary of the Karam of New Guinea, as discussed by Bulmer (1967), which has neither the feathers nor the brain of a bird; (3) creatures that morphologically belong to one class but have the habits of another class, for example, nocturnal antelopes, distinguished by the Lele from other antelopes on the basis of this habit; (4) creatures that morphologically belong to one class but stray into the habitat of another class, for example, the otter of the Thai, as discussed by Tambiah (1969), which invades the domestic fields in flood time. Bulmer (1967) also uses the habitat in his definition of anomaly.

Using both morphology and habitat, however, these four types of anomaly defined by Douglas become redundant. Thus, her types 1, 3, and 4 may all be seen to rest on one criterion – the mixing of more than one category, morphologically or otherwise. Her examples of the symbols for each type consequently show redundancy. For example, the pangolin, in the Lele view, is "an animal with the body and tail of a fish, covered in scales," and yet unlike a fish it climbs trees in the forest (Douglas 1975:33). In addition, the Lele perceive other features of anomaly in the pangolin. Unlike other animals it does not shun men, and it offers itself to hunters. Also, unlike other animals, but like men, it gives birth to one offspring at a time (Douglas 1975:33). Thus, although Douglas offers the pangolin as an example of the type 1 anomaly, this animal has characteristics of more than one category, not only morphologically but also in terms of habitat (lives in the forest instead of the river, although it looks like a fish), as well as in terms of behavior (does not shun men and reproduces like humans). Likewise, the otter of the Thai, as described by Tambiah, and offered by Douglas as an example of the type 5 anomaly, not only invades the fields in flood time but is viewed by the Thai as a revolting hybrid; it is a fish because it swims, but it has a head like a dog. In other words, the pangolin can be an example of types 1, 3, and 4 anomalies, and the otter can be an example not only of types 1 and 4 but also of type 3.

I offer here an alternative scheme for the typology of anomaly,[1] using no particular criteria such as morphology, habitat, or behavioral characteristics. In terms of morphology, habitat, behavior, or any other feature, a being (marked with an X in the Venn diagrams) is anomalous if:

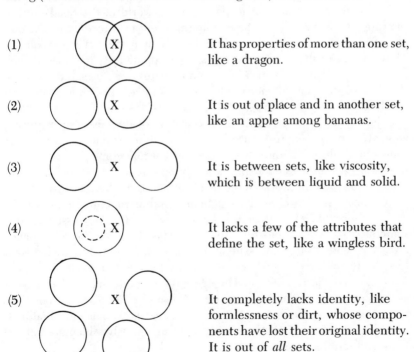

(1)   It has properties of more than one set, like a dragon.

(2)   It is out of place and in another set, like an apple among bananas.

(3)   It is between sets, like viscosity, which is between liquid and solid.

(4)   It lacks a few of the attributes that define the set, like a wingless bird.

(5)   It completely lacks identity, like formlessness or dirt, whose components have lost their original identity. It is out of *all* sets.

The first four types of anomaly may be seen to negate and defy a particular classificatory system. They do not obey the rules imposed by a given system. Among these four types, the first three may be seen to have the same structural principle in that they all represent a juxtaposition of categories of a given system. In contrast, beings symbolizing the type 4 anomaly may still be considered as members of a set, although marginal members; lacking some of the definitional criteria to be full-fledged members of a set, they are at the periphery. In contrast to the first four types of anomaly, type 5 is antithetical to all forms of structure, not to a particular classificatory system and its boundaries. It is like a vacuum or chaos.

All these types of anomaly are defined in relation to either a particular structure or structure in general. Here I am in agreement with Douglas, who emphasizes that the "dirt implies system" (1975:51). Like Turner's liminal, the type 5 anomaly is not structural contradictions but the essentially unstructured (e.g., 1967:98; 1969:96). But the notion of the unstructured presupposes the presence of a structure.

In the case of the Ainu, we have seen that the first type of anomaly is represented by the demon couple whose upper jaw touches the sky and whose lower jaw digs into the ground, cutting into two spatial sets – the sky and the ground. The musical instrument demons represent an anomaly of the second type. Their souls are out of place – that is, out of the body – and yet cannot rest in peace in the world of the dead musical instruments. They may also be seen to represent the fourth type of anomaly because they are demons only as long as their identity is not known. They are like orphans, who do not have kinship identity in a society such as that of the Ainu, in which kinship dominates one's social identity. In the case of the loom demon, only the out-of-place principle (type 2) is involved.

Other symbols involved in Ainu accounts of demons also represent anomaly. Thus, their residence is depicted either in mountain caves or somewhere offshore. The caves are abnormal topographical phenomena to which the Ainu assign a special symbolic value. Thus some caves are thought to reach the world of the dead Ainu at the other end. Just as the sacred bears stay in caves during their semihibernation, caves are the residences of the deities in myths. In other words, the Ainu assign special symbolic values of various sorts to caves. The offing, on the other hand, always belongs to demons. The appearance of demons is signaled by a bloody mist in the offing where demons are believed to reside (Kindaichi 1914; Ohnuki-Tierney 1969a). The offing is a spatially marginal area lying at the periphery of the Ainu universe. Because of its marginal position, the offing is the area assigned to demons, that is, anomalous creatures. The symbol of bloody mist also represents an anomaly – blood out of the body and formlessness.

Douglas (1966:37) sees little significance in differentiating between anomaly and ambiguity in their practical application, and Turner (1967:97) follows her interpretation. I should like to distinguish between the two by using the term *anomaly* to refer to the cognitive dimension of the unclassifiable and the term *ambiguity* to refer to the reaction of the members of a culture to an anomalous being, which is perceived as unclear and ambiguous. I prefer to reserve *marginal*, another term often used to refer to anomaly, for a particular kind of anomaly, that is, the type 4 anomaly in my scheme (which corresponds to type 2 in the scheme presented by Douglas). I follow anthropological custom in using the term *liminal* to refer to temporal anomaly.

In studying the concept of anomaly in a particular culture, I find it significant to include metaphysical or mythical beings, as I have done in Chapter 7. Douglas excludes the mythic beings of the Israelites, which often are hybrid beings such as the cherubim and the extraordinary being of Ezekiel's dream. She considers them not at issue because no face-to-face encounter in daily life was expected and "the rules of Leviticus II are concerned only with physical encounters" (Douglas 1975:315). For understanding the entire range of the concept of anomaly among the Israelites, however, it seems that mythical beings too should receive attention, especially because they are "not judged adversely" (Douglas 1975:315), whereas the anomalous beings encountered daily are abominable. As shown in Chapter 7, the Ainu case is the opposite. Thus, the Ainu demons, that is, mythic beings in Douglas's sense, represent anomaly *sui generis* and are the source of strong negative power, whereas "ordinary" anomalous beings, which are marginal symbols, can transcend the classificatory boundaries and exercise a positive power. By closely examining all possible symbols of anomaly, rather than only the dominant or key symbols, we may some day be able to engage in comparative work on different types of anomaly and characteristics assigned to each. Such meticulous examinations are important in that the concept of anomaly differs from culture to culture precisely because the classificatory system itself also varies. The types of anomaly, except the fifth, are defined in terms of a particular classificatory scheme.

Sperber's recent (1979) criticism of the assumption by Douglas that anomaly exists in most taxonomic systems brings to light another unfortunate confusion in symbolic anthropology. Sperber (1976:502) writes:

Her work on animal symbolism is built on the hypothesis that any taxonomic scheme cannot but generate anomalies. Yet the intensive work of ethno-zoologists over the past twenty years has shown on the contrary that folk-taxonomies are much more elaborate and regular than one might have thought, and that no locally known animal species is ever left out. There are no anomalies generated by the taxonomy, but, at best, species with "special taxonomic status."

Eminent cognitive anthropologists Berlin, Breedlove, and Raven (1974:26–7) point out that it is not uncommon to find "a number of classes of generic rank that are *aberrant*. . . and, as such, are conceptually seen as unaffiliated." The apparent confusion stems from the mixing of different stages of the perception, conception, and symbolization process. Taxonomic anomaly in ethnosemantics does not automatically lead to anomaly in the sense used in this book, because the latter notion represents the second-order symbolization process; taxonomic anomaly can remain unclassified without the ascription of further symbolic meaning. As Bulmer (1967:19) points out, it is futile simply to isolate the cassowary as a special taxon in the ethno-zoology of the Karam, because the symbolic meaning assigned to the animal does not derive simply from its strange appearance and behavior. According to Bulmer, the real symbolic meaning must be sought in the Karam cosmology:"So, for me, at least, 'special taxonomic status' is a function of something broader, a special status in culture, or cosmology, at large." (For further discussion on these points, see Ohnuki-Tierney in press.)

The confusion between taxonomic anomaly and symbolic anomaly is only an expression of the imprecision in the anthropological uses of the term *symbol*. There are several stages in the processes of human perception, cognition, and symbolization. Folk classification of ethnosemanticists deals with the initial stage of human perception and cognition of the external world. Here, a dog in the external world becomes a culturally defined dog, as opposed to other animals recognized by the culture. But the dog may acquire further symbolic meaning, such as a messenger of bear deities, as in the case of the Ainu. At the last or most abstract stage of symbolization, we encounter demons and other "mythical" beings, discussed earlier. These do not have reference points in the external world, although they can be given the most concrete form as icons. In an analysis of a symbolic system, it is vital to examine all of these symbols, including mythical beings, but it is also imperative to make clear distinctions among the different stages of the symbolization process. (For critical comments on the subject, see Barthes 1979:42; Sahlins 1976:120; a detailed analysis of the stages is presented in Ohnuki-Tierney 1981.)

Anomaly and power

Anomalous beings are prominent in anthropological literature not simply because the unclassifiable is intellectually fascinating but because a number of anthropologists believe that they often are important symbols with potent power. Furthermore, the power assigned to these symbols is not always negative, as discussed above; it is often positive. Eliade (1971:194) views an anomaly such as formlessness to symbolize beginning or a start of new creation. Turner eloquently describes the nature of liminal symbols as "unbound, the infinite, the limitless" and "a realm of pure possibility whence novel configurations of ideas and relations may arise" (1967:98, 97). Leach sees "the innate sacred-taboo quality of all boundaries" to derive from their ambiguity and claims that "power is located in dirt" (1976:71; see also 1967 c). In her 1966 publication, Douglas expounds on both the positive and negative powers of dirt, which in her discussion exemplify anomaly of the most potent kind. She explains that in the process of decay – the first stage – when the decomposing object has a half-identity, it is perceived as polluting and dangerous. At the final stage of decay, however, it no longer has any identity. It is at this stage that anomalies acquire positive power, as in the case of creative formlessness (Douglas 1966:160–1). Of the dangerous anomalies of the first stage, Douglas explains that they also can generate positive power if it is harnessed in a ritual context: "Those vulnerable margins and those attacking forces which threaten to destroy good order represent the powers inhering in the cosmos. Ritual which can harness these for good is harnessing power indeed" (Douglas 1966:161). Using the example of her favorite Pangolin cult of the Lele, she explains the nature of the power of anomaly harnessed by ritual:

By the mystery of that rite they recognize something of the fortuitous and conventional nature of the categories in whose mould they have their experience. If they consistently shunned ambiguity they would commit themselves to division between ideal and reality. But they confront ambiguity in an extreme and concentrated form. They dare to grasp the pangolin and put it to ritual use, proclaiming that this has more power than any other rites. So the pangolin cult is capable of inspiring a profound mediation on the nature of purity and impurity and on the limitation on human contemplation of existence. (Douglas 1966:170)

Thus she sees primitive existentialism in the pangolin cult that enables the Lele to exercise choice and thus to "escape from the chain of necessity" (Douglas 1966:178). Her typology of the power of anomalous symbols is schematically shown in Figure 8.3.

What is the precise distinction between the power generated by anomaly that has only partial identity but is ritualized, and the creative power generated by anomaly that is characterized by the total lack of identity? And where does the power of the pangolin fit? A pangolin is characterized neither by partial identity nor by total lack of identity; it is a type 1 anomaly in my scheme. From the structural point of view, the Lele pangolin, the Thai otter, and the Ainu demon couple all share the juxtaposition of properties of more than one category. Yet, the Lele pangolin generates creative power, whereas the other two have negative power.

My attempt to find systematic correlations in the Ainu symbolic system

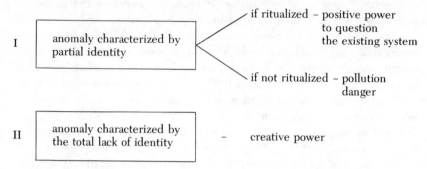

Figure 8.3. An interpretation of Douglas's concept of anomalies and their power.

between types of anomalies and types of power attributed to them has not been successful. The only clear-cut pattern I can discern is that the demonic anomalies are characterized by the juxtaposition of categories, whereas symbols that generate positive power are all marginal or type 4 anomalies in my scheme. Beyond this, there are numerous questions to be answered. For example, snakes and frogs are abhorred by the Ainu, who state that they are strange because they inhabit both land and water and are neither fish nor anything else. Thus, the Ainu perception of snakes and frogs is exactly the same, at least from the structural point of view, as the Ainu description of the demon couple that traverses both the sky and the ground. The demons are imaginary, whereas snakes and frogs are real. Is this the only explanation of why the demons are endowed with negative power, whereas the animals are assigned only negative meaning?

A similar question arises as to why *kawawe:* birds are mediators, whereas owls are deities in the Ainu symbolic system. Both owls and *kawawe:* birds are marginal members of the category of birds, whose activities are carried out during the day; both birds are active at night, the time allocated to deities and demons. Unlike owls, *kawawe:* birds lack visual identity; this seems to be the difference between them that the Ainu perceive. But I have no decisive Ainu answer as to why owls are placed upon the throne and *kawawe:* birds are not. In addition, ducks are anomalous in terms of spatial classification but are neither sacred nor demonic; they are mediators. Thus, all three species of birds (owls, *kawawe:* birds, and ducks) are anomalous, but owls symbolize the sacred, whereas the other two represent mediation.

Another set of questions arises when we examine the symbolisms of bodily dirt, which are seen to be not only dirty and polluting but also powerful in almost all cultures (Douglas 1966; Loudon 1975; Wilson 1957:232). Menstruation and excrement in particular are apt symbols of anomaly in many cultures (Douglas 1966:96, 121 et passim; Leach

1968:38; Lévi-Strauss 1973:255; Turner 1967: 96). Leach (1968:38, 37, 39) sees anomaly as a quality of the sacred: "The exudations of the human body are universally the objects of intense taboo. Whatever is taboo is sacred . . . supernatural beings of a highly ambiguous kind – incarnate deities, virgin mothers, supernatural monsters which are half man/half beast." The interpretation of anomaly by Douglas differs from that of Leach. We recall that according to Douglas, the negative cultural signifi- cance of bodily dirt is derived from the need of humans to distinguish themselves fron animals. Because humans see animals as not being able to control their bodily dirt, humans consider this to be the worst of all dirt and find it imperative to control it in order to distinguish themselves from animals (Douglas 1975:213–14). In the conceptual scheme of Douglas, bodily dirt is the greatest blasphemy and defiance of God, the creator of order. Although Douglas does not explicitly say so, her argument suggests that anomaly, symbolized by bodily dirt, should be equated with nature, which is the antithesis of the sacred. The Ainu case presents another type of symbolic association of anomaly. As noted in Chapter 7, I interpret the Ainu marginal symbols of menstrual blood and excrement, as used in medical rituals, as representing the most profane activities of procreation and consumption. Their power to expel deities and demons derives from the taboo of mixing categories; the profane (culture) cannot be mixed with the sacred (nature) or demonic anomaly. In short, bodily dirt is an almost universal symbol of anomaly, but its meaning and power may derive from the sacred, the profane, or something else, depending upon the symbolic structure of a given culture.

An examination of the typology of anomaly so far has not offered answers to the question of why only some of the unclassifiables are assigned mean- ing and others positive or negative power. In explaining food taboos among the Thai, Tambiah (1969) proposes that if an animal is anomalous in having properties of two categories, both of which consist of edible ani- mals, then the animal concerned will be auspicious as well as edible. On the other hand, if one category consists of edible and the other of inedible animals, then the animal concerned will be inauspicious and taboo to eat. Tambiah's scheme, however, does not explain the Ainu food taboo placed upon snakes and frogs, because both water and land animals are edible for the Ainu.

Since her 1966 publication, Douglas has increasingly sought answers for this question not in the conceptual categories themselves, but in the workings of the society. In her recent publications (1973, 1975, 1978), she takes the view that the social systems generate conceptual categories, including the meaning and power assigned to anomaly. This classical Durkheimian explanation focuses only upon the functions of conceptual categories and anomaly.

My contextual analysis of anomalous symbols presented in the next section differs from that of Lévi-Strauss, who also uses the context in which an anomalous symbol appears in order to determine the meaning and power assigned to the symbol. In explaining why menstruation has a positive significance in eagle hunting among the Hidatsa, during which the hunter assumes a low position in pits dug in the ground, in contrast to the high position of the eagles, he states (Lévi-Strauss 1966:52):

Menstruation acquires a positive significance from three points of view in a system of this kind. From a strictly formal point of view, since one hunt [ordinary hunting] is the reverse of the other [eagle hunting], the role attributed to menstruation is accordingly reversed. It is harmful in one case because its similarity is too great, but it becomes beneficial in the other where it has not only a metaphorical but also a metonymical sense: it evokes the bait as blood and organic decay and the bait is a part of the system. From the technical point of view the bloodstained carcass, soon to be carrion, which is close to the living hunter for hours or even days is the means of effecting the capture, and it is significant that the same native term is used for the embrace of lovers and the grasping of the bait by the bird. Finally, at a semantic level, pollution, at least in the thought of the North American Indians, consists in too close a conjunction between two things each meant to remain in a state of "purity." In the hunt at close quarters menstrual periods always risk introducing excessive union which would lead to a saturation of the original relation and a neutralization of its dynamic force by redundancy. In the hunt at a distance it is the reverse. The conjunction is inadequate and the only means to remedy its deficiency is to allow pollution to enter. Pollution appears as *periodicity* on the axis of successions or as *putrefaction* on that of simultaneities.

Lévi-Strauss thus places the interpretation in his basic frame of analysis – /symbol:sign::metaphor:metonymy::paradigmatic association:syntagmatic chain::harmony:melody/. (See also Lévi-Strauss 1969b:esp. 292–4.)

To recapitulate, anomalous beings and objects may be:
  A. Not ritualized
  B. Ritualized
    1. Endowed with meaning without power
    2. Endowed with power
      a. Endowed with sacred power
      b. Endowed with profane power
      c. Endowed with the power of mediation, which strengthens the existing structure
      d. Endowed with the power to create a new structure

Our task is to identify factors that generate each type of meaning or power. We need massive ethnographic evidence from many cultures before we can attempt to see some patterns in the symbolic treatment of anomalies in cross-cultural perspective. So far, the only thing we are sure of as a cross-cultural regularity is that beings and objects that are anomalous in a particular symbolic structure are more often chosen to symbolize various types of power than ordinary beings and objects. To assign any particular structural quality, whether sacred, profane, or any other, or to equate anomaly with a particular structural quality in toto (sacred = anomaly in Leach's scheme, or anomaly ≠ sacred in Douglas's scheme) does not seem to be validated in cross-cultural perspective.

Multiple symbolic systems: /public:domestic::men:women/

The last section of this chapter attempts to correlate symbolic oppositions discussed above with the activities of the people. It also attempts to elucidate further the taboo that results not from mixed categories but from the process of mixing them. Above all, it is an attempt to trace, at least in part, our quest for the contextual rules that determine the nature of the power and meaning assigned to anomalous symbols.

We recall from Chapter 7 that in the case of the Ainu there are at least two sets of symbolic systems. The group rituals officiated by men express the formalized and official ideology, in which the sacred is extolled and men occupy the central place. The shamanistic ritual, in contrast, expresses the ideology in which the power of the profane and that of women are symbolized. I think that the way in which the dualistic system of ideology/symbols is expressed is a correlate of the male occupancy of the public domain and the female possession of the domestic sphere.

Rosaldo (1974:23) defines the domestic in reference to women's sex roles of childbearing and rearing: "those minimal institutions and modes of activity that are organized immediately around one or more mothers and their children." The public refers to "activities, institutions, and forms of association that link, rank, organize, or subsume particular mother-child groups." Sanday's definitions (1974:190) of these domains emphasize authority in the public domain and power in the domestic domain. According to Sanday, the domestic domain is associated with "activities performed within the realm of the localized family unit," whereas activities in the public domain "take place or have impact beyond the localized family unit and . . . relate to control of persons or control of things." Authority is a legitimized power, whereas power is not. As Smith (1960:19) puts it, "authority is a derived or delegated right, while power is the possession of manifest or latent control or influence over the actions of persons including oneself." (For the distinction between authority and power, see also Peabody 1968; Weber 1947:esp. 152–3.)

It has been pointed out by many (e.g., Rosaldo 1974) that the /public:domestic:: men:women/ equation is a universal pattern in human society. Based upon this assumption, I suggest in Table 8.1 that we may also find in other cultures a dualistic system of thought similar to that of the

Table 8.1. *Spheres of activity and ideological systems*

	Domestic	Public
Activities	Domestic activities	Political arena
	Shamanistic and other individual rites	Group rituals
Ideological/symbolic systems	Nonformalized ideology	Formalized/public ideology
Politically peripheral (women and some men)	Authority	Power
	Clean and powerful	Polluting
Politically central (men)	(Power) ⟵————————— Authority
	⟵————————— Clean and powerful

Ainu. Significantly, the schema is not exactly symmetrical. First, as Sacks (1974:219) suggests, domestic power usually is not translatable into social or public power, whereas public authority is often translatable into domestic power. A man with high social status has that public role even at home; his domestic role of a husband or father is considerably influenced by his social status. This one-way movement of power is symbolically expressed by such taboos as the menstrual taboo and the absence of its equivalent for men. Menstrual blood is a positive symbol of women in the domestic domain, but it is taboo in the public domain. The function of the taboo is to separate the two domains and prevent the flow of domestic power into the public domain. Ethnographic studies seldom report taboos about men, such as taboos about semen. This phenomenon may be attributed in part to the lack of awareness of ethnographers. Buchbinder and Rappaport (1976:20) and Faithorn (1976:94) suggest that in the New Guinea highlands men too are potentially polluting in certain ways. With more ethnographic data on pollution by men, we will gain a clearer understanding of the situation. On the whole, my guess is that the lack of taboos about men relates to the translatability of public authority into domestic power, rather than simply a lack of ethnographic reports.

The second point about the asymmetrical nature of Table 8.1 is that the public ideology and the symbolic system expressed through group rituals are often consciously held by both men and women in the society. The people are likely to articulate the public ideology, and hence, it would be more frequently recorded by ethnographers. The domestic/nonformalized ideology, on the other hand, is apt to stay more or less unconscious, only vaguely perceived. Thus the basic meaning of the bear ceremony is well articulated by the Ainu, whereas the meaning of the shamanistic ritual is explained only in terms of its function – the healing of the ill. My idea here corresponds in part to Ardener's (1975:22) dominant and muted structures.

A model that may be applicable even to more stratified societies than hunting-gathering societies would be the opposition not between men and women but between the politically powerful and the politically peripheral, including some men, as noted in the parentheses in Figure 8.1. (For further discussion of the politically peripheral, see Chapter 10.) For example, the ideology supporting the societal hierarchy may be expressed in some rituals, whereas the power of the powerless or the ideology of egalitarianism and cummunitas may be expressed in other rituals, such as shamanistic rituals that are held during liminal periods.

Whether or not the schema presented in Table 8.1 applies to other cultures must be tested by others. The schema at least explains the multivocality of dominant symbols of the Ainu, such as menstrual blood. As noted at the beginning of this chapter, some of the dominant Ainu symbols have referents whose meanings are contradictory. This schema can explain a situation whereby the referents of a multivocal symbol have structurally opposite meanings in structurally opposed contexts. A model such as the one in Figure 8.1 also explains the simultaneous presence of any of the symbolic equations and their inversions.

Summary

This chapter is concerned with various theories and interpretations of symbols. Such universal oppositions as /sacred:profane/, /nature:culture/, and /men:women/ are discussed in order to elucidate how different meanings are assigned to these symbolic oppositions in various cultures. Such factors as a subsistence economy or the nature of religion are discussed as possible correlates, but not necessarily determinants.

The main purpose of a lengthy discussion of symbolic classification, however, is not simply to understand the classificatory system itself but also symbolic expressions of the unclassifiable – anomaly – because anomalous symbols hold the key to the understanding of Ainu illness perception. In Chapter 7, one set of anomalous symbols is personified as demons – which, in turn, are conceived as illness pathogens – whereas the other set of anomalous symbols appear in shamanistic healing rites as mediators. In order to decipher these two sets of anomalous Ainu symbols, I examined the problem of symbolic expressions of the unclassifiable in cross-cultural perspective. I attempted to classify different types of anomaly and analyzed the symbolic powers assigned to them. At this point, it seems best to conclude that beings and objects that have anomalous qualities are apt symbols of power; lack of classificatory confinements gives them freedom and power to transcend a given classificatory system. Various ethnographic data and their interpretations by scholars suggest that they can represent different types of symbolic power – the sacred, profane, nature, culture, or even anarchic anomaly. In other words, there seems to be no cross-cultural regularity about the association of anomalous symbols with particular types of symbolic meaning. For that matter, even within one culture, some anomalous symbols may, for example, represent the sacred, whereas others represent the profane.

In the last section of this chapter, I proposed that most cultures entertain more than one symbolic system and suggested possible models specifying contextual rules that generate various referents of a multivocal symbol.

9

Modes of perception and the classification of illnesses: a synthesis

After a long sojourn in the realm of symbolic interpretations of the Ainu medical system, we now return to the problem of Ainu modes of perception as revealed in their classification of illness. Although the cognitive dimension of perception receives the most coverage, the role of the emotive and sensory dimensions should not be neglected.

A larger aim of this chapter is to use the Ainu domain of illness in order to explore the problem of recognizing a structure, structures, or quasi-structures in a culture. Scholars differ in their views on this matter. Thus, whereas such scholars as Lévi-Strauss assume the presence of a single "Structure" in "Human Culture" or the "Human Mind," other scholars, such as Needham (1963:xix) and Conklin (1971), argue for the presence of more than one structure or mode of classification in a culture. Still others doubt whether a tightly delineated structure exists. Geertz (1973:407–8) opposes the structural approach in anthropology and sees cultural organization as follows:

The appropriate image, if one must have images, of cultural organization, is neither the spider web nor the pile of sand. It is rather more the octopus, whose tentacles are in large part separately integrated, neurally quite poorly connected with one another and with what in the octopus passes for a brain, and yet who nonetheless manages both to get around and to preserve himself, for a while anyway, as a viable if somewhat ungainly entity.

Needless to say, a comprehensive treatment of the subject is beyond the scope of this chapter. My discussion is confined to the problems that are most helpful in understanding the Ainu classificatory schema.

I begin by delineating the Ainu domain of illness and then compare two major groups of illnesses – habitual and metaphysical. The contrast between the tightly defined and classified habitual illnesses and the loosely conceived metaphysical illnesses leads to the problem of the degree of classification found in various domains or subdomains of a culture: Why are some areas of culture better delineated and classified than others? Next I explore different modes of perception, or more specifically, conceptualization, and the possibility that more than one mode of thought

133

may be present in a culture. The next section is devoted to two other dimensions of human perception – emotive and sensory. In the last section, the structural approach taken in this book is evaluated in relation to other approaches.

The domain of illness: problems of codification and subdivision

In Chapter 3, we saw the difficulties involved in the terminological approach to codifying the domain of illness. There is no one-to-one correlation between the Ainu term for an illness and the presence of a culturally prescribed illness. Some illnesses are recognized as such and yet are not habitually referred to as illnesses. Nor does a culturally prescribed cure indicate that a phenomenon is an illness; cuts, burns, and bruises with meticulously prescribed cures are not identified as illnesses. Of course, these two characteristics – the lack of terminological expressions for some illnesses and the presence of treatment for nonillnesses – are not peculiar to Ainu culture. In American society, for example, many phenomena such as colds, headaches, and stomach disorders are recognized as departures from health and medications are available, yet they are not always labeled as illnesses unless they are symptoms of something more serious.

A further complexity in the Ainu identification of illnesses is that a culturally prescribed cause determines whether or not a particular phenomenon is regarded as an illness. Thus a minor cut inflicted by a bear deity is considered a grave illness, whereas a cut that we might consider serious would not be classified as an illness. It is this symbolic causation as the primary criterion of an illness that justifies my emphasis upon the distinction between habitual and metaphysical illnesses; in the former there is no culturally prescribed cause, and in the latter the cause is even more important than the symptoms in illness identification. For instance, both the physical illness of smallpox and the mental illness of insanity accompanied by violence are caused by demons. I find it more meaningful, therefore, to define a category on the basis of a cause, for example, illnesses caused by demons, than to set up such categories as mental or physical illnesses. This does not mean, however, that the Ainu do not make the distinction; they distinguish between body and soul and between somatic and mental illnesses, just as most peoples do (cf. Obeyesekere 1970a). But the Ainu distinction is radically different from the distinction used in Western societies. In Ainu medicine, most of the metaphysical illnesses accompanied by somatic symptoms are in fact caused by nonphysical entities such as deities or souls. Therefore, to use the label *physical illness* for these illnesses of the Ainu is misleading.

By the same token, the severity of an illness as the Ainu would define it is different from our judgment of it. As noted above, a minor cut inflicted by a bear is a serious illness for the Ainu because it is caused by a supreme deity. The habitual illnesses in general are less serious for the Ainu because they do not involve serious causes, although some skin infections, for example, can be quite severe. Therefore, it seems necessary to look closely at a people's views of these categories before we conclude that the distinction between minor and serious illnesses is universal, as Sigerist (1951:126) suggests.

Likewise, to regard habitual illnesses as primarily empirical and metaphysical illnesses as symbolic, and to draw a sharp line between the two groups, is misleading. The dog in the dog headache is not the neutral *Canis familiaris* but the Ainu dog. Similarly, other materia medica used for habitual illnesses are not simply stones, herbs, and bones; they are endowed with symbolic meaning. Furthermore, as seen in Chapter 3, in the Ainu medical system the deities are ubiquitous; they are basically responsible for the general health maintenance of the Ainu. Thus, all Ainu illnesses are symbolically construed, and the habitual illnesses are only relatively more mechanical because they do not directly involve the supernatural or metaphysical agents. With this caution in mind, I now turn to general distinctions between the two groups of illnesses.

Contrasts between habitual illnesses and metaphysical illnesses

Perhaps one of the most exciting findings of the Ainu data is the fact that the habitual illnesses, which are often neglected in ethnography, are deeply embedded in the Ainu world view at the structural level. Although anthropological publications on non-Western medicine abound, the great majority of them focus on the so-called supernatural illnesses, or what I refer to in this book as metaphysical illnesses. This coverage is skewed for several reasons. Perhaps the most important reason relates to the history of anthropology. As noted in Chapter 1, anthropologists in the past did not pay serious attention to the medical systems of their host cultures, but they have long focused on the magico-religious dimensions of culture. For instance, shamanism has always received enormous attention, although again it was usually treated as a magico-religious rite rather than a healing rite. By the same token, witchcraft occupies a central place in the anthropological analyses of religion and, also importantly, of social control. As a by-product, we have information on supernatural illnesses.

Even when an anthropologist is interested in the medical system of his or her host culture, supernatural illnesses receive greater emphasis because they more readily clarify the point that among non-Western peoples illnesses are treated not as abstract biomedical things (Fabrega 1975) but as afflictions of both the body and the mind or soul. In addition, the supernatural illnesses include what we usually call mental illnesses, which are of great concern in most Western societies. All in all, habitual illnesses often seem uninteresting and also insignificant, not only for anthropologists but also for the people themselves. Even Ackerknecht (1946:478) and Hallowell (1963) – two prominent figues in early anthropological studies of illness – seem to share this assumption that habitual illnesses are insignificant: Hallowell (1963:276–7) states "[Ackerknecht] emphasizes the fact the indispositions of the former category [natural disease] 'are not important enough to theorize about...' My own observation of the Ojibwa confirms his position."

Valuable exceptions to this tendency to slight the ethnographic value of habitual illnesses include works by Frake (1961), Fabrega (1970), and Turner (1967). Frake's analysis of the skin illnesses of the Subanun of Mindanao treats these illnesses in depth, using the methodological approach of ethnosemantics (ethnoscience). Although he reveals some intriguing taxonomic principles involved in the classification of these skin illnesses, Frake's data relate the illness more to culturally construed social relations than to broader aspects of the Subanun world view. Although Fabrega does not make a distinction between habitual and metaphysical illnesses, the Zinacantan illnesses he investigated include what may be called habitual illnesses. The following criticism by Fabrega (1970:305) of ethnographic data on illness is especially relevant in this regard: "Exotic and 'peculiar' features or symptoms of illness which may or may not be intraculturally significant, however, often appear to receive more attention than the basic question of the bodily and/or behavioral elements that comprise the general model of illness in the culture..." Fabrega's own work corrects this situation. It is intriguing to find that such bodily and behavioral elements as "crying and sadness" or "quarrelsomeness and excessive hostility" (1970:308) included in the bodily disturbances serve to define Zinacantan illnesses.

Turner's analysis of the Ndembu Lunda medicine has yielded findings similar to mine on the Ainu habitual illnesses. He finds in the Ndembu treatment of headaches (1967:355) a systematic expression of basic values and color symbolism: "The treatment of headache thus reveals itself as a formal procedure controlled by religious ideas that are expressed in symbolic actions and symbolic articles: Whiteness/redness; above/below; strength/weakness; health/disease (a mode of blackness)..."

Similarly, the Ainu data illustrate that even seemingly minor ailments such as boils and headaches are intimately related to the basic perceptual structure of the Ainu. The dyadic structure seen in the classification of illnesses into aquatic and terrestrial thus corresponds to the /land:water/ dyad in the Ainu spatial classification of the universe. It appears then that the same binary opposition governs not only spatial perception, which is one of the most basic orientations in any culture, but also seemingly insignificant habitual illnesses such as headaches, throat illnesses, and boils. In addition, as noted previously, the temporal dyad seen in the classification of boils parallels the basic dyad in the Ainu temporal structure (Ohnuki-Tierney 1973c). Terrestrial boils have no openings and thus represent the first stage in the development of boils, whereas aquatic boils represent a later stage. The classification of the beings of the universe also consists of a dyad operative at several taxonomic levels (see Chapter 7).

Ainu space, time, beings, and illnesses are all classified using the principle of binary opposition and are at least partially aligned with each other, although the symbolic values of the sacred and the profane assigned to the dyads in the classification of space, time, and beings are not transferred to the illness classification. As Wallace (1970:143) succinctly puts it, a world view is "the very skeleton of concrete cognitive assumptions on which the flesh of customary behavior is hung" and "is implicit in almost every act." My Ainu data, Frake's data on the Subanun, and Turner's data on Lunda medicine all point to a possibility that if an investigator pays enough attention to so-called minor illnesses of the host culture, they may express basic symbolic values and powers assigned to space, color, time, and so on. The cultural content of these ailments may be as exciting as the much-studied supernatural illnesses.

Not only are the principles governing the habitual illnesses related to the structural principles governing the major domains of the Ainu world view, but these illnesses are meticulously classified, in some cases into several levels. Therefore, Ainu perception and cure of the habitual illnesses are not automatic reactions to natural phenomena; instead, their perception and treatment constitute an integral part of the Ainu cultural system. I also hope that my treatment of Ainu habitual illnesses has demonstrated the value of an analysis at a deeper or structural level, which may render seemingly unimportant ethnographic data systematic and coherent in meaning.

Whereas the habitual illnesses are related to a basic perceptual structure and world view, the metaphysical illnesses are closely linked with the narrow but well-articulated domains of religion and morality. Thus, at the most general level, metaphysical illnesses are classified in terms of the pathogens and etiologies involved: deities, demons, human actions, or souls. The metaphysical illnesses express the status of humans in relation to the deities, demons, and fellow Ainu.

In terms of classification, the metaphysical illnesses are defined in a manner radically different from that of the habitual illnesses (Table 9.1). Their classification is taxonomic only at the most general level discussed above. The principle of inclusion that characterizes any taxonomic classification is not involved in the classification of metaphysical illness at

Table 9.1. *Contrasts between habitual and metaphysical illnesses*

	Habitual illnesses	Metaphysical illnesses
Modes of classification	1. Taxonomic 2. Structural	1. Minimally taxonomic 2. Nonstructural
Diagnostic criteria	1. Physical symptoms 2. Standardized	1. Physical and mental symptoms plus causes 2. Not standardized
Causes (pathogens and etiologies)	1. Not important	1. Very important
Treatment	1. Materia medica 2. Standardized	1. Shamanistic healing rite; some use of materia medica 2. Individually determined
Degree of severity	1. Minor	1. Serious

more specific levels. Furthermore, whereas habitual illnesses are classified structurally, in the sense that a headache is defined in reference to other subcategories of headaches, definitions of metaphysical illnesses are not related to other metaphysical illnesses. In other words, different modes of classification may be involved within a narrowly defined domain of illness – a point I discuss further in the next section.

The differences in the conceptualization of metaphysical illnesses in contrast to habitual illnesses are not confined to the mode of classification; they are found in the diagnostic criteria as well. As shown in Table 9.1, whereas symptoms determine both identification and treatment in the case of a habitual illness, symptoms alone are rarely sufficient in identifying metaphysical illness. Even in the case of a metaphysical illness such as the arrow intrusion illness (*aymawko ahun*), which physical symptoms alone suffice to identify, the Ainu would not consider the identification complete until a shaman diagnoses a specific etiology. In other cases, the same biophysical symptoms may be interpreted as one type of illness or another, depending on the cause. In short, the diagnosis of habitual illnesses is standardized; and anyone can diagnose these illnesses, at least in theory. In contrast, a metaphysical illness must be determined each time by a shaman. This means that the Ainu place enormous trust in the judgment of shamans. Further, there is more room for variation in the diagnosis of metaphysical illnesses, as discussed further in Chapter 11.

It is significant to note here that although the notion of causation is vital in determining whether a cut is an illness or not, and also in identifying metaphysical illnesses, for habitual illnesses the Ainu are not at all concerned with causes (Table 9.1). When I first asked the cause of habitual illnesses, beings and objects in the analogy were pointed out. But further probing revealed that the notion of causality was not at all involved. Indeed, even the notion of what Jung (1971:505-18) calls *synchronicity* or "the occurrence of meaningful coincidences" does not seem to be involved. Nor does *inductivity*, which Porkert (1974) proposes as the principle characterizing Chinese science and as the complement to the notion of causality, seem to explain the situation. It appears that for these illnesses the Ainu simply do not seek pathogens and etiologies.

The mode of treatment between the two groups of illnesses shows a similar contrast (Table 9.1). The treatment of habitual illnesses is standardized, and materia medica alone usually suffice. Briefly stated, a set of symptoms is interpreted as analogous to a certain object or animal through a metaphorical association. The metaphor then provides a basis whereby a part of the object or being is used for treatment, the healing power deriving from a metonymic relation between the object/animal and its portion used for cure. (For the use of the terms *metaphor* and *metonym*, see Jakobson and Halle 1956; Leach 1976:15-16, 25-7; Lévi-Strauss 1966: e.g., 204-8; Turner 1975:151 criticizes the use of these terms by "current structuralists.")

The treatment for metaphysical illnesses involves a radically different procedure. Each case must be determined by a shaman, and depending upon the cause, the treatment differs from case to case even for the same illness. Although materia medica is often used in the treatment of a metaphysical illness, the shamanistic rituals are emphasized. Sometimes only an apology and offerings to an angered deity may be needed for healing. The nature of the treatment stems primarily from the prescribed cause of the illness, which is not automatically related to the symptoms. In the case of the arrow intrusion illness, a similar metaphoric and metonymic process seems to be involved in the choice of treatment – ground powder of an arrow. However, the perception of the cause of this illness – harsh words transformed into an arrow – is basic to the choice of an arrow in the treatment, rather than the symptom of an acute pain that simulates the feeling of an arrow being shot into the body.

For both habitual and metaphysical illnesses, there is a close relationship between diagnosis and treatment. In the case of a habitual illness, a set of symptoms indicates both the identity and treatment of the illness. For example, the nature of a pain indicates that it is, say, a bear headache, so the ground powder of a bear's skull must be used for its treatment. In the case of a metaphysical illness, when its pathogen or etiology is found, both its identity and treatment are determined. A close relation between diagnosis and treatment seems to be characteristic of medical systems in general, as Kleinman (1974:208) notes: "healing is not the outcome of diagnostic acts, but the healing function is active from the outset in the way illness is perceived and the experience of illness organized."

Degrees of subclassification

We have seen that there is a wide range in the classification of illnesses; some are tightly defined and others only loosely. Why are some illnesses, such as headaches and boils, not only meticulously defined but also finely subclassified? As an explanation of the case of the Subanun, Frake (1961:121) proposes that "the greater the number of distinct social contexts in which information about a particular phenomenon must be communicated, the greater the number of different levels of contrasts into which that phenomenon is categorized."

Skin abnormalities, upon which this conclusion is based, are much talked about among the Subanun, because in their climate they are not only common but also can constitute serious threats to health. Similarly, in the case of the Ainu, the frequency of occurrence may sometimes be responsible for an elaborate classification of certain illnesses. This would perhaps apply to headaches, which may occur alone or accompany other illnesses as one of the symptoms. However, it does not explain the meticulous classification of boils, for in the cold climate of the Ainu skin infections are fairly uncommon, at least among the Hokkaido Ainu.[1]

In the case of headaches, one may postulate that the Ainu emphasis upon the head as a body part calls for meticulous classification. The Ainu divide the body into upper and lower halves, with the lower end of the rib bone as the dividing line. The upper half is symbolic of the sacred and the lower half of the mundane, and the head symbolizes the upper half. However, my data indicate that not all the illnesses of the upper body parts are meticulously classified. Conversely, the illnesses of the stomach, belonging to the lower half, are well classified. Therefore, the correlation between the symbolic significance of a body part and the degree of classification of its illnesses seems weak.

Nor is the seriousness of an illness related to the complexity of its subclassification or the degree of its elaboration. In fact, there is almost a negative correlation between the two. The more serious the illness, in terms of either the gravity of its symptoms or the cultural significance of its etiological or pathogenic factor, the less articulated it is. Thus, the two most serious habitual Ainu illnesses, *hana* and *kemasinke*, are vaguely defined with numerous symptoms, only some of which indicate the occurrence of these illnesses at a given time. In contrast, relatively minor headaches, boils, stomachaches, and other habitual illnesses are highly articulated and meticulously subclassified.

Modes of perception

In addition to the degree of classification of an illness, different modes of perception may be involved in Ainu distinctions between habitual illnesses, classified taxonomically and structurally, and metaphysical illnesses, broadly defined only at the most general level. In this section, I present Ainu modes of illness perception in the broad framework of human perception and the role of cultural patterning. My interpretation is outlined in Figure 9.1.

My discussion starts with binary opposition, which seems to be the most pervasive classificatory principle of the Ainu. As noted earlier, binary opposition is the classificatory principle of habitual illnesses, such as headaches and boils, and also of metaphysical illnesses at the most general level; it is also used in other important domains, such as time, space, and beings. Let me now further explain how I understand this principle to operate in Ainu symbolic classification.

Although my adoption of the sacred and profane may have suggested the resemblance between Ainu dualism and classical Durkheimian dualism, the two are fundamentally different in that Ainu opposition is a classificatory principle. Significantly, the image of a domain governed by a classificatory principle such as binary opposition is not of a box with clearly defined boundaries. The resulting classification is not a domain completely sectioned, with pigeonholes in each section. As Needham (1973:117) states, binary opposition is "a mode of categorization which orders the scheme, not from the possession of a specific property by means of which the character or presence of other terms may be deduced." Unlike the Durkheimian concept of sacred and profane, Ainu opposition is complementary, not a dualism of mutually antagonistic forces (cf. Freedman 1969:7). Consider, for example, Ainu classification of the beings of the universe. When the context requires that human males be placed together with human females, and humans as a group be contrasted to the deities, human males assume a profane symbolic value as opposed to the deities, whose symbolic value is sacred. On the other hand, when human males are contrasted to human females in another context, the former is assigned sacred value and the latter profane value. By the same token, male deities assume sacred value and female deities profane value if the two groups of deities are contrasted. The context determines the nature of the opposition or contrast and assigns symbolic meaning to its parts. Therefore, a given classificatory structure that is governed by binary opposition, such as Ainu time, space, beings, and illnesses, can have many levels of classification in which equivocal symbols appear and reappear, governed by the univocality of each symbol on

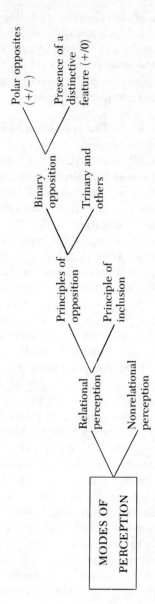

Figure 9.1. Modes of perception.

each level of contrast. (Cf. an eloquent explanation of the nature of binary opposition in Turner 1969:1–43.) This operation assigns both complexity and simplicity to the resultant symbolic structure.

Of the binary oppositions in Ainu symbolic classification, a predominant type is the opposition characterized by a distinctive feature, such as the sacred (superhuman) quality or the chill factor in habitual illnesses. Binary opposition characterized by polar opposites, that is, the contrast between (+) and (−), is not frequently used.

The findings so far suggest that binary opposition is persistent and pervasive in the Ainu classificatory system, as in the systems of many other populations. However, it does not preclude the possibility that some domains in Ainu culture hitherto unexamined may be classified by three, four, and so on. Durkheim and Mauss (1963, originally published 1901–2) assumed only one mode of classification to be present in a given culture. When more than one classification was present, they attributed this to the result of different modes of classification in an evolutionary progression. As Needham (1963:xviii–xix) aptly states, there is no need to assume that only one classificatory system exists in a given culture.

Leach (1967a:xiii) echoes Needham from a slightly different angle:

Not only does the human brain combine attributes of digital and analogue computers but the discriminating principles are multidimensional on a grand scale. Where an electronic computer has just two connections, one positive and one negative, to make a binary flip-flop, the human mechanism seems to be wired up with enormous varieties of redundancy, one hundred or more connections at a time. The messages that emerge from such an apparatus are hardly likely to be amenable to *simple* logical analysis.

Leach, like many others, believes that binary opposition underlies some mental processes, but that it is not the only mode of classification. Careful analysis is needed here, however, because, as the seminal work by Ortiz (1969) has successfully demonstrated, an apparent triad may be a variant expression of a basic dyad.

It is somewhat unfortunate that binary opposition has become, at least to some, synonymous with Lévi-Strauss, because its theoretical import has been diminished by other objections of scholars to this anthropologist. Many do not object to the proposition that binary opposition is a classificatory principle in some areas of a culture, but they doubt that it is the only classificatory mode of the human mind, or *esprit humain*. In an excellent summary of the field of symbolic anthropology, the first such treatise, Needham (1979) presents various forms of symbolic classification found the world over. They include the division into two, three, four, five, seven, and nine.

In short, we have sufficient evidence to assume that there are a restricted number of classificatory forms in human cultures, and that even within a single culture more than one structure exists.

Although binary opposition may operate in a taxonomic classification (a special type of classification that uses the principle of inclusion), it need not. In the case of Ainu metaphysical illnesses, binary opposition operates at the most general level, but these illnesses are not classified further to constitute a taxonomic classification. In some other domains of Ainu culture, such as time and space, binary opposition of the sacred and the profane governs the entire domain, with a resultant taxonomic structure of more than one level. In the case of headaches and boils, we have a slightly different situation; whereas taxonomic classification governs each domain (here, headaches or boils), the principle of classification used at each level is not the same. Thus, in the case of headaches, spatial division of the head classifies them at the most general level, but at the next level the division is based upon the spatial division of the universe into land and water. It is aesthetically more appealing to postulate that the /sacred:profane/ dyad underlies both the division of the head into the main part and the periphery and the division of the universe into land and water. Ethnographic data indicate that land is more sacred than water (Ohnuki-Tierney 1972), but such a distinction is not as evident in the division of the head. Therefore, the transformation of these dyads into that of the /sacred:profane/ is somewhat tenuous.

The prevalence of taxonomic structures in Ainu classificatory schema challenges Needham's claim (1979:67) that "one of the most interesting features of symbolic classification... is that characteristically it is not hierarchical." My feeling here is that if scholars in symbolic classification had focused upon a specific domain of culture, they might have found a greater prevalence of taxonomic classification. Somehow, the use of domain as the focus of analysis characterizes the approach in ethnoscience but not symbolic classification (cf. Chapter 10). We should remember that Durkheim and Mauss, the founders of symbolic classification, did insist that "primitive classifications" are "systems of hierarchized notions" (Durkheim and Mauss 1963:81).

The predominant mode of Ainu classification presented in this book is monothetic classification, in which a class is defined by the possession of at least one feature by all its members (cf. Needham 1975; 1979). The next question is: Is there any other type of Ainu perception, or human perception in general? Some anthropologists who are seeking alternative modes of human thought seem to find convincing the formulation presented by the late Vygotsky, who was recently "rediscovered." In the development of children's thought and speech, he (1970) discerns three types of thinking: congeries, complexes, and concepts. Congeries represent the child's first step toward concept formation and are a "heap" which consists of "disparate objects grouped together without any basis" (Vygotsky 1970:59). In complex thinking, individual objects are united both by the child's "subjective impressions" and by "concrete and factual" bonds existing between the objects. These bonds, of which Vygotsky discerns five subtypes, can be similarities, contrasts, or any other "perceptually compelling ties" between things (Vygotsky 1970:61-9). Although complex thinking is characterized by "the unification of scattered impressions," the concept presupposes more than unification. It assumes the ability "*to abstract, to single out* elements," which in turn must be viewed "apart from the totality of the concrete experience in which they are embedded" (1970:76; italics in the original). This combined ability of synthesis and analysis is absent in complex thinking, which instead is characterized by "overabundance, overproduction of connections, and weakness in abstraction" (1970:76). I believe that both Vygotsky's complex and concept thinking involve structural analyses in the sense that an object within a category is perceived in relation to others in the same category. Thinking in concept, however, involves a higher degree of analysis and synthesis – a type of thinking akin to the one involved in distinctive feature analysis. In apposition to the interpretation of totemism by Lévi-Strauss, Worsley (1967) proposes that the totemic distribution of the Groode Eylandt is founded either upon "congeries thinking" or "complex thinking" and not upon thinking in "concepts." Also under the influence of Vygotsky as well as Wittgenstein, Needham emphasizes polythetic classification, in which the members of a class do not share any one common feature but are grouped together by "having each a preponderance of the defining features" (1975; 1979:65).

Keesing is critical of the structural/relational mode of perception and classification itself. He thus criticizes the distinctive feature approach, which "classes things by what they are not, paying most attention to semantic *boundaries*. Yet increasing evidence suggests that we class things by what they are, not simply by the outer boundaries of categories," (1976:155). Later Keesing (1976:155) provides an example of how a witness sees the face and appearance of a bank robber as total patterns of features, whereas the police artist, like the anthropologist, demands that the witness pick out separate features, such as the nose and eyebrows, one after another. It seems to me that the witness's perception of the robber is not a satisfactory example of a human perception in terms of distinctive feature analysis. Distinctive feature analysis does not simply consist of perception in terms of component features; it entails a much higher degree of analysis and synthesis, as I described earlier using the example of the consonant system of American English. Furthermore, there is a possibility that even though the witness perceives the totality of the robber's face and appearance in one sense, this perception may also involve some comparison of the robber with other people whom the witness has encountered.

Nevertheless, the major point of these criticisms of binary opposition, or a structural approach in general, should be given serious consideration; it is likely that a nonstructural mode of perception is present in any culture. In the case of the Ainu, we have seen that binary opposition and taxonomic systems are seen in many domains or subdomains. On the other hand, we have also seen that metaphysical illnesses are classified only at the most general level. It is these metaphysical illnesses that require further deliberation from the point of view of classification and perception in general. The looseness with which the metaphysical ill- nesses are defined and classified challenges us to seek explanations, espe- cially because metaphysical illnesses as a group are more serious than habitual illnesses. Why then is there so much room for variation in the diagnosis, determined primarily by the shaman?

Let me first place this phenomenon of vagueness within a broader framework – a general tendency, as I see it, that the more loaded the intellectual and psychological content of a particular cultural phenome- non, the less articulated are the concepts involved. In Ainu religion, the power of the supreme deity, the bear, is defined only broadly; the bear protects the Ainu and provides them with general welfare. In contrast, the power of lesser deities, such as the fox or owl, is more articulated; the fox is the arbitrator and messenger among the deities, and the owl has the capacity to foretell future events. This tendency does not seem to be confined to Ainu culture. For example, in Christianity, God is almighty but his capacity is rarely spelled out, whereas each saint has a specified capacity, such as the protection of children by Saint Nicholas.

I think that the more complex or loaded concepts are, the less articu- lated they are because they involve more individual beliefs, which are different from collective representations. Therefore, they are often not amenable to an approach such as a distinctive feature analysis – a topic I discuss further in Chapter 10.

So far, my discussion has dealt with only some of the neatly classified and tightly defined habitual illnesses and broadly defined metaphysical illnesses. However, there are many illnesses that lie between these two in terms of classification and definition. Thus there are many ill- nesses, especially habitual illnesses that are not as meticulously defined and classified as boils and headaches but are better articulated than the metaphysical illnesses. They are the illnesses of the mouth, the stomach, and others that are presented in detail in Appendix A. Within the domain of illness, then, we have an entire range in terms of classification and definition.

Emotive and sensory patterns of perception

So far, our discussion has focused upon cognitive dimensions of the Ainu perception of illness. An increasing trend in anthropology is to include the emotive dimension of human behavior in the analysis. This is in part a reaction to ethnosemantics, with its emphasis on cognition, and also to such scholars as Durkheim, Mauss, and Lévi-Strauss, who did not really treat the emotive dimension of human perception, as discussed in Chapter 1. This emphasis on emotion, however, differs significantly from the earlier culture and personality approaches. These scholars are pointing to the importance of the emotive dimension of behavior or symbol perception, which also has a cognitive dimension, whereas only the latter has received much attention. Complementarity of the ethos and the world view of Geertz, discussed in Chapter 1, is a case in point. The emphasis on the fusion of the two dimensions of our behavior is also expressed in Turner's concept (1967) of evocative symbols and his acknowledgment of the emotional resonance of symbols.

For the study of the emotive dimension of human behavior, the domain of illness is most appropriate, because danger to health is perceived universally with strong emotions. People are often sad, angry, and fearful of illnesses, and by the same token, they rejoice with the recovery of health. These emotions are often reflected in the healing rituals of many peoples. Furthermore, emotions appear frequently in the illness pathogens and etiologies in many medical systems of the world. We saw in Ainu medicine that the anger of a deity or angry human words can constitute illness pathogens. Strong emotions are defined as illness pathogens in many medical systems, and one might almost speculate that these medical systems had linked the emotional state of the individual to ulcers and various other illnesses before biomedicine came to the same conclusion. This recognition is found not only in various humoral medicines but also in, for example, Mandari medicine, in which the illnesses and deaths caused by negative emotions expressed in quarrels and spiteful talks are defined as "verbal killing" (Buxton 1973:Ch.8). Such emotions as sadness and excessive crying or quarrelsomeness and hostility as symptomatic criteria of illness definitions are pointed out in Fabrega's insightful work (1970) on Zinacanteco concepts of illness. Even in Western medicine, doctors are now increasingly aware of the importance of the psychological dimension of illness.

Despite these perceptive findings and statements by anthropologists on the importance of emotion in symbols and human behavior in general, we have just begun to realize its importance; even such forerunners as Geertz and Turner have not yet provided us with sufficient methodological and theoretical directions. My data on Ainu perception and symbols are also weak on this point.

Of the three dimensions of human perception, the sensory dimension has received the least attention by anthropologists. Such scholars as Hall (1969), McLuhan (1964), and Segall, Campbell, and Herskovits (1966) have demonstrated that culture plays an important role in patterning the use of the senses. In symbolic analysis, Lévi-Strauss (1969b) discusses the "Fugue of the Five Senses" and introduces the opposition of noise and silence in his discussion of nature and culture. As noted in Chapter 8, he also points to the importance of vaginal odor, which symbolizes nature for the Brazilian Indians. Both Beidelman (1964, 1966) and Turner in his publications on Ndembu rituals (see, e.g., 1967:343–9) have made a unique contribution in this area by interpreting the references that symbols make to "basic physiological processes . . . which in turn are associated with the most basic *feelings* of physical security and gratification" (Beidelman 1964:386; italics mine). In general, however, anthropological treatment of symbols has not dealt with the sensory dimension in any systematic way. This may reflect our unconscious desire to distinguish "cultured" humans from animals, for which the biological senses are of primary importance in perceiving the environment.

In the case of the Ainu, to refresh our memory, the descriptions of minor ailments reveal that the Ainu not only see their universe but also feel, smell, touch, and hear it, and use different sense organs in perceiving the beings in its different spatial categories. Thus headaches with land animal labels (e.g., bear headaches) are characterized by the lack of a chill and by the nature of auditorily perceived pain; a bear headache aches like a bear's heavy footsteps. In contrast, sea animal headaches, which alone are accompanied by a chill, are perceived through the tactile sense; the pain of an octopus headache, for example, simulates the sucking of an octopus. Even when vision alone is used, beings are often perceived in motion – the walking bear, the galloping musk deer, the tree-pecking woodpecker, and so on. Likewise, it is not the wooden piece in the sled called *takapes* but its "painful" turning when the dogs pull the rope that provides the analogy for pain in the sides of the lower abdomen. Multisensory perception is also important in the Ainu notions of metaphysical illnesses. Not only is it involved in the causes of illness (for example, the auditory effect of words), it is also evident in the cures. The materia medica are full of smell, touch, and sound. A notable example is the beating of the drum, the most important ingredient in the Ainu shamanistic curing rite.

The multisensory perception of one's behavioral environment is not unique to the Ainu; it has often been shown to characterize the perception of peoples in many non-Western and nonindustrialized societies (e.g.,

Hall 1969:esp. 80–90). In particular, an emphasis on auditory rather than visual perception has drawn much attention from scholars. McLuhan emphasizes "phonetic literacy" [*sic*] as the causal factor in primarily visual perception; he claims that "primitive man" is "dominated by spoken words and by auditory media" (1964:esp. 144). A similar view is also found in Ong (1969). Recent works on the relation of the absence of writing to modes of thought (Colby and Cole 1973; Finnegan 1973) suggest that a systematic study of the importance of the auditory perception of nonliterate populations is in order. It should be noted, however, that English speakers, with what McLuhan calls a "phonetic alphabet" and a quantitative perception of time, experience the "pounding" of the head and "throbbing" pains, too. The Japanese, using nonalphabetical writing, have an extraordinary number of onomatopoetic analogies of pain and other bodily discomforts. Tsunoda (1971, 1974) proposes in his innovative studies that the unusual sensitivity of the Japanese auditory receptor be attributed to the effect of the Japanese vowel sounds upon cerebral dominance.

A study of the differential use of senses among populations is particularly important in ethnomedicine because not only is humoral medicine widespread in both the New and Old Worlds but basically most medical systems have a strong humoral element. Thus illnesses are often heard, smelled, and felt, in addition to being seen, even among populations with a well-developed biomedical tradition. We do not "feel" good, and you do not "sound" good.

Summary

The Ainu data suggest two tentative conclusions about the presence of structure(s), which was questioned at the beginning of this chapter. First, observable phenomena such as symptoms are not necessarily the key to identifying an illness, because a pathogen or an etiology can classify a cut, for example, as an illness or not. Second, there may be more than one mode of classification within a given culture; for example, there are at least two in the Ainu medical system. Habitual illnesses are generally neatly classified into taxonomic systems, whereas metaphysical illnesses are loosely defined and only basically related to each other. In addition, there are a number of illnesses that lie between the two extremes. If we can get away from the notion that structure or classification implies a box with grids, and recognize that the presence of a structure indicates an ordering by the principles of classification, then we may be more willing to recognize the presence of a structure or structures in a given culture. On the other hand, there are areas of culture that are less meticulously or only vaguely classified. It seems best to view a culture, or at least Ainu culture, as a generally but not exhaustively classified system governed by more than one principle of classification.

There is an urgent need for anthropologists to discover theoretical and methodological tools with which to examine the emotive and sensory dimensions of human perception, in addition to the cognitive dimension. These two dimensions are just as important in our perception of the universe, if not more so.

10

Language and cognition: theoretical and methodological problems in arriving at perceptual categories

In the preceding chapters, I followed the general procedure of ethnosemantics without strictly using monolexemes. I also used the Whorfian hypothesis. In addition, I followed the usual practice in symbolic classification using general ethnographic methods. In short, in attempting to arrive at the perceptual structures of the Ainu, I combined these radically different approaches without explicitly stating my theoretical and methodological reasons for their use. In this chapter, I briefly explain my approaches by comparing the theoretical bases of ethnosemantics and the Whorfian hypothesis (two approaches in anthropology that attempt to arrive at cognitive structures through language), along with a symbolic classification using general ethnographic information. My comparison focuses upon the problem of what constitutes evidence for the presence of a conceptual form – a core problem in the relationship between language and cognition.

After briefly summarizing some of the major premises of ethnosemantics, I discuss the problem of covert taxonomies – conceptual forms without lexical representation. In order to consider language and cognition further, I next examine the problem of how the same set of lexemes yields more than one classificatory system. A brief discussion of the Sapir–Whorf hypothesis is followed by a consideration of what so-called conceptual forms represent; here I stress the need for a clear distinction between individual beliefs and culturally construed concepts. The distinction also allows us to understand that some concepts have more tangible evidence for their presence.

Ethnosemantics

Curiously ethnosemantics has seldom been compared with symbolic classification, which has a long tradition in anthropology, in spite of the fact that the two approaches show striking similarities and basic differences. Most importantly, they both deal with folk classification. Both are concerned not simply with pigeonholing categories but also with discovering classificatory principles that produce a given categorical system.

On the other hand, there are two major differences. First, scholars in ethnosemantics start their analysis by codifying a domain and trying to see how it is categorized by finding classificatory principles. Scholars in symbolic classification focus upon finding principles that govern various aspects of a culture. The second major difference lies in the premise of ethnosemantics that lexical labels are both methodologically and theoretically important. On the other hand, scholars interested in symbolic classification (e.g., Beidelman, Douglas, Durkheim, Leach, Lévi-Strauss, Mauss, and Needham, to name only a few) do not believe that there must be a particular type of tangible evidence for the presence of a concept – a stance that invites critics to accuse them of not having a rigorous methodology.

In this chapter, I focus on the implications of the second difference between the two approaches by examining some of the premises of ethnosemantics. Frake (1971:74) states the objective of ethnosemantics as "the formulation of an operationally explicit methodology for discerning how people construe their world of experience from the way they talk about it." He further explains the major assumption of ethnosemantics – its focus upon the analysis of lexemes (1971:75):

The analysis of a culture's terminological systems will not, of course, exhaustively reveal the cognitive world of its members, but it will certainly tap a central portion of it. Culturally significant cognitive features must be communicable between persons in one of the standard symbolic systems of the culture. A major share of these features will undoubtedly be codable in a society's most flexible and productive communication device, its language. Evidence also seems to indicate that those cognitive features requiring most frequent communication will tend to have standard and relatively short linguistic labels.

For the purposes at hand, three major issues may be discussed here. How do we determine that a feature is "culturally significant"? Are all culturally significant features expressed linguistically? If so, in which linguistic structure(s) can we expect to find them?

The question of what constitutes culturally significant features includes some preliminary issues. For example, what is the relative significance of concepts underlying the so-called infrastructures and those expressed through suprastructures? Should significance be judged from the point of view of the people concerned or according to the so-called culture-free scales applied by outside analysts? Consider, for example, plant food with low cultural value but high nutritious value or quantitative significance (see Flannery [1968] for various types of food value). Which do we consider to be culturally significant, economic value (etic evaluation) or symbolic (emic) evaluation? An even more complex problem is, what constitutes cognitive features? Do they refer to the concept of "God" with its culturally prescribed definition as stated by the people? Or do they refer to the classificatory principle, such as the sacred and profane binary opposition that generates a category such as "gods"? This is the level of abstraction I addressed in Chapter 7 with Ainu material, and then in Chapter 8 with cross-cultural data. Cognitive features may even mean the mode of classification – binary versus trinary or taxonomic versus nontaxonomic. This is the level of abstraction discussed in Chapter 9. In short, there are at least three levels of abstraction to which the concept of cognitive features may refer.

Ethnosemanticists state explicitly that they elicit emic principles – principles unconsciously held by the people themselves. They may also compare emic classifications from a number of cultures according to the etic (culture) scale, as exemplified in the study of color classification by Berlin and Kay (1969).

Although the taxonomic principles and paradigms are considered by ethnosemanticists to be culturally significant, there are many other culturally significant principles that do not yield to ethnosemantic analysis. As we discussed in Chapter 9, there may be other modes of classification and perception.

The assumption of ethnosemantics that culturally significant features are expressed linguistically has ironically been contradicted by discoveries of the ethnosemanticists themselves, who found that some conceptual forms are not lexically expressed. As Goodenough (1956:209) noted, "there may be conceptual systems within a culture whose categories are not all represented by lexemes." His answer (1956:210) to the question of the incomplete paradigm is: "It is significant for the study of cultural forms that our analysis should enable us to get at concepts which are not lexically objectivized through those which are." Goodenough (1956:210) suggests that lexical expression of all the conceptual forms results in a superfluity of lexemes far beyond the need for communication among the people concerned. In his discussion of kinship studies (1956:210), he does not find the lack of lexical expression of some conceptual forms to be of major importance:

Why only certain conceptual variables are utilized, why only certain combinations of their values are symbolized in lexemes, are questions which have challenged many students of social organization, but they are not our concern here.

Although Goodenough dismisses the problem, Berlin (1976), Berlin, Breedlove, and Raven (1968, 1974), Keesing (1972), and many others have seriously tackled this problem of *unnamed classes, covert categories*, or *unlabeled taxa*, as this phenomenon is referred to by various terms. (For good bibliographical information on the works in which unlabeled taxa are discussed, see Berlin, Breedlove, and Raven 1968:297–8, note 3.)

A frequently reported finding is the absence of monolexemes for broader categories in non-Western languages. In one of the earliest and best studies in ethnosemantics, Conklin (1955) notes that there is no lexeme for the domain of color in Hanunoo. Likewise, the absence of a monolexeme for the domain of eating is reported by Landar (1964) and Berlin (1967). A major finding of Berlin, Breedlove, and Raven (1968, 1974) is the absence of labels for mid-level taxa in the Tzeltal plant classification. In Ainu, there are no lexemes for the domains of plants, animals, minerals, space, and time, although each constitutes a distinct and important domain. Yet there is little question for the Ainu whether a being in nature, as we would put it, belongs to the category of plants or animals, with the latter distinguished from the former by such features as mobility or possession of a soul. Furthermore, each of these domains is meticulously classified and taxa within them are all lexically expressed, not always with monolexemes, however. Even mid-level taxa are often lexically expressed. Thus, the Ainu talk about *mun* (useless grass), *kina* (useful grass), or *ni:* (trees and bushes). Or they engage in *kimun koyki* (mountain going = hunting) or *atuy koyki* (sea going = fishing) and talk about *kam* (meat), *čeh* (fish), or *čikah* (birds). Yet there is no term for animals or for plants as a whole. The domain of illness is somewhat different. As we discussed earlier, the term *araka* seems to be the lexeme for the entire domain of illness, although it can also mean simply pain. *Araka* is not always used as a collective noun; sometimes it is also used as a noun or a verb. It is also used in such expressions as "so-and-so became ill" or "a bad illness is going around."

The absence of lexemes for these higher-level taxa or for the domains themselves is related to the ethnographic finding that ethnoscience is applicable only to a fairly small number of domains in any culture, as Keesing (1972:307–8) summarizes:

The new ethnographers have been unable to move beyond the analysis of artificially simplified and delineated (and usually trivial) semantic domains, and this has discouraged many of the originally faithful. Ethnoscience has almost bored itself to death. This is one answer to the question, What ever happened to ethnoscience?

Nevertheless, ethnosemantic endeavors did make a significant contribution, in my view – the discovery that only some culturally significant features are amenable to lexical analysis. These include the classificatory principles involved in such domains as color, kinship, animals, plants, and a few others. As noted earlier, some categories of illness are also included. Although there is a problem in defining the criteria that determine what is culturally significant, in general, domains that are cognitively and emotively less loaded are more amenable to ethnosemantic treatment in most cultures. My finding that the less serious habitual Ainu illnesses yield to ethnosemantic analysis seems another example of the general feeling about the utility of ethnosemantics.

Both the weaknesses and strengths of ethnosemantics can be explained once we note that it deals with the initial stage of cultural identification of external things and phenomena. That is, whatever ethnosemanticists attempt to study, they must deal with concrete things and phenomena that have names. When we remember that the vast realm of symbolization with which anthropologists are concerned lies in a process beyond this initial stage of cultural identification, we see why and how ethnosemantics has a very restricted application. Ethnosemantics deals with a culturally defined lion in relation to other animals in the domain of animals. However, it cannot deal with a lion that has further symbolic meaning, such as the King of Beasts, because at this stage we encounter a second-order symbolization process. Thus, as noted earlier, ethnosemanticists can deal with the concrete, but the more complex and abstract cultural concepts elude them. This is where symbolic classification comes in, with more general ethnographic observations and statements as its data for interpretations. (For further discussion on this point, see Ohnuki-Tierney 1981.)

Another problem in the relationship between language and cognition highlighted in ethnosemantic studies is that one linguistic form may represent more than one conceptual form. This is the problem: The same terminological system has been shown to produce alternative semantic structures. As noted in Chapter 5, although I used the wet/dry opposition in interpreting the underlying perceptual structure of habitual illnesses, other classifications are possible, using the number of loci of pain involved or other features of pain. I suggest that the presence of alternative structures should not in itself discredit ethnosemantic findings. In fact, alternative structures reinforce the interpretation that a conceptual form consists of a bundle of distinctive features, each feature being chosen for articulation in different contexts. In the case of Ainu illnesses, in some situations the presence of a chill is of primary importance in identifying an illness as a water animal headache as opposed to a land animal headache. In other situations, the headache is contrasted to other water animal headaches rather than land animal headaches; hence the multiple loci of pain receive attention. Using as an example the exchange of money in the United States, Conklin (1971:88-91) not only illuminates the distinction between the analysis of semantic structure and the presentation of an arbitrary arrangement but also notes that features such as color or engraved human figures have cognitive significance in the identification of coins and bills, although these features are not involved in their classification.

In short, it seems that some cognitive features are expressed as the principles of a classificatory structure and others as those of an alternative structure. Still others are not expressed in either form but are recognized, implicitly or explicitly, by the people.

Besides lexical structures, there are other structures of human communication that express conceptual forms. Possibilities exist in other linguistic structures, structures of nonverbal communication, or structures of other symbolic expressions. In verbal communication, for example, some concepts may be simply communicated in phrases and sentences. Besides this possibility, two nonlexical linguistic structures have received serious attention by scholars interested in the relation of language to cognition; they are the grammatical structures suggested by Whorf and Sapir, and the "deep structure" or generative semantics of Chomsky and post-Chomskian linguist–semanticists. My discussion here concentrates on the Whorfian hypothesis, because the findings of generative semantics do not seem to relate to a treatment of a particular culture and its cognitive structure at this point.

Sapir–Whorf hypothesis

The so-called Sapir–Whorf hypothesis had a relatively short life in American anthropology. It not only sees correlations between the structures of the world view of a people and the grammatical categories of their language but it also claims that the latter determine the former. According to Sapir (1964:128), language "actually defines experience for us," and he points to the "tyrannical hold that linguistic form has upon our orientation in the world." Similarly, Whorf (1952:5) explains language, especially grammatical categories, as "the shaper of ideas." The ill fate of this hypothesis, which Keesing (1976:161) calls "exciting partial truths," is largely due to what is regarded as lack of proof: "Does Whorf mean that it is the grammatical framework that structures thought? How can you find out because both are in the realm of ideas which is by definition unobservable?" (Keesing 1976:160).

Keesing's criticism of the Whorfian hypothesis, based on the unobservable nature of grammatical structures and conceptual form, brings us back to the starting point of this chapter – the difference between ethnosemantics and symbolic classification, both of which seek folk classification. In my interpretation, ethnosemanticists set out to objectify unobservable conceptual forms in the lexical structures. When they fail to do so in certain areas, some at least concede that conceptual forms are not always lexically expressed, although their presence is clearly discernible. The realization by ethnosemanticists that lexemes are not absolute proof of the presence of conceptual forms is also seen in their reliance upon other ethnographic information gathered through ordinary ethnographic methods for determining which of the alternative semantic structures should be chosen as the dominant one.

In contrast to scholars in ethnosemantics, scholars in symbolic classification have always sought evidence for the presence of conceptual forms in richly contextual ethnographic data based upon informants' statements and/or observations of their behavior. It is therefore not just coincidence, but a reflection of similar intellectual backgrounds, when Needham (1972:128-9), a major figure in symbolic classification, points out:

According to Whorf, the most impressively penetrating logical discriminations in some African and North American languages are often those that are revealed by analysing to the covert or cryptotypic level; and such "covert categories," more-over, are "quite apt to be more rational than overt ones" . . . If the concept can exist as a covert category, then the absence of an overt denotation in the form of a separate word is not evidence that the concept itself is lacking.

In this context, it is meaningful to note that Kuhn (1962), who calls attention to the culturally patterned nature, as it were, of science and who allows a significant place in science to "tacit knowledge" and "intuition" (1962:191-8), notes his encounter with Whorf's work (1962:vi).

As for the Ainu, intriguing concordances between the grammatical structures of the verbs, and the classification of habitual illnesses (Chapter 5) and time classification (Ohnuki-Tierney 1969b, 1973c), seems convincing enough for me not to discard the Whorfian hypothesis. I refrain, however, from claiming that the grammatical structure of a language is the determinant of thought processes. Furthermore, because the unit of analysis of the Whorfian hypothesis is the grammatical categories, and these categories are limited in number in any language, the hypothesis, like ethnosemantics, has a very limited applicability.

Meaning of conceptual forms

An important clarification remains: What is meant by conceptual forms and, in particular, conceptual forms expressed through structural features of linguistic forms? Put simply, I think they represent culturally meaningful features of concepts that are minimal requirements for fascinating communication among members of a society. Most importantly, they are not the same as an individual's belief or total thinking.

Major credit in clarifying this idea must go to Wittgenstein (1968), whose work has been most influential in contemporary anthropology. He emphasizes that words are not a "description of a mental state" but merely a "signal" (1968:73). Needham (1972), who is intellectually indebted to Wittgenstein, explains the issue as an anthropological problem: "There is no point, that is, in speaking of collective representations, or dogma which are true of a culture as a whole, as 'beliefs' if it is not implied that the individual human beings who compose the social aggregate in question actually and severally believe them" (1972:6). A belief is "an inner state which can pertain only to individual men" (Needham 1972:6). It should be clearly separated from conceptual forms, expressed in words or without words, which are cultural constructs utilized by the members of a society for their communication.

In a sympathetic and constructive criticism of Lévi-Strauss, Yalman (1967) also cautions against taking conceptual categories derived from myths as individual thought:

On the philosophical side an important objection remains: myths, like poetry, conform to standardized local conventions. They are not simply equivalent to "thought". . . Can these myths be seriously treated as an accurate reflection of the reasoning of these tribesmen? (Yalman 1967:83–4)

But what does this analysis show about the thinking processes of the tribes in question? What indeed is the relationship between the relatively formal myths and the rest of the mental activity of the tribes? Can the myths be taken as an accurate reflection of their thought even in religious matters? And, finally, what is the relationship of the many formal patterns indicated by the analyst to the expressed customary attitudes of the people? Are some conscious and the others unconscious? (Yalman 1967:86)

The last portion of Yalman's statement leads us to another important point. Just as the structural features of the world view or cognition of a people remain unconscious, so do the structural features of the grammar and lexical system of their language that show concordance with the structure of their world view.

In short, rather than claiming that we can tap the central portion of the speakers' cognitive world (Frake 1971:75), a more humble proposition would be that anthropologists, through either a standard ethnographic technique or any form of linguistic analysis, can get at the features that are minimal requirements for communication within the society. Most ordinary communication does not involve a speaker's thoughts and feelings, and the real cognitive world or the inner experience of the speaker is often veiled. What anthropologists have been able to arrive at as a cognitive structure or thought process may simply be the skeleton hidden under the flesh. Despite its limitations, however, the discovery is meaningful because this skeleton is necessary for culturally meaningful communication among the members of the society.

I think that this distinction between individual beliefs and culturally shared conceptual forms is a major key to understanding the relationship between language and cognition, or more broadly, conceptual forms and concrete evidence of their presence. It enables us to understand why some conceptual forms are better articulated than others – the point raised in Chapter 9. As noted earlier, minor illnesses of the Ainu are better defined and more articulated than the more serious illnesses. The conceptual difference between the two types of illness is an example of a common phenomenon – the more loaded the concept, the less articulated it is. Thus God is only vaguely defined, whereas the saints are better delineated. This phenomenon becomes intelligible when we consider that the more serious or more loaded concepts are those in which there is room for individual beliefs. For these concepts, the collective representation stays at the bare minimum, and the members of a culture communicate with one another about these concepts while also entertaining their own beliefs.

The same logic enables us to understand why ethnoscience has been applicable to relatively insignificant domains of culture, and why we must rely upon the traditional ethnographic method to study more complex domains such as religion. Likewise, covert categories are found at higher or more generalized levels of classification.

Similarly, the distinction advances our understanding of the role of grammatical categories in the Whorfian hypothesis. According to Hoijer (1968:407), language is "a way of directing the perceptions of its speakers and it provides for them habitual modes of analyzing experience into significant categories." This role is played primarily by "the category of habitual, frequently used, and relatively simple structural-semantic devices" (Hoijer 1968:410). If we replace Hoijer's "habitual modes" of thinking or experience with collective representations, the role of grammatical categories becomes better elucidated. The grammatical categories both reflect and direct the collective representations of the Navaho and the Yana peoples, for example, about shape distinctions (cf. Sapir and Swadesh 1964:103–4); they neither reflect nor direct the beliefs of individual Navaho or Yana.

There may be a functional advantage in defining phenomena vaguely. When the intellectual and emotional content of a phenomenon is only dimly perceived, there is the advantage that it can be embraced by more people with diverse backgrounds than when its components are spelled out. My interpretation here is somewhat similar to what Turner proposes as the characteristic of the dominant multivocal symbols. These symbols, according to Turner (1975:155), enable a wide range of groups and individuals to relate to the same signifier-vehicle in a variety of ways because these dominant symbols are simple at the level of *signans* (the signifier or a word), complex at the level of *signata* (the signified), and various in the modes of *signification* (the relationship between the signifier and the signified).

Summary

This brief discussion of some of the assumptions and findings of ethnosemantics and the Whorfian hypothesis indicates that only some of the conceptual forms are represented in linguistic structures, and that no particular linguistic structure – be it lexical, grammatical, or syntactic – may have an exclusive claim for their representation. Thus, a particular set of cognitive features may be expressed lexically, another set through grammatical structure, and yet another syntactically. For that matter, certain features may be expressed nonverbally. We cannot afford to throw away the baby with the bathwater just because a particular method falls short of producing God's truth. These investigations of perceptual structures through linguistic structures should be used when possible, as long as we clearly evaluate their merits and limitations. We should, however, also note that every conceptual form does not have a particular expression or concrete or observable evidence; for the study of those more abstract conceptual forms, a general ethnographic method is the only form of investigation. In the case of the Ainu, there is at least partial concordance between the principles governing the lexical structures of some illnesses, those governing the grammatical structures of the verb, and those of symbolic structures of space and time identified through symbolic classification.

The perceptual structures of a people that anthropologists decipher through these studies should be clearly distinguished from the beliefs, inner thoughts, and experiences of individuals. In general, conceptual forms that do not involve the beliefs of an individual tend to be better articulated, either through linguistic structures or other more tangible expressions such as symptoms.

11
Illness, the individual, and society

Leaving the topic of the relationship of illness to perceptual structure and culture in general, this chapter explores the relationship of illness to Ainu society. As with many hunters and gatherers, there are no full-time specialists among the Ainu, whether political, religious, or medical. The mode of life in this small foraging society requires every adult Ainu to know the basics of diagnosis and cure at least of the habitual illnesses, for a hunter may become sick while alone in the mountains, or a woman may fall ill while gathering plants alone. Or a woman may have to give birth when others are not around. Yet, some individuals are well informed about the diagnosis and cure of illnesses, whereas others may possess only the minimal knowledge. On the whole, women tend to know more about the treatment of habitual illnesses than men, because the majority of items used as materia medica (see Table B.1), such as plants and shellfish, are gathered by women. Indeed, learning how to identify and gather not only edible but also medicinal plants, shellfish, and other items is crucial to becoming an adult woman in Ainu society. It should be emphasized here that a large portion of Ainu plants, of which Chiri (1953) recorded 472 kinds (see also Table B.1), are medicinal; the task of learning to identify these plants, let alone other medicines, is enormous, as I witnessed in the field. As noted earlier, in the case of metaphysical illnesses, which are usually more serious, the Ainu must resort to shamans, part-time medical specialists, who alone can diagnose and cure these illnesses.

The aim of this chapter is to examine the Ainu medical system and the role of shamans in relation to the individual concerned and to society at large. I begin by presenting ethnographic data on the social identity of Ainu shamans and the nature of their power. Next, the multiple roles of Ainu shamans are discussed in order to portray the complexity of the shaman's role. The next section deals with the shaman as the healer of social ills and as a covert politician – the shaman's most important role for the topic of this chapter. Next, I examine the nonformalized power a shaman can exercise and relate it to the marginal status of many shamans in society. A brief comparison is made with the shamans in Ainu societies in other times and places in order to seek further evidence that would link

161

the politically peripheral, especially women, with the shamanistic career. After presenting data to support the hypothesis that some Ainu shamans are victims of a psychobehavioral disorder called *imu*: in Ainu, I discuss the relationship of the shaman's personality to psychobehavioral disorders in a cross-cultural perspective. I explore possible causal factors for them and also the function of the shaman's role as a cultural mechanism that not only resolves frustrations but in fact endows the afflicted individuals with a special power. Unlike other chapters, this one includes information on shamanism and shamans from other Ainu societies, especially those on the east coast of Sakhalin. These comparative data help us to understand the shamanism of the northwest coast Sakhalin Ainu.

Shamans and their power: a description

Shamanistic practitioners, regardless of sex, are called *tusu aynu* (*tusu* = shamanistic rite; *aynu* = human being), *nupuru aynu*, or *nupuru kuru* (*nupuru* = holy; *kuru* = person). The term *nupuru*, as in the last two designations, refers to the properties of the Ainu deities, in particular to the power they enjoy over humans. These designations thus imply that shamans are thought to possess some superior power that ordinary Ainu lack. Pilsudski (1961:185) reports the same term, *nupuru*, in describing the abilities of shamans on the east coast.

Not just anyone can become a shaman, nor can one become a shaman simply by wanting to be one. Although most of the powerful shamans are older, many receive their "call" during their teens and start their careers quite early in life. Usually a person starts by experiencing a strong feeling over which he or she has no control. Most shamans have this experience during their early teens, around the time of puberty, although for some it may occur even earlier. Some years later, often at the time of some life crisis, they may perform their first shamanistic rite, often while unconscious, as the following examples indicate. It may take several years before they become full-fledged shamans who can perform rites upon request rather than only when seized by the uncontrollable desire to do so. Information from the Sakhalin Ainu on the east coast confirms this general picture. Thus in oral tradition from the east coast Sakhalin Ainu, a powerful female shaman is referred to as a deitylike "little" (= young) woman (Kindaichi 1914:103), and Pilsudski's observation (1961) confirms that a shaman's career may start at an early age.

My key informant, Husko, at about fifteen years of age started to feel every day at mid-afternoon a strong desire to sing out loud about anything that came into her mind. At the same time, it seemed to her that a strong wind was eddying around inside her body. Her elders told her that she was feeling the desire to perform shamanistic rites. Her first actual performance of a rite did not come, however, until she was thirty-eight years old, when her daughter drowned in a lake at Rayčiska. At the sight of her daughter's dead body caught in a fishnet, she fainted and was carried back to her home. Here she regained consciousness, but her body started to shake vigorously. Those present gave her the necessary equipment with which she performed her first rite. Not until her son died several years later, however, did she perform the rites regularly.

A woman in her late fifties, with whom I became well acquainted during my fieldwork in 1964 at the Wakasakunai settlement, also first started to engage in "religious performances," as she put it, when her daughter died. At the time of my encounter with her, she had been, at least officially, converted to the Nichiren sect of Japanese Buddhism and observed its rituals. However, her account of her performance of these rituals and my observations of her work strongly indicate a high degree of syncretism between this sect of Japanese Buddhism and Ainu shamanism. For example, as she beats her drum of the Nichiren sect, which resembles in shape and sound the drum used by the Sakhalin Ainu shamans, she goes into a trance and speaks "words of the deities." Although she denies knowledge of Ainu, she talks in Ainu during these rites.

In the above two cases, a personal crisis was the catalyst that caused the women to become shamans. Pilsudski (1961:184–5) cites two examples of how a person became a shaman on the east coast of Sakhalin. In both cases, the shaman started by experiencing an inexplicable and uncontrollable feeling, but in neither case was a personal crisis the precipitating cause.

The Ainu do not regard a shamanistic predisposition as a psychological abnormality or a sign of mental illness. Nor do they regard shamans as cunning or mysterious. As their terms for *shaman* indicate, the Ainu consider shamans ordinary human beings with a special ability to deal with the deities because of their ability to be possessed by spirits.

Although the position of a shaman as such is not considered hereditary, the disposition to be a shaman is thought to run in the family. Husko's family provides a good example. Both of her parents were shamans. Her father's half-brother, Sirimoysuye, was one of the greatest shamans in the Rayčiska settlement; he is said to have begun his career while still a child and to have continued after he lost his eyesight at around twenty years of age. Two of Husko's maternal uncles and some of their offspring are also shamans. Husko's own brother is a shaman, and one of her daughters has recently started on a career. The mother of the shaman at the Wakasakunai settlement was also a shaman at the Tarantomari settlement on the southern coast of Sakhalin. Pilsudski (1961:183,185–6) reports that, although the position of shaman is not hereditary, the Ainu on the east coast believe that shamanistic power is passed on from father to children.

In contradiction to this statement, Kubodera (1960:105) claims that among the east coast Sakhalin Ainu, as well as the Saru Ainu of Hokkaido, shamanistic ability is believed to be transmitted through the female line. Nagano, Ishibashi, and Nakagawa (1966:15) likewise report a strong tendency for shamans to come from particular families.

In the case of the northwest coast Ainu, there seems to be no necessary relationship between a person's social or economic position and his or her status as a shaman. Thus either a headman or a poor member of the community may be a shaman. Also, despite a certain amount of economic gain, shamanistic practice alone does not bring a fortune to the practitioner. The goods that the client brings are considered to be offerings to the deities and not payment to the shaman. They may consist simply of food. Full-scale shamanistic rites, often involving more than one shaman, are held only at the time of major life crises. Offerings at such times may vary in quantity as well as quality, but even then the amount of the offerings is determined by the socioeconomic position of the client rather than by the ability of the shamans. The only occasions on which a sizable amount of wealth is involved occur when one of the few wealthy members of the community chooses to consult the shaman about an illness or some other problem. On such occasions, however, if the client is male, he may offer sheets of leather, shoes, mats, wooden bowls, or even lacquer ware obtained from the Japanese. A wealthy female may offer such items as necklaces with beads acquired from the Nanay or shoes of harbor seal skin. The absence of economic gain by shamans is also reported from the east coast (Pilsudski 1961:188).

There are both male and female shamans. Until recently, they were about equal in number, but presently female shamans far outnumber male practitioners. This may be a result of the more rapid acculturation of the male Ainu. Although either men or women may become shamans, there seems to be a subtle distinction in the nature of their work. Thus, miracle performances seem to be a specialization of male shamans, as we will shortly see, although males also engage in healing the sick. Male shamans are said to be more powerful. They can perform a rite in a grand fashion, for example, beating the drum more dramatically than can female shamans, who must perform their rites more modestly and also must begin by seeking forgiveness from Grandmother Hearth for performing a rite. Pilsudski (1961:185–6) reports a slightly different situation on the east coast, where he met 8 shamans out of a population of 1,360; only 2 were women. He reports that, although these two women were condemned by their people because they were evil shamans, female shamans were often considered more powerful.

The Ainu feel free to deal with shamans other than those in their own settlement. The local shamans not only do not resent this but often perform jointly with visiting shamans. Also, a sick person may, if able, travel to another settlement where a famous shaman resides. Flexibility in the choice of shamans is consonant with the fact that the Ainu are often willing to try even foreign methods of cure and foreign practitioners when sick.

A brief description of why and when a shaman is consulted should provide us with information about the nature of the power that the Ainu see in shamans. The power of shamans seems to consist of two basic types. First, shamans can deliver messages from a deity or an ancestor, which may take the form of information, instructions, or an expression of the intentions of these beings. Because the majority of shamanistic performances are healing rites, these messages usually consist of diagnoses and curing methods. It should be emphasized here that although the messages are to come ultimately from the deities, shamans engage in a long talk with their clients, asking them about their dreams, thoughts, and so on, either before they perform a rite or between rites if more than one is necessary to obtain the diagnosis and cure from the deities. The shamans also seek information from the deities concerning their intentions. When a child is born, for example, a shaman may ask the deities whether they have some special purpose in mind for the child or what the child's holy name should be (an Ainu usually has both a holy name and a nickname). This rite need not be held immediately after birth; it may be postponed for several years.

Another type of information frequently sought from the deities is the location of a missing object or person; the latter is often diagnosed as a case of fox bewitchment. At the Wakasakunai settlement, an elderly man frequently became lost. When repeated searching through a nearby wood failed to locate him, the aforementioned woman was consulted.

Second, Ainu shamans can resolve certain situations that call for extraordinary actions, or "miracle performances." For example, a shaman may revive a dead bear or a deceased human being by going to the world of the dead and fetching back the departed soul; of course, only the shaman's soul is involved in these trips. Sirimoysuye, the famous shaman of the Rayčiska settlement, was once asked to recover a mouthpiece of a pipe that was lost in a storm during a seal hunt at sea. During his performance, it is told, a mouthpiece suddenly fell into his drum from the sky window; the audience packed in his house heard only the sound of its hitting the drum. However, when Sirimoysuye asked for more wood to be added to the hearth to increase visibility, the people saw in his drum a turquois mouthpiece covered with wet sand from the sea. Other examples include a shaman driving a knife into his chest without harming himself and another miraculously creating the sea and walking on it with a cane.

Some of the reported miracles were performed by legendary shamans now long deceased. Whether in legend or in actuality, these miracle performances serve to reinforce the belief in shamanistic power.

In my examples, all the miracle performances are done by male shamans; female shamans specialize in curing.[1] Ainu shamanism completely ignores such matters as fertility and sexual problems, except in covert forms.

Shamans often demonstrate, during their rites, skills that they do not ordinarily possess and that are attributed to the actions of their spirits. My key informant, Husko, for example, would stretch her legs, something she ordinarily could not do because of an injury to her hip. As previously noted, shamans may consume extremely salty potions, eat lethally poisonous aconite roots, or talk in a language that they claim not to know.

Shamanistic power does not work at all times. Shamans advance a number of circumstantial reasons to explain their failure. For example, the shaman at Rayčiska, Sirimoysuye, used to blame the presence of a menstruating woman in the audience, whose odor prevented good deities and spirits from coming to his assistance during the performance.

Multiple roles of Ainu shamans: an interpretation

The above description indicates that shamans in Ainu society have multiple roles, some formalized and others nonformalized. In a brilliant study of role analysis, Chiñas defines these two sets of roles (1973:93-4):

Formalized roles are... defined as those given formal status and recognition by the members of the society. That is to say, every adult member of the society recognizes the existence of the role and has a fairly clear concept of the rights and duties the role demands... Nonformalized roles are those which are not so clearly perceived or rigidly defined by the members of the society... Only the observer becomes aware eventually that nonformalized roles exist, an awareness occasioned by observing repeated instances of similar behavior by many different individuals in many different contexts.

Chiñas combines these two types of roles with two other analytical concepts – covert and overt roles and domestic and public domains – which together comprise a complex system. Among the covert nonformalized roles, it is possible to differentiate roles covertly recognized by the people and those recognized by outsiders, that is, anthropologists, although this distinction is not always easy to establish. For our present purpose, I use only the distinction between formalized and nonformalized roles.

The above description of Ainu shamans and their power indicates that shamans may be considered religious specialists, health care specialists, theatrical performers, and covert politicians. Of the four roles, only the first two are formalized. In this section I discuss shamans as religious specialists, health care specialists, and theatrical performers briefly in order to convey the complexity of the shaman's roles. The role of covert politician is examined in detail in the next section, because this role relates most significantly to our topic of illness and society.

Shamans as theatrical performers have received much attention recently in anthropological literature (e.g., Beattie 1977; several articles, especially one by Leiris in Beattie and Middleton, eds., 1969; Firth 1966–7). Indeed, Ainu shamanistic rituals are the only type of regular communal entertainment for which almost everyone gathers at the beat of the shaman's drum that announces the commencement of a rite. Miracle performances in particular must have a large theatrical element. In the past, this element could have been more prevalent in Ainu shamanism, because battles in Sakhalin Ainu oral tradition from the east coast are often "magical contests" between shamans (Kindaichi 1914). I have no evidence for this, however, among the northwest coast Ainu.

As religious specialists, shamans are unimpressive. They are passively possessed by spirits, which are minor members of the Ainu pantheon. They perform the curing rites only as individuals for single patients in a house. Their humble status becomes obvious when contrasted to that of a male elder, a politico-religious leader of the community, who holds an elaborate ceremony for the supreme deity, the bear. Not only the entire community but also members of adjacent and even distant east coast communities are invited to participate in the ceremony, which lasts for several days. The elder, acting as a host, is much admired by all the participants for his generosity in holding the ceremony, as we saw earlier.

As health care specialists, Ainu shamans are much different from physicians in biomedical practices, but they share many features with shamans and other health care specialists in nonbiomedical traditions. Of these features, four are by far the most important for an appreciation of shamanistic medical practitioners in Ainu society and elsewhere. First, although the diagnosis and cure are believed by the Ainu to derive from the deities, the diagnosis is actually an identification of the illness agreed upon by the shaman and her patient; this agreement is reached while the two discuss the patient's dreams, memories, thoughts, and feelings. During the conversation, the shaman finds out what things have been bothering the patient and, with the aid of her own knowledge of the client and fellow Ainu, she synthesizes the picture – the diagnosis. Note that the main focus of shamanistic diagnosis is that of culturally construed pathogens and etiologies – the causes – which in turn identify the illness. It thus becomes clear why the metaphysical illnesses, for which shamanistic diagnoses are requested, do not have standardized symptoms for identification; the causes, pathogenic or etiological, determine their identification.

This aspect of shamanistic diagnosis as one mutually agreed upon by shaman and patient provides a dramatic contrast to biomedical diagnoses. As Fabrega (1975:973) points out, in biomedicine a patient often believes himself to be ill, whereas the doctor does not find anything wrong. Or, conversely, an individual feels fine, but the doctor proclaims that he has a disease.

The second point of importance about Ainu shamans as medical practitioners is a corollary of the first: Shamans treat all illnesses as psychosomatic. As Bidney (1963:154) notes, "the medicine man treated his patient as a person, as a psychosomatic unit." Shamanistic treatment, then, is essentially psychotherapy, which uses such mechanisms as confession and suggestion most effectively. (Anthropological discussions of this subject abound: e.g., Hallowell 1963; Kiev 1964.) For this reason the Ainu relate how much better they feel after the performance of a rite for them. My informant, Husko, even performs a rite for herself if she has not been feeling well for some time.

The third point relates to the source of authority or authenticity of shamans as medical practitioners. Needless to say, the process described, whereby shamans and patients come to agree upon a diagnosis, would not be acknowledged by the Ainu; in the Ainu's view, the diagnosis is given by the deities via shamans because of the shamans' superhuman power. As the Ainu see it, possession by the spirits and the possession trance during which shamans transform their identities into those of the spirits is pivotal; this is the proof of the authenticity of the shamans' power and consequently of their diagnoses. In other words, the competence of shamans as medical doctors comes from their special ability to become possessed and enter a trance, rather than from the personal knowledge of disease that is so important for biomedical doctors. Thus, the basis of a shaman's competence is the culturally standardized performance. In this connection, we should note the interpretation by Lévi-Strauss (1967:174) that Quesalid, a Kwakiutl shaman, "did not become a great shaman because he cured his patients; he cured his patients because he had become a great shaman."

The fourth and last point about shamanistic healing is that it is a communal event; almost all the people from the settlement gather at every shamanistic performance. As many anthropologists have already pointed out, community involvement is a major source of moral encouragement for the patient, who can see and feel that others are concerned about his or her well-being. Needless to say, it provides a marked contrast to the practice of biomedicine in the United States, where doctor and patient are alone behind a closed door in the examination room.

Shamans as healers of social ills
and as covert politicians

The power of Ainu shamans to heal individual patients is not the only power they possess. In fact, the dramatic importance of a shaman's power becomes much more apparent when we look at the Ainu definition of illnesses for which shamans are consulted. They are asked to diagnose and cure illnesses characterized by the involvement of the most important members of the Ainu universe – demons, deities, souls, and spirits – either in the etiology, as pathogens, or as a source of cure. We saw that *kamuy iramohkari* (punishment by the wrath of a deity) strikes when an Ainu engages in some form of disrespectful behavior toward a deity, and *aymawko ahun* (entrance of the spirit of an arrow) takes place when one person utters angry words about another in the community. These illnesses are usually not characterized by a standard set of symptoms, and only shamans can identify and provide the cures. Even when a set of symptoms immediately identifies the illness, a particular etiological factor that led to this instance of the illness must still be identified by a shaman, who then can provide instructions for the cure.

The definition of these illnesses clearly indicates that they are seen as expressions of disjunction in the social network of the beings of the universe, a disjunction caused by human misconduct (cf. Fabrega and Silver 1973:81 for a similar interpretation of illness). In other words, the Ainu consult shamans for social ills, in addition to individual illnesses. This aspect of shamanism becomes even more evident when we recall that the person who falls ill may not necessarily be, and indeed is often not, the one who violated the Ainu moral and social codes. A wrongdoing by a member of the settlement is translated into a collective breach of the code, which in turn expresses itself by afflicting an innocent victim.

The role of the shamans is to examine the behavior and interpersonal relationships of their fellow Ainu in order to locate the cause of these social ills, that is, the seat of these disjunctions. As judges of the moral and social behavior of their fellow Ainu, however, shamans cannot be autocratic. Before reaching a diagnosis, shamans ask their patients about their dreams, feelings, and thoughts about themselves and others, as noted above. They may also receive information pertinent to a diagnosis from others in the community. When a shaman reaches a diagnosis, it must be convincing not only to the patient but also to the rest of the community. This means, then, that shamans' diagnostic abilities rest heavily on their knowledge of the behavioral patterns and personalities of the members of the settlement and the interpersonal relations among them. For example, anybody who is ill-tempered, apt to provoke others verbally, or generally antisocial is a likely suspect in the case of *aymawko ahun*, the illness caused by harsh words. For shamans to blame some other type of person is not convincing, and may cause the loss of their credibility and even their profession. Therefore, although shamans are assigned the special role of diagnosing the pathogens and etiologies of illnesses, they often must find out the consensus of opinion in the community and express it. At the very least, the members of the community have much influence in the shamans' decision-making processes. This finding that Ainu shamans are social analysts *par excellence* is not a unique or new discovery. It is paralleled in Turner's observation of the Ndembu doctor (1967:359–93), Elliott's observation of the Chinese soul raiser (1955:134–40), and others.

Seen in this light, the shaman's role is not simply that of a healer of an individual's illness. Shamans heal the individual while they heal a social ill. As Turner (1975:159) most eloquently puts it: "Here health represents restoration of wholeness both to person and group; *mens sana in societate sana.*"

It follows then that as healers of social ills, Ainu shamans play important roles in the area of social control. First, they are the judges of the moral and social behavior of their fellow Ainu. Second, their presence in the community and their power act as deterrents against moral and social misdemeanor. Everyone must behave well toward the deities, other Ainu, and the soul-owning beings of the universe, lest someone be afflicted with illness and someone else be forced to take the blame. Thus the Ainu medical system in general, and illness definition and the nature of the shaman's power in particular, work as effective means of social control. This aspect of the medical system takes on even greater significance when we consider the absence of an elaborate system of legal codes and a well-developed political structure, which are corollaries of ecological and demographic factors of this semisedentary population (Ohnuki-Tierney 1976a). In other words, when crimes, that is, legally defined breaches of codes, are not well articulated, there is greater room for taboo. The breach of taboo then becomes the focal point of the shamanistic trial, which serves as a nonformalized legal system.

It should be recalled, however, that as a method of social control, the Ainu medical system is nonpunitive, in contrast to that of many other societies. First, the essence of the Ainu health care system is that if someone violates a rule, a fellow Ainu will become ill; thus, everyone must behave properly at all times. There is no element of personal retribution, in contrast, for example, to the Ojibwa medical system (Hallowell 1963:264–6). Second, the pathogens of the worst illnesses, epidemics, and severe cases of insanity are demons. The Ainu do not seek human causes of grave human misfortune.

The next question is, do all shamans simply play the passive role of analyzing the social situations of their fellow Ainu? I think not. Although I do not have empirical evidence, I believe that some are likely to play a more positive role, subtly directing the course of events in the community by revealing the past misconduct of others, thereby influencing the behavior of the offenders and even of others who are reminded of the outcome of misconduct. If we recall that the authenticity of the shamans' power rests with their ability to enter a possession trance, rather than with so-called medical knowledge, we appreciate that as a shaman's reputation increases, she or he becomes more independent of the opinion of the people. Rather than passively identifying a consensus of popular opinion, such powerful shamans may indeed become opinion leaders. As such, their power can be considerable.

For that matter, patients, too, are in a position to influence others. For example, when my informant, Husko, became sick, she had her father, who was visiting a co-wife in another settlement, return and take her all the way to the east coast, where famous shamans were visiting from Hokkaido. Because this woman had been unusually close to her father, it seems reasonable to interpret that her motivation – perhaps unconscious – in this illness episode was to gain her father's attention. A similar example is provided by Good, who meticulously illustrates, with the case of an Iranian woman, the fact that an illness episode has an important instrumental value for the patient as an actor who can "negotiate changes" in the behavior of others through "the rhetorical use of illness language" (1977:49).

In short, both shamans and patients in Ainu society, as well as perhaps in many other societies, are covert politicians who are in a position to manipulate their social environment if they so desire.

To label shamanistic rites as individual rites, then, is misleading. Although Ainu shamanism requires essentially two actors, a shaman and a client, the entire community is in fact intensely involved. The shaman's patients are usually not family members but members of the settlement, all of whom are interested in the shaman's ability to diagnose and cure their fellow Ainu. A shaman with a good reputation may even have clients from another community or may be induced to travel to a distant settlement to heal the ill. In other words, contact between shamans and their clients may constitute one of the few means of intersettlement communication. Earlier I described the bear ceremony as the only Ainu ritual on a supracommunity scale. Yet, seen in this light, shamanistic ritual may also be considered to have a supracommunity scale and sphere of influence. The difference is that, whereas the communal and supracommunal nature are institutionalized for the bear ceremony, they remain nonformalized for the shamanistic ritual.

The politically peripheral, nonformalized power, and shamans

The shamanistic career, open to anybody regardless of sex or kinship status, provides unlimited potential for the exercise of nonformalized power to those who choose it. This is of vital significance in interpreting the role of women in Ainu society. In contrast to some anthropologists' view that hunters and gatherers are egalitarian, the ideological and behavioral norms in Ainu society place women in a low status. Numerous restrictions are placed upon them; they are barred from hunting, fishing, officiating in group rituals, and any leadership roles in formal sociopolitical activities. These are the crucial activities in Ainu society that endow men with the formalized power of authority. Women's activities are confined to the domestic domain, and their sphere of influence is limited to the members of their family. Yet this one area of shamanism is open to women, who set aside their role as wife, mother, or grandmother and take on a professional role, thereby reaching far into the affairs of the community and beyond. Needless to say, male shamans enjoy the same position and power. As with many other societies (Lewis 1971:100–5; Mair 1969:216; Needham 1973, 1976; Turner 1967:371; Worsley 1968:ix–xxi), Ainu men who are somehow barred from following the regular routes to political success are also attracted to this profession. For example, a noted shaman of the Rayčiska settlement was blind and therefore could not engage in hunting, fishing, and other male activities that provide the means for males in Ainu society to achieve power.

In Ainu society, where one's social position is determined largely by sex, age, and kinship (cf. Ohnuki-Tierney 1974a:84–5), it is the shamanistic career that creates opportunities for the politically peripheral, which categorically includes all women.

Table 11.1 summarizes the formalized and nonformalized structures of Ainu society that have been discussed so far. It should be compared with Table 8.1 because the concepts represented in both share a similar interpretation.

By accommodating the politically peripheral and those who are not in the main stream of society due to personality and other difficulties, by providing them with the role of healer, Ainu society endows them with a strong nonformalized power that complements the authority of the politically central and powerful. Similarly, just as the community depends upon male elders for their ability to recite the sacred oral tradition to prevent epidemics, it must depend even more upon women, whose menstrual blood and its symbolic substitute of red bog moss are the only antidote for smallpox. The community also depends upon women to col-

Table 11.1. *Formalized and nonformalized structures*

Formalized	Nonformalized
Bear ceremony	Shamanism
Political structure	Medical system
Crime and legal trial	Taboo and shamanistic trial
Authority	Power
Politically central	Politically peripheral

lect herbs and other materia medica such as shellfish. We recall also that weak infants have clothes made from a woman's undergarment, or they are named after the term for the undergarment. In short, the Ainu medical system provides mechanisms that require able hunter-fishermen to rely upon the old, the disadvantaged, and women.

Shamans in other Ainu societies

In order to shed additional light on the relationship of the role of shamans to the politically peripheral, I now briefly examine information about shamanism in Ainu societies other than those of the northwest coast Sakhalin Ainu during the ethnographic present. There are some indications that, in the past, the cultural valuation of shamanism was higher than at present, not only among the northwest coast Ainu but also among other groups. In a tale from the oral tradition of the northwest coast, two brothers, who lived at the Rayčiska settlement at the beginning of the world and are regarded by the Ainu as their great ancestors, are said to have been powerful shamans. One of them was married to the Goddess of the Sun and Moon and could travel to the sky while performing a shamanistic rite (Ohnuki-Tierney 1968:248–9). In a sacred tale from the east coast, the culture hero, during his battle with female demons, is saved by a woman whom he subsequently marries. She is depicted as a deitylike young woman with shamanistic ability (Kindaichi 1914:103–4). In another story, also from the east coast, the culture hero himself is described as being a powerful shaman (Pilsudski 1912:149–55). The story implies that he is expected to excel in miracle performances rather than in the ordinary cure of illnesses. Chiri generalizes and proposes a hypothesis that the culture hero represents Ainu headmen, who necessarily were shamans in the ancient Ainu society (Chiri 1953:90; 1960:111). In the northwest coast Ainu society up to the ethnographic present, shamanistic ability has remained a most desired and desirable quality in a person.

Very little information is available on Hokkaido Ainu shamanism, past or present, due in part to the insignificance assigned to shamanism by both the Ainu and outsiders (see Chapter 6, note 24). Scholars point out that Hokkaido Ainu shamanism is not as well developed as Sakhalin Ainu shamanism (e.g., Hanihara et al. 1972:178; Kindaichi 1944:299). Among the Hokkaido Ainu, all shamans are reported to be women (Kindaichi 1961:45; Segawa 1972:192), although in the past there were some male shamans (Chiri 1973b:23; K. Wada 1971:19). Batchelor (1927:275-85), on the other hand, notes that he met both male and female shamans. Hokkaido shamans too enter into a possession trance. In sharp contrast to the Sakhalin Ainu shamans, a Hokkaido Ainu shaman becomes possessed only if a male elder induces it in her by offering prayers to the deities (Kindaichi 1961:45; K. Wada 1971:18-19). In the past, the primary role of Hokkaido Ainu shamans was to deliver instructions from the deities in regard to political, economic, and other decisions that men were about to make. At that time, the shamanistic ability of a wife, sister, mother, or any other close female relative was essential for the success of a male who was or who strived to be politically successful (cf. Kindaichi 1961:45-6). In the recent past, major decisions were made by the males without consultation with shamans, thus diminishing the importance of shamans in Hokkaido Ainu society. Hokkaido Ainu shamans also engage in the diagnosis of illnesses. However, their function is confined to diagnosis, after which male elders take over the healing process (Munro 1963:10; Uchimura, Akimoto, and Ishibashi 1938:36).

Available information on Hokkaido Ainu shamanism, then, suggests two major features that distinguish it from Sakhalin Ainu shamanism. First, it is the exclusive territory of women, at least during the ethnographic present. Second, a much more minor role is assigned to Hokkaido Ainu shamans, who are no more than assistants to male elders and not autonomous or full-fledged specialists in medicine or religion, although their nonformalized power can nonetheless be great.

The minor role of Hokkaido Ainu shamans should be viewed against the background of Hokkaido Ainu society. As noted elsewhere (Ohnuki-Tierney 1974b, 1976a), the Hokkaido Ainu, especially the Saru Ainu, among whom most of these scholars worked, have a larger population with permanent settlements, and their sociopolitical structures are well developed. Their bear ceremony is a far more elaborate venture, with important political functions, than is its counterpart among the northwest coast Sakhalin Ainu, among whom shamanism has a greater cultural significance than Hokkaido Ainu shamanism. Although we do not have any systematic study of the status of men vis-à-vis women in Hokkaido Ainu society, scholars note that men as a group enjoy a much higher status than women in Hokkaido (Kindaichi 1961:44), and that the difference in status between men and women is greater among the Hokkaido Ainu than among the Sakhalin Ainu (e.g., Chiri 1973b:153).

The above comparative data from other Ainu societies seem to provide some basis for speculation that when a society is small, as in the case of the ancient Ainu societies both on the northwest coast and elsewhere, shamanism occupies a central place in the culture and functions as a politico-religious institution. In these societies, shamans may at the same time be political leaders; thus shamans are often males. When a society becomes larger and a group religion or an institutionalized religion develops, as in the case of Hokkaido Ainu society in the recent past, the group religion, for example, the bear ceremony, takes over political functions and shamanism loses its high cultural valuation. In a large and complex society, the distance between the public and domestic domains is great, with the public domain receiving a much higher cultural valuation. The allocation of activities often starts to follow the sex line more strictly, with public activities being given exclusively to men. As a corollary, the role of shaman is assumed by the politically peripheral, including women, whereas men claim the leadership in group religions that lie in the public domain. The relationship between the role of shaman and the politically peripheral is further analyzed in the next section, where I discuss the personality of Ainu shamans.

Individual personality: *imu:* and shamans

I now turn to the issue of the individual personalities of shamans. Are shamans individuals with psychological disorders? There is no consensus among anthropologists on this question. Although many scholars, such as Lebra (1964, 1969), Lévi-Strauss (1967:161–80), and Spiro (1977), suggest that pathological thinking and acting are seen among the shamans they have examined, Kennedy (1973:1151) asserts that there are enough data "on shamans with stable, strong personalities and no evidence of disordered episodes or deviance."

Are all Ainu shamans healthy and normal, with politically peripheral status as their only peculiarity? In order to answer this question, I must briefly introduce a psychobehavioral disorder referred to as *imu:* in Ainu. It has drawn much attention from anthropologists, psychologists, and psychiatrists, and the Ainu term for the disorder is used in the literature. I discuss the details of my findings and those of others in Appendix C and focus here on those points relevant to the subject matter of this chapter (see also Ohnuki-Tierney 1980b).

According to the northwest coast Ainu, there are two distinct categories of *imu:*. The first category is a mild state in which an individual becomes surprised, but not necessarily frightened, and mumbles nonsensical phrases. The second category is a more severe state in which the individual loses touch with reality and has no self-control. In this state, which lasts only a few moments, the individual will often do whatever he or she is told to do, no matter how dangerous the act may be (manifested automatic obedience) or imitate whatever he or she hears or observes (echolalia and echopraxia).

The Ainu do not classify *imu:* as an illness or a sign that the individual may be sick. They simply regard the behavior during an *imu:* seizure as amusing. If a respected shaman or a political leader happens to be a victim of *imu:*, it in no way affects the respect he commands; the others laugh at him only during the seizure.

Imu: among the Hokkaido Ainu is similar in some respect to *imu:* among the Sakhalin Ainu. They too regard it as an amusing act rather than an illness. B. Wada (1956:45) notes that whereas manifested automatic obedience characterizes the Sakhalin Ainu *imu:*, the Hokkaido Ainu *imu:* is characterized most strongly by negative automatic obedience – doing the opposite of what one is being told to do. Other symptoms of the Hokkaido Ainu *imu:* include echolalia, echopraxia, mentioned above, and coprolalia and copropraxia – the involuntary utterance of obscenities and performance of obscene behaviors. Whereas the precipitating factor for the Sakhalin Ainu *imu:* is mild shock, for the Hokkaido Ainu it is almost always the sight of a snake or an Ainu word for it. Other types of stimulus include a frog, an octopus, a crab, a metal washing pan introduced by the Japanese, and neon signs that an *imu:* Ainu saw while visiting Tokyo (Uchimura, Akimoto, and Ishibashi 1938:29).

On the basis of etymological analyses and information from the oral tradition of the east coast Sakhalin Ainu and the Hokkaido Ainu, Chiri (1952) and K. Wada (1965b) convincingly argue that in the past the Ainu saw a close association between *imu:* and shamanism. However, present-day Ainu, either in Sakhalin or Hokkaido, do not consciously relate *imu:* to the personality of shamans. However, when I checked a list of individuals who were victims of *imu:*, more than half of them were also shamans. Of the thirteen Hokkaido Ainu shamans and one Sakhalin Ainu shaman whom Uchimura, Akimoto, and Ishibashi (1938:39) investigated, nine, including the Sakhalin Ainu, were also *imu:* victims. Uchimura, Akimoto, and Ishibashi also report that for 20% of their sample the initial occurrence of *imu:* was related to shamanism, in that during a major illness these individuals consulted a shaman who diagnosed the cause of the illness to be possession by a snake. In each case the individual was cured by an elder on the condition that she would eventually become an *imu:* sufferer, as they indeed started to periodically experience *imu:* shortly after the recovery (Uchimura, Akimoto, and Ishibashi 1938:35–6). Among the Niputani Ainu of Hokkaido, Munro (1963:161–3) records two prayers that attempt a "transmutation of an incapacitating or distressing neurosis to *Imu* [sic]" and two other prayers that aim at "transmutation to *tusu* shamans in case of a severe neurosis where *imu* [sic] could not be obtained."

It is noteworthy that among the Sakhalin Ainu there are some male *imu:* victims just as there are some male shamans, although a higher percentage of both *imu:* victims and shamans are women. In contrast, among the Hokkaido Ainu, both *imu:* victims and shamans are exclusively women. (For details, see Appendix C.)

In order to understand the relationship between Ainu *imu:* and shamanism in their sociocultural context, let me first attempt to interpret the occurrence of *imu:* among the Hokkaido Ainu. Recent studies indicate that certain psychobehavioral disorders, many of which are culturally sanctioned, are prevalent among the members of a social group for whom culturally important rights and positions are not accessible. Such studies as those of Foulks (1972), Kenny (1978), Lewis (1971), Obeyesekere (1970b), Rubel (1964), and Spiro (1977) demonstrate the prevalence of psychobehavioral disorders among women in societies in which women, regardless of their ability and personality, not only are deprived of rights and privileges of high cultural esteem but are expected to meet strict and rigorous role expectations. Thus one can speculate that low status in a society can result in psychological stress beyond the individual's capacity to resolve it, but that the culture provides a way for these individuals to resolve it in a culturally sanctioned manner such as *imu:*, *latah* (a so-called culture-bound syndrome found in Malaysia and Indonesia), and demonic possession. Culture thus provides simultaneously both pathogenic/ etiological agents and healing agents (cf. Wallace 1970).

Such sociocultural factors as the marginal position of the individual or strict role expectations provide at least a partial explanation for the *imu:* occurrence among women in Hokkaido Ainu society. The fact that negative automatic obedience, coprolalia, and copropraxia are characteristic behavioral patterns of the Hokkaido Ainu *imu:* but are not symptoms of the Sakhalin Ainu seems to support this interpretation. As noted earlier, there is a greater distance between men and women in Hokkaido Ainu society than in Sakhalin Ainu society, and women's modesty, especially in regard to their body, is strongly emphasized. Also of importance here are some of the stimuli. The snake, the primary precipitating factor for Hokkaido Ainu *imu:*, is not a consciously perceived phallic symbol, according to Chiri's information on snakes among the Hokkaido Ainu (1962:223–8); instead, a turtle is called *ečinke* (one whose head looks like a penis) in one of the Hokkaido Ainu dialects (Chiri 1962:223). Although the snake may or may not symbolize a threat posed by men, Japanese washing pans and neon signs are clearly symbols of the threat of the Japanese to Ainu society (cf. Murphy's 1976 interpretation of *latah* as a response, at least in part, to new European overlords). Note that Japanese washing pans became the major stimulus for *imu:* in the Tokachi district of Hokkaido when they were first introduced to the Tokachi Ainu (cf. Uchimura, Akimoto, and Ishibashi 1938:29). Thus, there is at least partial evidence that *imu:*

among Hokkaido Ainu women is linked to their marginal status vis-à-vis Ainu men, who form the dominant group in Ainu society, and also vis-à-vis the Japanese, who constitute the dominant group in a larger universe of the Ainu, who have become a minority group in Japanese society. Even in the case of the Sakhalin Ainu, such stimuli for *imu:* seizure as a domesticated cat of the Japanese or raw fish eating introduced by the Japanese (see Cases 2 and 3 described at the end of Appendix C) suggest that their *imu:* too may be related to the minority status of the Ainu in Japanese society.

The next question is, how do we explain that in societies in which the status and role of an individual are fairly rigidly defined, we find shamanism and mental disorder in the same social group or in the same individual? Here the role of the possession trance, either of a shaman or of the afflicted, looms large. During a possession trance, individuals are not held responsible for their behavior. Thus, they can assume the identity of that which has possessed them – a demon, a god, a general, a deceased patriarch, and so on. Possession therefore serves as a culturally sanctioned mechanism that has a definite therapeutic function for the individuals who, either because of their personality or role constraints, cannot otherwise express themselves in a manner that is possible during a possession trance. As Spiro (1965) eloquently stated, religion serves as a "culturally constituted defense" and provides a "nonpathological resolution of the conflicts" (Spiro 1965:107). In discussing Burmese shamans, Spiro (1977) successfully demonstrates that the availability of a variety of *nats* makes it possible for these Burmese female shamans, who have different personality types, to resolve their various frustrations through the *nat* possession. Similarly, using the eloquent example of a case of demonic possession in Sri Lanka, Obeyesekere (1970b) illustrates how the role resolution is accomplished through a culturally sanctioned means of temporarily deviating from the norm. He (1970b:102) states:

The adoption of a new status, and its attendant role, which utilizes and acts out the psychological problem of the individual in a positive matter, would be considered a normal way of "coping."

A similar reasoning is behind Wallace's (1970) explanation of the process of becoming a shaman as one example of mazeway resynthesis, during which a confusing and anxiety-provoking world starts to make sense. Lewis (1971:31) likewise explains:

For all their concern with disease and its treatment, such women's possession cults are also, I argue, thinly disguised protest movements directed against the dominant sex. They thus play a significant part in the sex-war in traditional societies and cultures where women lack more obvious and direct means for forwarding their aims.

In contradiction to the sex-war interpretation of Lewis, Wilson (1967) asserts that illness and possession are caused by tensions and frustrations between the members of the same sex arising from competition for the same goals and rewards, such as competition for the husband's attention among co-wives; according to Wilson, they are not due to tension between the sexes. It seems to me that Wilson's interpretation in fact reinforces that of various scholars, including Lewis, which links sociocultural deprivation to possession, illness, and various culturally normative departures. If cultural rewards and goals are narrowly defined for women, then competition becomes sharper and thus causes greater anxiety for the individual.

In short, whether they occur in the healer or the patient, these culturally normative altered states of consciousness have a very positive therapeutic function. They are also effective without causing the individuals concerned to be labeled as abnormal.

Marginal status as a cause of these phenomena, however, should not preclude a possibility that, as Bourguignon (1973b:328) suggests, the therapeutic function of these cultural institutions resolves not only "deprivation resulting from low social status or lack of power" but also "deprivation in personal satisfaction." Thus, whereas the presence of *imu:* individuals and shamans among Hokkaido Ainu women may be explained as related largely to the social position of women in their society, there should be other shamans and *imu:* individuals for whom the cultural institutions resolve conflicts arising from personal difficulties, as perhaps is the case with many Sakhalin Ainu *imu:*.

Although I have presented the view that some shamans may be individuals with psychological difficulties, I must emphasize here that this interpretation should in no way preclude the possibility that some shamans are stable, healthy individuals without major psychological problems, as Kennedy (1973) suggests. Given the complexity of the multiple roles that shamans carry out, and given the fact that at least half of the population, that is, women, are politically peripheral and have only a marginal status in society, we must allow room for perfectly healthy individuals to become shamans for other reasons, such as the exercise of nonformalized power. A female sorcerer in pre-Communist China who became an eloquent village representative (Yang 1969:132; also quoted in Wolf 1974) is an example of a healthy and strong-minded magico-religious practitioner who, given the opportunity, would have used a legitimate route to achieve authority.

Symbolic power and sociopolitical power

We now leave the topics of the individual personalities of shamans and functional analyses of shamanism and conclude this chapter by returning to the relationship between culture and society.

In Chapter 7 we saw that there were two sets of symbols in the Ainu shamanistic ritual – the profane symbols representing women and cooking and the marginal symbols representing mediation. The symbols representing women and cooking are interpreted to be profane because women represent the profane half of human society and men the sacred half. We saw in this chapter that shamans are profane religious practitioners, in contrast to the sacred male elders who officiate in group rituals.

As social persona, shamans often are marginal persons – women and/or men not in the mainstream of their society. Furthermore, the possession trance, which is the essence and the seat of authority for shamans, is a state during which the shaman's identity is lost and is replaced by that of a spirit. Thus, just as the state of illness (Table 7.2) is anomalous, the possession trance is also an anomalous state in which the shaman's identity is merged with that of a spirit.

It is in the shamans, who are marginal in several ways, that the power to cure is entrusted. Just as profane but marginal symbols have the power to cure structural ailments produced by anarchic anomaly of demons, women and shamans heal not only the ailments of an individual but also social ills. Similarly, just as the marginal symbols mediate between conceptual categories by transcending categorical boundaries, shamans mediate between families and settlements as they heal patients from different social groups, and women mediate between social groups through marriage, establishing kinship ties among families, patrilineal groups, and settlements that are otherwise unrelated to each other. For both the marginal symbols in the rituals and shamans and women in Ainu society, their power and freedom to transcend and mediate between conceptual categories and social groups respectively derive from their symbolic and social marginality (see Table 11.2).

As Kleinman (1974:208) perceptively notes, health care systems "may crudely be characterized as expressions of the cultural loci of power which they [people] utilize to explain and control illness" (cf. a similar observation in Turner 1967:343–50). In the case of the Ainu, nonformalized

Table 11.2. *Symbolic power and sociopolitical power*

Symbolic power	Sociopolitical power
Profane symbols	*Shamans and women*
Healing of structural ailments	Healing of individual and social ills
Marginal symbols	*Shamans and women as the politically and socially peripheral*
Mediation between categories	Mediation between social groups

power rests in the hands of politically peripheral members of the society; on the conceptual side, it rests in the process that is identified as the Ainu way of life and is represented in medical rituals by profane symbols.

I began writing this book in order to understand the Ainu view of health and illness. As I reach the end, I cannot but be impressed by the good fit between an illness as a liminal period for the individual, the healing power of anomalous and profane symbols in the medical rituals, and the nonformalized power of the politically peripheral in Ainu society.

Summary

The Tungic term *saman* has long been with us in anthropology and other disciplines in Western academia. During the first half of the twentieth century, however, *shamans*, as the term became anthropologized or Anglicized, were regarded primarily as "primitive" magico-religious specialists who carried out individual rituals. They were regarded as less important or impressive than monks, priests, and other religious specialists who represent the people of a religious institution and who officiate in elaborate rituals. From the standpoint of individual personality, shamans were often regarded as mentally ill, although anthropologists were quick to recognize that many of the technologically less advanced peoples were more tolerant than their highly industrialized neighbors in that they did not ostracize their deviants but instead provided them with a culturally sanctioned role.

With a resurgence of interest in native health care systems as part of the rapidly growing field of medical anthropology, anthropologists are re-examining the phenomena of shamanism and shamans. Recent anthropological observations and interpretations of shamanism and related phenomena point to a need to recognize that shamanism is a highly complex phenomenon with various facets. We realize now that shamans have multiple roles, some formalized and others not, and the position of shaman may be occupied by individuals with various personality types. In order to understand the dynamics of shamanism in its many varieties throughout the world, we should take a dual approach, examining both the personality of shamans and a number of sociocultural factors.

I speculate, as a gross generalization, that when a society is small, shamanism often receives high cultural valuation and shamans are not confined to certain personality types, certain statuses in the society, or one sex. In a larger society, shamanism is culturally insignificant and consequently is an arena for the socially marginal, including women. As a corollary, a greater number of shamans are individuals with psychological difficulties. These difficulties are resolved through the experience as shamans, and in particular, through the possession trance. A shamanistic career also provides the means to exercise nonformalized power for those who are otherwise powerless. Relevant sociocultural factors in these larger and more complex societies that are responsible for this form of shamanism include such institutions as an established religion, social stratification, a great distance between the public and domestic domains, ascribed statuses, strict role allocation, rigid role expectations, and several other related factors. The shamanism of the northwest coast Sakhalin Ainu in the past is that of a small society in which shamanism was an important cultural institution; in contrast, the shamanism of the Hokkaido Ainu typifies that of a large and complex society. Northwest coast Ainu shamanism during the ethnographic present is a type that falls somewhere between these two.

Originally I set out to write this chapter in order to find an answer to a question: How do we account for a seeming discrepancy between the strong representation of women and their roles of cooking and reproduction in the medical symbols, and their lack of sociopolitical power and low status in Ainu society? I found a key to an understanding of this phenomenon in anthropological theories about nonformalized power and nonformalized methods of social control, on the one hand, and the presence of multiple symbolic structure, on the other. Once we realize that shamans and women are endowed with strong nonformalized power, then we begin to see a concordance between symbolic power and sociopolitical power. The healing power that is assigned to the profane and anomalous symbols in the Ainu shamanistic ritual presented in Chapter 7 corresponds to the nonformalized power of shamans and women presented in this chapter.

Details of Ainu habitual illnesses

In this section I provide details of some Ainu habitual illnesses. Of the 106 illnesses that I recorded in the field, many are eliminated from the present description in order to conserve space. The description of each illness starts with its Ainu label, followed when possible by an English approximation in parentheses. The word order in English approximations follows the one in Ainu labels. Occasionally there is another English substitute if it gives a better idea of the nature of the illness. It should be kept in mind, however, that the English translations and substitute terms are not exact equivalents. The illness label is then followed by information about (1) diagnostic criteria and (2) treatments. The numbers 1 and 2 indicate this respective information. For convenience, I use the following abbreviations in describing standard methods of treatment with medicinal substances:

A   Making an amulet from the substance and hanging it over the affected area, often from the neck or the hip.

C   Making a compress with the substance and applying it to the affected area.

CE   Cooking and eating the substance.

E   Eating the substance.

D   Making a decoction by boiling the substance in hot water and having the patient drink this liquid.

GA   Grinding the substance and applying the powder to the affected area.

GP   Grinding the substance, adding water, and applying the resulting paste to the affected area.

P   Applying the substance to the affected area.

SA   Soaking the substance in water and applying the water to the affected area.

SD   Soaking the substance in water and letting the patient drink the water. This differs from D in that the substance is not boiled in water.

Ainu medicine often utilizes animals and plants. The primary sources of identification of Ainu animal and plant names are by Chiri (1953) for plants and Chiri (1962) for animals. When some animals and plants in my data are not identified in Chiri's work, other sources are consulted. Chiri, an Ainu scholar of Ainu culture, was the first to articulate an important ethnobotanical fact regarding Ainu identification of plants (see Ohnuki-Tierney 1973b). In contrast to Latin identification of a plant, which refers to the whole plant, in the Ainu system different lexemes are often applied to different parts of a plant. Furthermore, parts of a plant deemed useless by the Ainu are left nameless; only edible roots, medicinal leaves, and so on are labeled, whereas flowers are often left nameless. I attempt here to specify which part of a plant is specifically referred to by each Ainu term.

A. Body-part illnesses

As noted in the text, when a category of body-part illnesses is further classified, it is either subdivided in terms of the subsection of the body part affected by the ailment or other disorder, or it is differentiated into single illnesses based on the nature of the disorder. In some cases of the first type of subdivision, the lexeme specifying the body part, for example, *sapa* (head), is either replaced by an entirely different lexeme designating a part of the head, such as *kistomoho* (forehead), or receives a modifier, for example, *ariki* (half). In other cases, however, such as with three illnesses of the lower abdomen, the location of the abnormality at a subsection of a body part is not terminologically expressed. Whereas the lower abdomen is called *hopana* and the illnesses in this area are referred to as *hopana araka*, the three illnesses of the lower abdomen are referred to as *okuy eskari*, *čuhkes araka*, and *takapes araka*, without bearing the term *hopana* in their lexical construction.

More frequently, the illnesses occurring within the same body part are differentiated in terms of the abnormality, that is, the nature of the pain involved or the appearance of the affected part. In these cases, an additional lexeme specifying the nature of the abnormality is added to comprise an illness label. Thus, in the case of *iso sapa araka* (bear headache), the term *iso* (bear) is added to the general term for headache, *sapa araka*, because this particular headache reminds one of the heavy footsteps of a bear.

I. *Sapa araka* (head illness)

I.1. *iso sapa araka* (bear headache) – 1. The head pounds like the heavy footsteps of a bear. 2. A bear skull (GP). The paste is put in a bundle of ritual shavings and placed on the forehead. Because bears are the supreme deities of the Ainu and it is taboo among the northwest coast Ainu to keep bear skulls at home, several elders make a special trip to an altar in the mountains where the bear skulls are enshrined and there make a small amount of powder from a skull. The religious significance of a bear as the supreme deity, however, does not seem to play a role here.

I.2. *seta sapa araka* (dog headache) – 1. The head aches like a dog gnawing on something hard. 2. A dog skull (GP). Dogs, used both to pull sleds and for food, are not deified but are considered servants of the bear deities and are sacrificed during the bear ceremony and sometimes in shamanistic rituals.

I.3. *ni:nah čikah sapa araka* (woodpecker headache) – 1. The headache feels as though a woodpecker were pecking a tree. 2. Feathers from the head of a woodpecker (P). For this purpose the Ainu usually keep at hand a skin, with feathers attached, from a woodpecker head. The bird is not deified, and the Ainu use it only for medicinal purposes.

I.4. *opokay sapa araka* (musk deer headache) – 1. The headache resembles the galloping steps of a musk deer. 2. A musk deer skull (GP).

I.5. *ahkoype sapa araka* (octopus headache) – 1. The head aches like the sucking motion of an octopus and feels as if an octopus is crawling on one's head. When it feels as if the creature has slipped off the head, then the headache temporarily ceases. 2. (a) Slime from an octopus (P). (b) A dried octopus (SA). The Ainu do not treasure octopi, but when they are available, they eat them or dry them for eating and medicinal uses. They have a fear of giant octopi, which are believed to strangle fishermen to death.

I.6. *takahka sapa araka* (crab headache) – 1. The headache resembles the incessant but small bites of a crab. It feels as if cold water is touching one's head because crabs belong to the sea. When it feels as if the crab has slipped off the head, then the headache temporarily ceases. 2. A crab shell (GP). The Ainu eat crabs if available, but they assign neither high food value nor symbolic meaning to them.

I.7. *ikurupe sapa araka* (lamprey headache) – 1. The headache resembles a lamprey digging into a rock. 2. Dried lamprey (GP). For this purpose the Ainu keep the head of a lamprey handy, slit in half and dried. As a "long thing" lampreys are much disliked by the Ainu, who abhor snakes, the most representative of the long things.

I.8. *kasuh sapa araka* (ladle headache) – 1. The headache moves gradually to the part of the head next to the neck. The analogy here is the shape of a round ladle and its handle to the human head and neck. 2. The "neck" part of a *kasuh* (wooden ladle) (GP). Because a wooden ladle is believed to have a soul, before shredding it to make powder one must decorate it with ritual shavings made into a circular ring.

I.9. *kistomoho araka* (forehead ache) – 1. The headache is confined to the forehead area. 2. Also *kasuh* (GP).

I.10. *sapa ariki araka* (head-half ache; pain on one side of the head) – 1. The pain is confined to the right or left half of the head (migraine?). 2. None.

General cure for all headaches. A plant called *keyoro kus kina* (not identifiable), with white flowers and yellow roots, is considered effective for any type of headache. It can be made into a headdress or a pillow, or simply placed on the head of the patient or between the head and a pillow.

II. *Sis araka* (eye illnesses)

Included in the *sis araka* category are abnormalities of the eyeball, the eyelids, the space between the eyes, and the rest of the area surrounding the eye. Blindness, however, is not considered an illness. The blind, both those who are born blind and those who become blind after birth, are believed to receive special favors from the deities and are often considered to have special talents. For example, much of the power of a famous shaman named Sirimoysuye on the northwest coast was attributed to his blindness and consequent favor from the deities; blind women are supposed to be good at sewing and embroidery. Although the Ainu recognize *oheros sis koro aynu* (a cross-eyed person) and *yu:pohkuste aynu* (a person who has a nervous habit of looking up from below; vertical squint?), these abnormalities of the eyes are not considered illnesses.

Of the following eight eye illnesses, three (1, 2, and 3) are specifically identified as *sey sis araka* (shellfish eye illnesses) because of the great amount of fluid discharged.

II.1. *kaywantahpo sis araka* (*kaywantahpo* shellfish illness) – 1. The eyeballs protrude, looking like *kaywantahpo* shellfish (not identifiable); this appearance is accompanied by acute pain and much tearing. 2. (a) Shell of this shellfish (GP). Apply around the eyes. (b) Heated empty shell (P). Apply over the eyelids while the eyes are closed. (c) Slime from the shellfish (P).

II.2. *takahka sis araka* (crab eye illness) – 1. The pain feels as though a crab were crawling on the eyeball, and there is excessive tearing. 2. Dried eyeballs of a crab (GP).

II.3. *ikurupe sis araka* (lamprey eye illness) – 1. A great deal of tearing, accompanied by acute pain, as if a lamprey were digging into a rock. 2. The eyeball of a lamprey (SA).

II.4. *hu: saranpe araka* (red garment illness) – 1. The white of the eye turns red. 2. (a) Apply water with a piece of *saranpe*, which is an imported Japanese silk garment treasured by the Ainu. (b) *Hu:re nupotoh* (red sphagnum) (SA). Use fresh plants in summer and dried ones in winter. It could very well be that this curing method was the traditional one before the introduction of Japanese garments, which might have changed the illness label as well. Wada, in the early 1940s, recorded an eye illness named *kosontosis'araka* [sic] with identical symptoms (K. Wada 1964:104). *Kosonto* is a borrowed word from the Japanese *kosode* and is used to refer to the red Japanese silk garment that the Ainu also descriptively call *hu: saranpe* (red garment) – the terms used in the label for this illness.

II.5. *maysikah* (growth of a spot; *may* = spot; *sikah* = to grow) – 1. A sore spot on the pupil that looks like a lead bullet. The term *may* refers to an abnormal growth on the eyeball perhaps corresponding to a leukomatous spot. 2. Place a bullet, an imported item, on the hand and recite, while gently moving the hand in a circular fashion, "*May ru:, may ru:* (Spot melt! Spot melt!)."

II.6. *impiri* – 1. A small swelling at the edge of the eyelid (sty?). 2. Charcoal made from a burnt stem of *mačahči* (an unidentifiable grass) (P).

II.7. *siki oaka asin* (eye posterior-ridge gets out; *siki* = eye; *o* = posterior; *aka* = the back of a fish or the ridge of a mountain; *asin* = to exit) – 1. Swelling around the eyes. 2. No special cure.

II.8. *sikuturuke araka* (between-the-eyes illness) – 1. Pain at the glabella. 2. (a) A tuft of hair from the same spot on a dog (P). (b) A seal's glabella (GP). To use this, one must grind the bone at a *keyohniusi*, an altar where seal bones exclusively are enshrined. It is owned communally and is located at a place overlooking the sea.

General cures for all eye illnesses. (a) Berries or wood shreddings from the stalk of *iso mawni* (*Rosa rugosa* Thunb. [Chiri 1953:123–4]) (SA). *Mawni* is the term for the stalk of this plant, and *otaruh* refers to its berries. (b) Shredded root of *ikema* (*Cynanchum caudatum* Maxim. [Chiri 1953:41]) (P). This root is also used extensively as a charm against evil spirits. (c) The leaves of *oyaw kina* (*Ammodenia oblongifolia* Rydb. var. *maxima* Nakai [Chiri 1953:153]). The term *oyaw kina* means snake grass. The eyes are closed, and the leaves are then rubbed all over the face. Some Ainu wipe their face with the leaves even when healthy so that their eyes will stay strong.

III. *Čaru araka* (mouth illnesses)

Included in this category are illnesses of the interior wall of the mouth (the hard and soft palates), the tongue, the gum, and the lips. Illnesses 3, 4, 5, and 6 may be identified more specifically as *aw araka* (tongue illnesses). The *imah araka* (tooth illnesses) are considered to be separate from the mouth illnesses. The term *čapus epehtuy* is used to refer to both the harelip and the lip cracked in the middle due to dryness; however, neither are considered illnesses.

III.1. *ekaytama čaru araka* (snail mouth illness) – 1. The hard and the soft palates become swollen, looking like a snail, and much saliva is produced. 2. Slime from a snail (P).

III.2. *uhkurači čeh čaru araka* (sturgeon fish mouth illness) – 1. An x-shaped boil forms on the interior wall of the mouth. 2. The boil is rubbed with the skin and/or bone of a sturgeon. Sturgeon was not commonly found on the northwest coast, so the Ainu occasionally obtained the fish from farther north, especially from the Santan traders, and kept the skin and bones when available.

III.3. *otah čaru araka* (shark mouth illness) – 1. Small white growths, referred to in Ainu as *tetara enukuki*, form on the tongue, and the mouth acquires a foul odor. 2. Sliced dried tongue of a shark (SD or SA). Apply around the throat. For this purpose, the Ainu remove the tongue from a shark and dry it on a skewer for future use.

III.4. *erekus čaru araka* (codfish mouth illness) – 1. Small white growths form on the tongue, but there is no foul odor. The inside of the mouth looks like that of a codfish. 2. A dried tongue of a codfish (SD or SA). Apply on the interior surface of the mouth.

III.5. *arakoy čaru araka* (*arakoy* smelt mouth illness) – 1. Small white growths on the tongue characterize this illness, but there is no foul odor. The inside of the mouth looks like that of an *arakoy* smelt rather than that of a cod; this seems to be the only difference between this illness and *erekus čaru araka*. 2. A dried tongue of this fish (SA or SD).

III.6. *parakinači čaru araka* (*parakinači* mouth illness) – 1. Formed on the tongue are small yellow growths, like the pollenia of *parakinači* (*Lysichiton camtschatense* Schott var. *japonicum* Makino [Chiri 1953:216]). 2. Juice from the leaves of this plant (P).

III.7. *epasiču:* or *apahču araka* (meaning of these terms not clear) – 1. The lips swell and assume the color of *toy su:*, clay pots. 2. Potsherds (GP). Clay pots were commonly found at archaeological sites near the Ainu settlements. The Ainu believe that these pots were made by their ancestors, who were small in stature and lived at the beginning of the world.

III.8. *osukeh čaru araka* (hare mouth illness) – 1. A swollen gum. 2. A dried gum or a dried scalp of a hare (GP or SD).

IV. *Rekuči araka* (throat illnesses)

Included in this category are abnormal conditions of both the interior and exterior walls of the throat. Illnesses 5 and 6 are specified as illnesses of sea creatures.

IV.1. *iso oypepuy rekuči araka* (bear cage window throat illness) – 1. The throat (inside) becomes swollen, and the patient is unable to eat or drink; there is no change of color. There is a small opening, called *iso oypepuy* (bear cage opening), in the bear cage through which the Ainu feed a bear in captivity. The opening is made so small that the bear cannot put his snout through it even to eat or drink, so that its keeper is protected from being bitten. The inability of the bear to open its mouth while it is in the cage opening must have contributed to the name of this illness. 2. (a) Sawdust is taken from a log comprising a window of a bear cage. A small amount of it is placed in ritual shavings, sprinkled with water, and applied around the throat. The rest of the sawdust is soaked in water, which the patient drinks. (b) A dried thyroid cartilage of a bear, which is either ground and applied or hung from the throat on a string. For this purpose, the Ainu boil a cartilage and dry it to keep on hand. The religious significance of the bear as the supreme deity does not seem to play a role in the perception of this illness.

IV.2. *hay rekuči araka* (nettle throat illness) – 1. The inside of the throat becomes swollen; there is no change of color. This condition is less severe than *iso oypepuy rekuči araka*. The throat looks like "the throat (*rekuči*) part" of the plant *hay* (nettle; *Urtica Takedana* Ohwi [Chiri 1953:162–4]), which is the part at the very end of the stalk, next to the root. 2. A root of nettle (D). The Ainu use this plant extensively to make threads for garments. The fresh plant, when in contact with human skin, produces itching.

IV.3. *moawetuh* (small-tongue-protrudes) – 1. The small tongue (*mo* = small; *aw* = tongue), that is, the uvula, becomes swollen (*etuh* = sticks out). 2. *Ya:kara kem* (a wooden or bone needle for fishnet making) (GP). Apply around the throat or prickle the uvula with it.

IV.4. *kučisah araka* (throat absent illness) – 1. The throat dries up and one loses one's voice. 2. A twig of *hu:reni:* (*Hydrangea paniculata* Sieb. [Chiri 1953:129–30]) (D). Also, the throat may be rubbed with this decoction.

IV.5. *otasuh rekuh araka* (sandy-beach throat illness) – 1. An excessive discharge of saliva. 2. Sand from the beach (SA).

IV.6. *otaka: ris rekuči araka* (shore throat illness) – 1. An excessive discharge of saliva. The distinction between this illness and the above is not clear. 2. An empty shell of some kind. No information about the method of its application is available.

IV.7. *kurukituh* (the lymphatic vessel protrudes) – 1. The lymphatic vessel (*kuruki* in Ainu) swells. (The gill of a fish is also called *kuruki*.) 2. (a) The patient's throat is rubbed with a bundle of plants called *kuruki kina* so that the juice from the plants will work on the throat. This plant, with small wine-colored flowers, is not identifiable. (b) Broiled *erekus* (cod) or *supun* (dace). (c) The slime from a fresh cod or dace (P). Apply to the throat.

General cure for all throat illnesses. A piece of a woman's underwear, called *raunkuh*, is wrapped around the throat, although one must not expose it because it is something nobody should see. The *raunkuh* is believed to have extremely potent power to expel not only demons or evil spirits but also deities when they endanger humans. (See the story of a dragon deity expelled by an elderly woman with a *raunkuh* in Ohnuki-Tierney 1974a:104.) The Ainu also wave it when threatened by fire. A hunter usually carries with him a piece of his mother's or, if married, wife's *raunkuh* as a general protection against demons and deities. (For the relationship of the *raunkuh* to the matrilineal exogamous rule among the Saru Ainu of Hokkaido, see Ohnuki-Tierney 1976b:315.)

V. *Honihi araka* (stomach illnesses)

The Ainu term *honihi* refers to the abdomen in the most general sense, including both the internal organs and the exterior wall. When the internal organs alone are to be specified, the term *ramorihi*, which collectively means all the internal organs, or specific terms for each internal organ, such as *kinoh* (liver), are used. The term *honihi araka* is used in three ways: as a general label for the category of illnesses relating to the abdomen, as an ordinary stomachache (V.1), or as a labor pain (V.5). Thus, it should be noted that labor pains and menstrual cramps are at least terminologically referred to as stomach illnesses. There are many beliefs and behavioral taboos connected with pregnancy, parturition, and miscarriage, but the following account covers only the medical treatment of actual illnesses. Illnesses 1 to 9 are considered to be problems of the abdomen in general, whereas illnesses 10 to 12, collectively called *hopana araka* or *tuy honkes araka*, refer more specifically to the illnesses of the lower abdomen. The terms *hopana* and *tuyhonkes* are synonymous and refer to the lower abdomen.

V.1. *honihi araka* (abdomen illness) – 1. Severe stomachaches without any other symptoms, such as diarrhea. 2. (a) *Apa turu*, that is, grime (*turu*) accumulated at the doorsill (*apa*) (P). Apply on the stomach. While scraping grime from the doorsill with a knife, one must recite, "Grandmother doorsill, because this girl (or whoever is sick) has a stomachache, give me the medicine. I will get the medicine from you, and so please quickly cure her stomachache." (b) The root of *ikema* (*Cynanchum caudatum* Maxim [Chiri 1953:41]) is chewed. (c) The leaves and stalks of *tukara kina* (not identifiable) (D). For this purpose, the Ainu gather the plants during the summer, when they are blooming, and dry and store them. (d) Dried and shredded bark of *sikereni:* (cork tree – *Phellodendron amurense* Rupr. var. *Sachalinense* Fre. Schm. [Chiri 1953:102]) (D).

V.2. *huhteh yamuhu honi araka* (spruce leaf stomach illness) – 1. The stomach aches as if leaves of *sunku* (spruce – *Picea jezoensis* Carr [Chiri 1953:236–7]) are prickling it. The term *huhteh* means a branch of either Yesso spruce or Sakhalin fir, but my informant, Husko, specified the use of a spruce branch in this case. 2. A branch of spruce is heated over the hearth (C).

V.3. *seta honkah honi araka* (dog stomach skin stomachache) – 1. Severe stomachache. It is not clear how this condition differs from other stomachaches. 2. Take a piece of skin or a tuft of hair from the stomach of a female dog, wrap it in a piece of material, and tie it to the patient's stomach. Because dogs have souls, when taking out the skin or hair, one must place a necklace made of ritual shavings around the dog's neck.

V.4. *eha: honi araka* (*eha:* [plant] stomachache) – 1. No details known. 2. The root of *eha:* (*Boschniakia rossica* Hutt. [Chiri 1953:34]) is chewed.

V.5. *tuye ikoni* (guts ache) or *honi araka* (abdomen ache) – 1. Labor pain. 2. Before parturition: small amount of ground dried umbilical cord (SD). For this purpose, a woman would usually keep an umbilical cord from her own or someone else's previous childbirth. At the time of parturition, a bonfire is made outside the house; leaves of *yayuh* (fir – *Abies sachalinensis* Fr. Schm. [Chiri 1953:233–6]) are warmed over it and put over the stomach of the woman in labor. Postparturition treatment: (a) Steamed leaves of *yayan hamičan kina* (a *Cirsium* plant [Chiri 1953:13–14]) (C); or a dish containing this plant, a leek, a fish, and some root crop (CE). (b) A plant called *kina tesma* (an unidentifiable creeping vine) (D or C). The leaves are steamed, put in a bag, and used to warm the woman's stomach. (c) *orahnu* (an unidentifiable plant) or *seta kina* ("dog's grass" – *Arctium Lappa* L. [Chiri 1953:11]) (CE). Either one of the plants is cooked until soft, and then root crops such as lily bulbs and leeks are added.

V.6. *honi čiseku araka* (abdomen swelling illness) – 1. Swelling of the abdomen. 2. A dried stomach of a fish called *nanuwen čeh* (*Hemitripterus villosus* Pallas [Chiri 1962:16]) (SA or SD).

V.7. *niteh kara kina araka* (violet illness) – 1. Sudden stomachaches accompanied by the vomiting of yellow water. 2. *Niteh kara kina* (*Viola kamtschadolorum* Beck. et Hult. [Chiri 1953:75]) (SD). Use hot water or rub the stomach with it. A person suffering from this illness is called *niteh mawko ahun aynu*, a person into whom the spirit of a tree branch has entered (*niteh* = tree branch; *maw* = spirit; *ahun* = to enter). The connection between this illness and the plant is not clear; the plant bears purple, rather than yellow, flowers.

V.8. *opičahse* (diarrhea) – 1. This is listed as a stomach illness, perhaps because of the pains accompanying diarrhea. 2. Either fresh or boiled *tuhku* (root of *Polygonum Weyrichii* Fr. Schm. [Chiri 1953:158]); its stalk is called *irure* (E). This root is a favorite ingredient for a category of dish called *čikaripe*, which is made from various cooked vegetables, often mixed with fish eggs but never with grown fish or the meat of land animals.

V.9. No Ainu term for this illness recorded – 1. Stomachaches accompanied by greenish stool. 2. (a) Plant called *siwkina* (a carrot family plant – *Angelica ursina* Benth. et Hook [Chiri 1953:59–60]). The grass is put into hot water and then used to rub the stomach. The plant is greenish blue, as is the stool in this condition. (b) Plant called *ičarapo* (*Anthriscus nemorosa* Spreng. [Chiri 1953:61]) (C). (c) Dried young plant of *tukara kina* (not identifiable) (E). Put in gruel and feed to the patient.

V.10. *okuy eskari* (the pubic region urine gets blocked) – 1. One suffers from pain in the lower abdomen and is unable to urinate. 2. (a) Dried *etetara* (SD; SA if the vulva or penis is also affected). *Etetara* is the name of the plant *Petasites japonicus* Miq. (Chiri 1953:17–18) in its early stage, that is, when it is still ball-shaped just after coming out of the ground in early spring. *Ruwe kina* refers to its stalk and *koriyam* to its leaves. It is a very valuable plant for the Ainu. The Ainu of northern Hokkaido and Sakhalin distinguish between male and female in this plant, although their identification is the opposite of the one in our biology. This reversal of the sexes is noted to be widespread (Chiri 1953:17). (b) *Kito* (leek – *Allium Victorialis* L. var. *platyphyllum* Makino [Chiri 1953:195]). A large amount is put into a dish (CE) or rubbed on the vulva or penis if they are affected (D). The *kito* is another important plant that the Ainu spend much time collecting and drying for year-round use. It is frequently used in cooking and also as an offering to the deities. The medicinal use of this plant is explained in terms of its potency; when one consumes a great deal of leek, one's urine and excrement take on its smell.

V.11. *čuhkes araka* (lower abdomen illness) – 1. Menstrual cramps in the lower abdomen. The term *čuhkes* is the same as *hopana* and means the lower abdomen. 2. Treatment is the same as for *okuy eskari*.

V.12. *takapes araka* – 1. A sudden attack of sharp pain at the sides of the lower abdomen. The pain is felt thrusting downward toward the legs, although confined to the sides of the lower abdomen. The term *takapes* refers to the part of a dogsled that connects the body of the sled to a rope pulled by dogs. The designation for this type of stomachache is based on the similarity, as perceived by the Ainu, between the pain and the pressure on the *takapes* when the dogs pull the sled; the rope gets twisted at the *takapes*, and its appearance suggests the nature of the pain. 2. A chip from a *takapes* (A). It is wrapped in a piece of material and then hung.

VI. *Nius araka*

This category of illnesses is characterized by sudden sharp pains at multiple loci.

VI.1. *ahsere nius araka* – 1. The pain is located at *ahsere*, the sides of the thorax just above the iliac crest.

VI.2. *niusi takuh araka* – 1. The pain is located at *takuh*, the shoulder.

VI.3. *rampokisikayus* – 1. The pain is located at the lower part of the chest (*rampoki* = the lower part of the chest; *sikay* = wooden nails; *us* = get stuck in abundance). This illness can be referred to as a *nius araka*.

A general cure for all *nius araka*. Someone must simulate the motion of pounding a wooden skewer, nail, or drill into the ailing part of the patient.

B. Skin abnormalities

I. *Huhpe*

Included in this section are only the subcategories of *huhpe* that are identified primarily as *huhpe*, rather than associated with the skin covering a particular part of the body; some of the latter subcategories have been presented in the section on body-part illnesses. In addition to those listed below, there are three other *huhpe*, for which no information other than the name is available: *esaman tasumpe* (otter pain), *erumu tasumpe* (mouse pain), and *ečisintamu tasumpe* (shrimp pain).

I.1. *keputenka huhpe* (bat boil) – 1. A boil causing pain similar to the cry of a bat. 2. A tuft of hair from a bat (P) or the dried meat of a bat (GA). The Ainu attach no special meaning to bats, which they classify as birds on the basis of their ability to fly.

I.2. *ni:na čikah huhpe* (woodpecker boil) – 1. A boil with pain like the pecking of a woodpecker. 2. Sawdust made by a woodpecker in a tree trunk (P). The sawdust is believed to hasten the process by which the boil forms a head that issues dark, bloody pus.

I.3. *uriri huhpe* (cormorant boil) – 1. A boil surrounded by a black ring. Except for a very small amount of blood, there is no discharge from this kind of boil, which distinguishes it from the *ikurupe huhpe* discussed below. 2. A few feathers from a cormorant (P).

I.4. *tomakači huhpe* (bee boil) – 1. A large boil with numerous small openings, resembling a beehive. 2. A beehive (SA).

I.5. *sumari huhpe* (fox boil) – 1. A boil with the reddish color of a fox. 2. Pieces of fox fur (P).

I.6. *ikurupe huhpe* (lamprey boil) – 1. The largest and most dangerous of all the boils. It can erupt on any part of the body and is very painful, as if a lamprey were digging into it. It is accompanied by a foul odor and a great deal of dark, bloody pus, which is somewhat foamy. It is also often referred to as *ikurupe tasumpe*. 2. (a) A rock in which a lamprey has made holes (GA). Use the part of the rock around the hole. (b) The dried head of a lamprey (SA).

I.7. *tekahka huhpe* (crab boil) - 1. A boil with the bright red color of a crab. It aches as if a crab were biting at it and is often itchy too. 2. A crab shell (GA).

I.8. *ahkoype huhpe* (octopus boil) - 1. A boil with the color of an octopus, that is, a darker red than that of a crab (see the crab boil discussed above). It is also accompanied by the discharge of much pus, and by pain simulating the sucking motion of an octopus. 2. (a) Slime from an octopus (P). (b) A dried octopus (SA).

I.9. *hewnay huhpe* (sea anemone boil) - 1. A boil as red as a *hewnay* (sea anemone - *Actiniaria* [Chiri 1962:135; Chiri records the pronunciation as *heunnay*]), accompanied by pus and a large swelling with a great deal of pain like the sting of a sea anemone. It can erupt on any part of the body. 2. Dried outer skin of a sea anemone (GA).

II. *Asispe*

II.1. *yoasis* - 1. The skin breaks out all over the body and itches. The Ainu were much concerned about this *asispe*, although they caught this illness only when visiting settlements on the east coast; it was not indigenous to the northwest coast. 2. (a) Crushed berries of *etuhka tureh* (*Skimmia repens* Nakai [Chiri 1953:104]) (P). The juice is rubbed into the skin. This is the most effective treatment. The name of the berries, *etuhka tureh*, means "crow berries" in Ainu; crows like these berries – hence the designation. These berries are available only in winter. (b) Dog's fat and sawdust (P). (c) The bark of the *kikini* tree (cherry tree – *Prunus Padus* L. [Chiri 1953:119]) (D). The decoction is used to wash the affected area but is not for the patient to drink. (d) Menstrual blood (P).

II.2. *keyčima* (meaning unclear) - 1. Formation of a number of scabs on the head that later leave permanent bald spots (head scabs?). It is taboo among the Ainu to ridicule a bald person or one who has bald spots caused by this illness because certain deities who reside in the mountains are portrayed as bald-headed (cf. Ohnuki-Tierney 1974a:98-9). 2. (a) *Tetara sinrus* (white lichen). This lichen is burned and the resultant charcoal, mixed with herring oil, is rubbed on the affected spots. The analogy is between the appearance of the infected spots on the head and the way this lichen grows on the ground. (b) Use a *mas* (sea gull), *kopeča* (duck), or *hočom* (a bird similar to the sea gull but not identifiable). After the meat of such a bird, which is treasured by the Ainu, is eaten, the skin of the breast with its thick layer of fat is put over the head like a cap, fastened by material tied under the jaw. The next day, the skin is removed and the head is washed. Then dog fat, bear fat, or herring oil is applied, and the head is covered with a leaf of *ruwe kina* (butterbur – *Petasites japonicus* Miq. [Chiri 1953:17-19]) tied with a piece of material to the head.

II.3. *imukina tasumpe* (*"imu:* grass" pains) – 1. Blisters covering the entire hand and the joints of the fingers. The hand would thus look like a plant called *imukina* (*Impatiens Noli-tangere* L. [Chiri 1953:81–92]). (The name of this plant comes from the resemblance between the behavioral disorder of a person suffering from *imu:*, details of which are presented in Appendix C, and the way the pods of this plant crack open when touched.) Much pain is involved. 2. Dried pods of this plant (GA).

C. Other illnesses

I. *Kemasinke* – 1. For the symptoms, see the text. 2. For both types of *kemasinke*, the following plants are used (D): *čiray kina* (*Botrychium robustum* Under. [Chiri 1953:243–4]); *seta kina* (*Arctium Lappa* L. [Chiri 1953:11]); *uyta:ni* (*Juniperus conferta* Parl. [Chiri 1953:232–3]); *utukoyni:* (*Malus baccata* Borkh. var. *mandshurica* Schneid. [Chiri 1953:116–17]); *ayusni:* (*Kalopanax ricinifolius* Miq. [Chiri 1953:70]); *umew kina* (*Conioselinum kamtschaticum* Rupr. [Chiri 1953:62–3]); *kamuy noya* (*Artemisia iwayomogi* Kitam. [Chiri 1953:8–9]); *učičiw* (*Lathyrus maritimus* Bigel. [Chiri 1953:106–7]). In the case of *učičiw*, the berries are used, and for *uyta:ni*, the leaves or branches with berries. For the rest, the leaves are used. Both *seta kina* and *čiray kina* may also be used in cooking and eaten by the patient. Also considered effective are berries called *katam* (cranberries – *Vaccinium Oxycocus* L. [Chiri 1953:54]), which are eaten raw.

II. *Čirayetehka araka* – 1. For the symptoms, see the text. 2. *Raykara kina*, a plant with numerous thorns (unidentifiable), is used. The leaves of this plant are put into a cloth bag and crushed. The joints are rubbed with juice from this plant as it runs from the bag. The entire body of the patient may be cleaned and rubbed with the leaves.

Beings and objects used in the cures of
habitual illnesses

As noted in the text, each of the illnesses has several alternative cures, making the number of healing techniques for the habitual illnesses extremely large. Table B.1 and the following list provide a general picture of the types of beings and objects used in these cures. (There are six illnesses for which I have no information regarding remedies.)

Following the Ainu classificatory schema, a snake is classified in the land animal category, because it is not singled out in a separate category. Likewise, a bat belongs to the category of birds. When sawdust made by a woodpecker is called for, I counted this cure in terms of the woodpecker, because in this case the symbolic value of the treatment derives from the woodpecker rather than from the sawdust per se. Likewise, the use of sawdust from a bear cage is listed in the bear section, and powder made from the hole that a lamprey has dug in a rock is tabulated under lamprey.

In the following listing, the first number in parentheses represents the number of parts of the same being used; the second number in paren-

Table B.1. *Frequency of the use of beings and objects in treatments*

Beings and objects	No. of species and items	Frequency of use
Terrestrial beings		
Land mammals and amphibians	10 (8.6)	36 (19.4)
Birds	5 (4.3)	12 (6.5)
Shellfish	10 (8.5)	17 (9.1)
Fish	7 (6.0)	14 (7.5)
Other water beings	6 (5.2)	13 (7.0)
Plants	61 (52.6)	74 (39.8)
Objects	16 (13.8)	19 (10.2)
Other (menstrual blood)	1 (0.9)	1 (0.5)
Total	116 (100)	186 (100)

Note: Numbers in parentheses are percentages.

theses represents the number of times that particular animal, plant, and so on is named in cures. For example, "bear (5) (5)" indicates that five different parts of the bear (in this case, part of the bear cage is counted as part of the bear, as noted above) are used for cures, but each part is used only once. In the case of a hare, however, three different parts are used four times in all, indicating that the use of one part appears twice.

Land and sea animals – ten species
bear (5)(5); dog (14)(14); musk deer (1)(1); seal (2)(2); hare (3)(4); mouse (2)(4); wildcat (1)(2); fox (2)(2); otter (1)(1); snake (1)(1)

Birds – five species
woodpecker (2)(2); seagull (1)(2); *hočom* (a marine bird related to the seagull) (1)(3); cormorant (1)(1); bat (3)(4)

Fish – seven species
sturgeon (2)(2); shark (2)(2); cod (3)(2); dace (2)(2); herring (1)(3); smelt (1)(1); *nanuwen čeh* (*Hemitripterus villosus* Pallas [Chiri 1962:16]) (1)(1)

Shellfish – ten species
kaywantahpo (unidentifiable) (2)(2); *ekaytama* (snail) (2)(3); *askiteh* (scallop) (1)(1); *ikayuhsey* (unidentifiable) (1)(1); *warawahsey* (unidentifiable) (1)(2); *sahpesey* (unidentifiable) (1)(1); *maspohka* (unidentifiable) (1)(1); *pipa* (*Unio margarritiferns* Linne [Chiri 1962:121]) (1)(1); *ninči* (a *Buccinum* shell [Chiri 1962:127]) (1)(2); *ka:nisuma* (abalone) (1)(1)

Other water beings – six species
octopus (2)(3); crab (2)(3); lamprey (3)(4); sea anemone (1)(1); sea cucumber (1)(1); *kero* (a *Placophora* animal [Chiri 1962:118]) (1)(1)

Plants – sixty-one species
For reasons of space, I have eliminated a complete list of the species of plants used in cures. I have the English common names for only some of them; I was able to identify many of them in Latin and Japanese, following Chiri (1953); for others I have only Ainu names.

Objects – sixteen items
With the exception of beach sand and wooden drill, the rest appear only once.
beach sand (2); wooden drill (2); ladle; lead bullet, red garment traded from the Japanese; potsherds; needle for making fishnets; cooking pot and black thread; wooden nail; red pebble; grime at the doorsill; umbilical cord; *takapes* (part connecting the sled to the rope); turquoise beads traded from the Santan; beehive; water from a mountain spring.

Imu:

A temporary psychobehavioral departure from the norm, referred to in Ainu as *imu:* is described in detail here. The meaning of this Ainu word is not clear (Chiri and Wada 1943:67; for other interpretations, see Uchimura, Akimoto, and Ishibashi 1938:9–10).

As discussed in Chapter 11, there is at least a partial overlap between the individuals who become shamans and those who are victims of *imu:*. I also noted in Chapter 11 the value of comparing the Sakhalin Ainu and the Hokkaido Ainu in regard to the three related phenomena of the role of shamans, the personality of shamans, and *imu:*. The relationship of these phenomena to the society and culture in which they occur provides clues to understand them. For this reason, I include in this appendix a fair amount of information about *imu:* among the Hokkaido Ainu. This information should also be helpful for non-Japanese, because despite brief references to *imu:* even in introductory textbooks in psychological anthropology (e.g., Barnouw 1973), details of findings are published primarily in Japanese.

Original systematic field investigations of *imu:* are very limited. They include the work by Jimbo (1901), Munro (1963), Suwa et al. (1963), and Uchimura, Akimoto, and Ishibashi (1938); some information is also published in Uchimura (1935). All of these investigations were carried out among the Hokkaido Ainu, except that of Uchimura, Akimoto, and Ishibashi, who included five Sakhalin Ainu. Munro, a medical doctor, examined twelve cases of *imu:*, but only a summary of his observations and four prayers have been published (Munro 1963, presented by Seligman). In the summer of 1977, I combed through all the manuscripts, photos, and letters written by and to the late Munro (Munro n.d.) that were originally entrusted by Munro's wife after his death to S. Fosco Maraini and now are housed at the Royal Anthropological Institute in London (cf. Munro 1963:xvii, 159), where Seligman describes the circumstances related to the field material left by Munro. I found very little information about *imu:* or illness in general.

The work by Uchimura, Akimoto, and Ishibashi is by far the most comprehensive. Their field investigation was carried out between 1931 and 1935 at various settlements in Hokkaido, where they examined eighty *imu:* cases. In addition, they collected descriptions of thirty-one cases. The report is thus based upon a total of 111 cases, among whom only 5 were Sakhalin Ainu. Seven photos of various *imu:* conditions and seven additional pictures of individuals with *imu:* but not during seizures are also included in the publication. These photos were taken when the investigators intentionally created an *imu:* condition in the individuals for the purpose of observing and photographing it – a questionable field method.

The following description is based upon nine cases of Sakhalin Ainu *imu:* described to me by my informants. Because the information pertains to the Sakhalin Ainu of the northwest coast, it is referred to as the Sakhalin Ainu or Sakhalin Ainu *imu:*, unless otherwise specified. The information on Hokkaido Ainu *imu:* comes primarily from Uchimura, Akimoto, and Ishibashi (1938), although pertinent information from other sources is also included.

The individuals with an *imu:* seizure are called *imu: aynu* (*aynu* = human beings) or *imu: kuru* (*kuru* = person). The Sakhalin Ainu dealt with in this book do not regard *imu:* as an illness. Thus neither a cause nor a cure is sought for *imu:*. Among other Sakhalin Ainu, however, *imu:* is said to be caused by possession by a spirit called *imu: kamuy* (*kamuy* = deity) (K. Wada 1964:112). The Niputani Ainu of Hokkaido under Munro's investigation also link *imu:* with possession by a snake. Thus an *imu:* victim would usually consult a shaman, and "a frequent diagnosis is that the illness is due to possession by an evil snake spirit" (Munro 1963:161). It is somewhat unclear whether *imu:* is identified as an illness by the Niputani Ainu or was so called by Munro himself.

Although the Sakhalin Ainu do not regard *imu:* as an illness, they do take much interest in the condition, are vividly aware of who has it, and remember the patterned behavior of each *imu:* Ainu during his or her seizure. They often make fun of them in a good-natured way and encourage a person to be seized or one already seized to carry out acts that are even dangerous to others, as the cases presented at the end of this appendix illustrate. The Hokkaido Ainu investigated by Uchimura, Akimoto, and Ishibashi are also reported not to regard *imu:* as an illness and to make fun of the individuals who have it (1938:10). This attitude is thus similar to the Eskimo attitude toward *pibloktoq*, which they regard as a natural ailment, like a broken limb, without assigning a supernatural agent to it; they too attach no stigma to the person afflicted with *pibloktoq* (Wallace 1972:374, 379).

The Sakhalin Ainu see two distinct categories of *imu:*. The first category involves a mild state in which an individual becomes surprised, but not necessarily frightened, and mumbles meaningless sounds. Each *imu:* Ainu, when surprised, almost always utters the same nonsensical phrases, such as "Ačikapahse," which has no meaning in Ainu. While in the field, I once stood up, bumped my head on a bare light bulb hanging from the ceiling, and uttered an English exclamation, "Oops." Those Ainu present thought that I was experiencing an *imu:* state, because they had never heard the expression, which was of course meaningless in either Ainu or Japanese. In fact, this incident precipitated a series of discussions on *imu:* that provided rich ethnographic information. The manner in which an *imu: aynu* reacts to a mild shock is seen as analogous to the way in which a seed pod of a certain plant snaps open and expels the seeds; this plant has been identified by Chiri (1953:81) as *Impatiens Noli-tangere* L. The plant is thus named *imu: kina* (*kina* = grass in Ainu). Although individuals with an *imu:* tendency seem to become *imu:* whenever they are surprised, one informant stated that she became more susceptible when she was tired.

The second category of *imu:* is a more severe state during which the individual loses touch with reality and has no self-control. The Sakhalin Ainu refer to these individuals "who do *imu:* in a grand way" as *sikutu* and terminologically distinguish them from the milder *imu:* Ainu. Each individual exhibits a definite pattern during the *imu:* seizure (see the three cases described at the end of this appendix). According to B. Wada (1956:45), the Sakhalin Ainu *imu:* is characterized by manifested automatic obedience – doing what one is told to do. In the samples listed by Uchimura, Akimoto, and Ishibashi (1938), the compulsive imitation of what one observes (echopraxia) and compulsive imitation of what one hears (echolalia) are also noted.

The symptoms of the Hokkaido Ainu *imu:* are more varied. According to B. Wada (1956:45), the Hokkaido Ainu *imu:* is characterized by negative automatic obedience, thus contrasting sharply to the Sakhalin Ainu *imu:*. Although Uchimura, Akimoto, and Ishibashi (1938:13) report one case of manifested automatic obedience among their Hokkaido Ainu samples, their description of symptoms is so incomplete that it is hard to affirm or deny Wada's statement conclusively. Other symptoms include echolalia and echopraxia, as well as copropraxia and coprolalia – involuntary utterances or behavior that is obscene or sexual. Chiri's examples of coprolalia include "A filthy looking person had diarrhea," or "Let your penis have a drink" (Chiri 1952:56; 1953:84-5). Uchimura, Akimoto, Ishibashi (1938:26) report that coprolalia and copropraxia take place usually at a drinking session. (For further discussion of symptoms, see Tsuboi 1889:457-8; Uchimura, Akimoto, and Ishibashi 1938:19-28; K. Wada 1965b:264-5; Winiarz and Wielawski 1936:184.)

In regard to the precipitating factor or stimulus, there is a marked difference between the Sakhalin Ainu and the Hokkaido Ainu. In the milder form of *imu:* for the Sakhalin Ainu, the stimulus seems to be a mild but unexpected shock caused by various phenomena and objects. In the more severe *imu:*, sometimes a verbal suggestion alone suffices to bring on the *imu:* state. For example, a male (Case 2 below) who initially became an *imu:* at the sight of a writhing reindeer that he had shot immediately entered this state when someone asked, "What happened to the reindeer you shot?" In contrast, the precipitating factor for the Hokkaido Ainu *imu:* almost always seems to be the sight of a snake or the Ainu word for snake, that is, *tokoni*. Thus, for all of the seventy-seven Hokkaido Ainu *imu:* individuals listed in Table 1 by Uchimura, Akimoto, and Ishibashi (1938:10–13), the stimulus was hearing the word *tokoni* or seeing a snake, a toy snake, or a picture of a snake. Uchimura, Akimoto, and Ishibashi (1938:28, 46) report a case of a male Hokkaido Ainu who talked about a snake by referring to it as "a long worm" or "an abominable worm" without falling into an *imu:* state until one of the investigators asked if he meant *tokoni*, using the Ainu term for snake, upon which he became seized with *imu:*. As noted in the text, other items that serve as a stimulus to some Hokkaido Ainu include a frog, an octopus, a crab, a metal washing pan introduced by the Japanese, and neon signs that an Ainu saw while visiting Tokyo (Uchimura, Akimoto, and Ishibashi 1938:29).

The Sakhalin Ainu do not regard *imu:* as sex linked. However, out of nine cases described to me, seven are women. On the other hand, the two males had severe cases of *imu:*. This situation again contrasts to that of the Hokkaido Ainu, among whom Uchimura, Akimoto, and Ishibashi (1938:29) found no male *imu:* Ainu, although they do refer to other scholars' observations that indicate very infrequent cases in the past. Jimbo (1901:1) also states that *imu:* afflicts only women. It should be pointed out that one of the two males in my sample had originally come from Hokkaido when he was young, perhaps before his first seizure of *imu:*. Thus it seems that although *imu:* affects some men, especially in Sakhalin, it affects women with a much higher frequency in any Ainu group.

Those who suffer from *imu:* are elderly. In fact, the mental picture that the Sakhalin Ainu have is that of individuals in their late fifties or sixties. When individual *imu:* Ainu were examined, however, some seemed to have begun their seizures as early as their forties. Among the Hokkaido Ainu at Hidaka, out of forty-five cases seventeen were in their fifties, fourteen were in their forties, and ten were in their sixties, although the onset of *imu:* is predominantly in the twenties and thirties (Uchimura, Akimoto, and Ishibashi 1938:33). According to Jimbo (1901:7–8), out of twelve individuals under his investigation, three experienced the first seizure in their teens. Evaluation of Jimbo's information is somewhat difficult because his investigation is fairly limited in scale and depth.

My data are too inconclusive to provide meaningful speculation about the percentage of *imu:* in the total population of the northwest coast of southern Sakhalin. The investigation by Uchimura, Akimoto, and Ishibashi (1938:15) shows the highest frequency of 3.91% at the Piratori settlement in the Hidaka district, 2% elsewhere in the Hidaka area, and less than 1% outside of the Hidaka area of Hokkaido. The Hidaka district has the highest density of Ainu population in Hokkaido, and its Piratori settlement is referred to as the Ainu capital because of its large Ainu population and strong retention of the Ainu way of life in the community.

As the highest frequency of *imu:* at the Piratori settlement suggests, there seems to be a definite correlation between frequency of occurrence and the degree of integrity of the Ainu way of life. The retention of the Ainu way is often facilitated by the great distance of the settlement from a Japanese city, as in the case of the Piratori settlement (Kumasaka 1964; Uchimura, Akimoto, Ishibashi 1938:13–14). As a corollary, with the rapid process of Ainu acculturation into the Japanese way of life, *imu:* is quickly disappearing, at least in its classical form, just as in the case of *latah* and *amok.* When Suwa and his colleagues carried out an investigation in 1958, they located only four *imu:* Ainu in the Niputani settlement in the Piratori district (Suwa et al. 1963).

Although not included in the text, multiple etiology, as suggested by Foulks (1972) as an explanation for the polar Eskimo *pibloktoq*, is another useful tool of interpretation. In particular, a biochemical basis of psychological disorders such as calcium deficiency (Foulks 1972; Wallace 1972) should be taken into consideration. In the case of *imu:* studies, however, no intensive nutritional, environmental, and psychiatric studies have been made so that we can engage in a meaningful discussion of *imu:* etiology along this line.

The following three cases illustrate the *imu:* state among the Sakhalin Ainu. Six additional cases of *imu:* described to me by the Sakhalin Ainu will not be presented here because information about them does not contradict the basic pattern of *imu:* behavior as seen in these three cases.

Case 1: The pattern of *imu:* behavior exhibited by this middle-age woman was dangerous; she attempted to stab people with a knife or threw objects at them. At the time of the trout run in spring, people from nearby settlements annually came to the Hurooči settlement to engage jointly in trout fishing and drying, the latter for winter supply. As observed by my informant, Husko, when she was still small, a nephew of this woman who was known to like to joke once asked her, "Aunt, aunt, why don't you stab me with your knife?" This woman, who was cleaning trout with a knife, fell into an *imu:* state and threw her knife at him. The knife barely missed this young man and landed on the ground instead. She then realized what she had done and scolded the nephew for inciting this reaction. Others present also reprimanded him for his unwise act. During another trout fishing/cleaning session, other women who were working next to this woman jokingly told her to stab the dogs that were eating the trout they had just cleaned. She again fell into an *imu:* state and started to stab the dogs. This woman usually came out of *imu:* when a person, or a dog in the second instance, became injured and screamed. She always regained consciousness with a loud shout.

Case 2: During a reindeer hunting trip a man at the Čiray Yohnay settlement shot a reindeer, which fell to the ground and writhed in agony. At this sight he was seized with *imu:* for the first time and started to imitate the motion of the animal, whereupon other men in the group laughed heartily. Ever since this incident, whenever someone purposely asked him how this reindeer behaved, he went into an *imu:* state and imitated the writhing motion on the ground. He usually regained consciousness after a few minutes and became angry with the one who had incited him, at times throwing things at the person, but not while he was in an *imu:* state.

This man also exhibited another pattern of *imu:* behavior that involved eating raw fish. After he had finished his share, if someone told him to look at those who were still eating, he would grab a fish bone and imitate the motion of eating. As noted in the text, food for the Ainu means food cooked for a long time; raw animal meat is abhorred, although raw fish was eaten in the recent past, perhaps as a result of Japanese influence.

Case 3: This middle-age woman had once traveled to the east coast of southern Sakhalin and saw Japanese domestic cats. Traditionally the Ainu never kept cats as pets and dreaded wild cats. After seeing the domestic animals for the first time, this woman became seized with *imu:* whenever someone asked what the cats did on the east coast. She would then imitate not only the crying of cats but also their behavior during mating season. When people harshly scolded her, she emerged from the *imu:* state with a loud shout.

Biological, cultural, and linguistic identity of the Ainu

The problem of Ainu identity can be approached in several different ways. Here I present the endeavors of scholars in various fields, grouping them in three categories: early scholars who attempted to solve the problem from the standpoint of Ainu relationships to the aboriginal populations of the Japanese archipelago; those who attempted to identify the Ainu in terms of racial classification; and those who attempted to relate Ainu cultural and biological characteristics to those populations represented in each of the archaeological stages on the Japanese archipelago.

During the second half of the nineteenth century, Japanese scholars were concerned with identifying the aboriginal population of the Japanese archipelago. John Milne was the first to claim in 1882 that the aboriginal population was not the Ainu but the *koroppokuru* – the "small people" who were reported to appear in the Ainu oral traditions as early as in 1808 in *Watarishima Hikki (Report on Hokkaido)*. S. Tsuboi advanced this theory forcefully. He argued that the *koroppokuru* were the Stone Age people of the Japanese archipelago, occupying Honshu (the Japanese main island) as well as Hokkaido and manufacturing pottery and stone implements. He thought that the Ainu, who did not have such technological knowledge, later moved into the Japanese archipelago and drove the *koroppokuru* out of their original habitat. He believed that the latter were driven north through the Kuriles, Kamchatka to Greenland, and that the present-day Eskimo are derived from this *koroppokuru* population (this paragraph in Serizawa 1963:89–91).

Tsuboi's theory was challenged by R. Koganei, who claimed in 1893 that the Ainu were the true aborigines of the Japanese archipelago. He argued that they were later pushed north by the ancestors of the historic Japanese, who had come to the island from the Asian continent. He based this argument on the similarity of the skeletal material of the Jomon people to that of the recent Ainu and its dissimilarity to the historic Japanese (in Hasebe 1956:101–2; Serizawa 1963:91–2).

The *koroppokuru* theory of Tsuboi was overthrown for good, however, by his student, R. Torii, whom Tsuboi sent to the northern Kuriles and Kamchatka in 1899. Torii found that until recently the Kurile Ainu had been using bone and stone implements, pits, and Naiji pottery. This pottery is characterized by handles attached to the interior surface of a pot; it had been found at many archaeological sites. Torii therefore argued that the *koroppokuru* were the Ainu and that the Hokkaido Ainu had once been at the same technological stage, although the introduction of metal implements from the neighboring peoples had eliminated the use of pottery, and they eventually forgot that they had once used it (Torii 1903:177–200; 1919:280–9).

K. Kiyono suggested a third major theory. He postulated that the aborigines of the Japanese archipelago, of unknown origin, were the population from which both the recent Ainu and the historic Japanese were derived. He believed that the Ainu resulted from a mixture of the aboriginal population and the people who later migrated to the islands from northeastern Siberia, whereas the historic Japanese are a mixture of the aborigines and the people who later came from the south (Kiyono 1925:5–11). E. Morse held a similar opinion (in Serizawa 1963:95).

K. Hasebe, on the other hand, had argued for a long time that the ancestors of the historic Japanese are the Jomon people, who came from south China to Kyushu and then moved north on the Japanese islands either at the end of the diluvial epoch or the beginning of the alluvial epoch, that is, at the end or right after the Würm, whereas the ancestors of the Ainu came from the north to Hokkaido (Hasebe 1956:101–5). (For details of opinions of early Japanese scholars, see Kiyono 1949:27–65 and Serizawa 1963:89–100.)

The second approach to the problem of Ainu identity is to determine it primarily on the basis of the biological characteristics of both the living Ainu and the skeletal material identified as that of the recent Ainu because of burial goods and other evidence. Some of the early scholars who pursued this type of investigation assigned a racial classification – an approach that often obscures the complex manner in which the distribution of genes cross-cuts the rigid racial label.

Scholars' opinions on this matter have always been sharply divided. It was A. S. Bickmore who first proposed that the Ainu belonged to the Caucasoid race on the basis of their distinct physical characteristics such as widely separated eyes, small cheekbones, and abundant beard growth (Bickmore 1868, cited in Levin 1963:266). This hypothesis was supported by E. Baelz (1883), who claimed that the Ainu were derived from the ancient Caucasoid population of eastern Asia, and also by A. C. Haddon (1925:102–3), G. Montandon (1928–1937), and Von Eickstedt (1934) (Montandon and Von Eickstedt, cited in Levin 1963:267–9).

Other early scholars, such as M. Dobrotvorskiy (1870:26; 1876:321) and Dönitz (1874) (both cited in Levin 1963:266), identified the Ainu as a Mongoloid population. Still others, such as D. N. Anuchin and L. I.

Shrenk, pointed out the diversity in physical types within the Ainu population and concluded that some showed European features whereas others showed more Mongoloid features (in Levin 1963:266–7).

The Ainu racial affiliation with the Australo-Oceanic peoples was first proposed by Vivien de Saint-Martin (in Levin 1963:269). Other early proponents of this theory include A. Tarenetzkiy (1890:4), Giuffrida-Ruggeri (1912), J. M. Dixon (1923) (all cited in Levin 1963:269–70), and R. Koganei (1927). L. Sternberg pushed this theory forcefully by bringing in additional cultural, linguistic, and archaeological data (Sternberg 1929; also referred to in Levin 1963:271–3). Pilsudski likewise supported this theory with folklore and other ethnographic data that he considered as proof of the southern origin of the Ainu (Pilsudski 1911:165–6, 228–9). An Ainu affiliation with the Australo-Oceanic peoples still has a strong hold on Soviet scholars. After reviewing existing theories, Levin concludes that despite insufficient facts to solve the problem, "the idea of genetic kinship of the Ainus and types of the Equatorial racial stem seems to agree best with the present state of our knowledge" (Levin 1963:270).

Recent studies, especially in Japan and the United States, tend to regard Asiatic or Paleo-Mongoloid (ancient Mongoloid) affinity as more convincing. Although earlier serological studies are available (Ninomiya 1925, Grove 1926, Furuhata 1941 – all cited in Kobayashi 1952:93–5 – and Kobayashi 1952), Spuhler's more recent work (1966) is most significant in this respect. He systematically compared ten genetic systems of Hidaka Ainu of Hokkaido with those of other populations in order to determine the phyletic position of the Ainu. He concluded that the Ainu have a closer phyletic affinity with their geographical neighbors in northeastern Asia, especially the Japanese, Chinese, Koreans, and possibly certain peoples of northeastern Siberia, than with the peoples of either Europe or Australasia (Spuhler 1966). Thus, he sees the Ainu affinity as being closest to the Mongoloid peoples in the Far East. Omoto's serological analysis (1974) too presents the same interpretation.

A most comprehensive report, published recently in English, on the Ainu morphological and genetic characteristics and physiological functions is found in Watanabe, Kondo, and Matsunaga, eds. (1975:225–333). In this publication, Hanihara, Masuda, Tanaka, and Tamada (1975:256–62) present an interpretation that strongly favors the derivation of the Ainu from Mongoloid stock and a possible common ancestry with neighboring populations such as the Japanese, Eskimos, and native Americans. These scholars explain that the differences in physical characteristics between the Ainu and their Mongoloid neighbors are not necessarily indicators of a certain racial stock but are archaic characteristics of human populations. According to them, the arctic Mongoloids acquired their highly adaptive characteristics to cold during the maximum stage of the last glaciation. The Ainu, whose abundant body hair and lack of body fat are not favorable characteristics in an extremely cold climate, may have been derived from the same racial stock as the neighboring peoples, but the others changed in their physical characteristics through climatic adaptation, whereas the Ainu did not. A major problem in the studies of Ainu biological characteristics has been that with a long history of inter-marriage between the Ainu and other populations, especially. the Japanese, it has been difficult to isolate and identify "pure" Ainu biologi-cal characteristics.

The third approach to the problem of Ainu identity and their relation-ship with other peoples is to trace the Ainu, as a genetic population as well as a culture, step by step through archaeological stages on the Japanese archipelago. Let me first outline the major interpretations and then present those of representative scholars. As shown in Table D.1, there are significant differences between the prehistory of the main island (Honshu), where agriculture was introduced, and that of Hokkaido and Sakhalin, where the heart of the Ainu homeland is located. The Hokkaido and Sakhalin archaeological sequence, shown in the right-hand column of Table D.1, is established primarily on the basis of Hokkaido archaeology, because due to the political history of Sakhalin, we have little information about Sakhalin prehistory. Many scholars believe that southern Sakhalin was basically in the cultural sphere of Hokkaido, with some significant influences from the Asian continent (Yoshizaki 1963:145).

As shown in Table D.1, the major portions of the islands were first occupied, possibly around 30,000 B.C., by a nonsedentary hunting-gathering people, or more likely peoples in small scattered settlements. Unless there was a migration of people around 10,000 B.C., which seems unlikely, these inhabitants became the earliest known pottery makers in the world, although they remained ignorant of agriculture for a long time. Because their pottery had *jomon* or cord-marking designs, they are called the Jomon people. By 300 B.C., but possibly as early as 600 B.C., rice agriculture was introduced to the southwestern part of the main island, perhaps by way of the Korean peninsula, with a possible origin in southeast Asia. We are not sure whether the agricultural technique alone was intro-duced or whether it was accompanied by migration of people. In either case, at its inception rice agriculture penetrated neither into the north-eastern half of the main island nor into Hokkaido and Sakhalin. The cold climate in the latter two areas and some cultural factors that were not receptive to a shift of the economic base to agriculture are generally held to be responsible for the nonpenetration of agriculture to these areas. In any event, in the areas where agriculture was introduced, the life of the people started to change dramatically, shifting to denser and permanent settlements, which eventually led to the formation of states and the

Table D.1. *The Ainu and archaeological stages on the Japanese archipelago*

	Main island		Hokkaido and Sakhalin
30,000–10,000 B.C.	Preceramic culture (hunting and gathering)	20,000–5000 B.C.	Preceramic culture (hunting and gathering)
10,000–300 B.C.	Jomon ceramic culture (hunting and gathering)	5000–100 B.C.	Jomon ceramic culture (hunting and gathering)
300 B.C.–A.D. 300	Yayoi culture (agriculture)	100 B.C.–A.D. 700–800	Post-Jomon culture (hunting and gathering; metal use)
A.D. 300–500	Kohun period (state formation)		
A.D. 500–present	Historic period–Japanese nation	A.D. 800–1300	Satsumon culture (hunting and gathering; pit dwelling; hearth; cooking fire; ironware) (Okhotsk culture)[a]
		A.D. 1300–present	Historic Ainu

[a] The Okhotsk culture, which appeared and disappeared rather suddenly and enigmatically, is considered by many scholars as an intrusive culture. It overlaps with the Satsumon culture in terms of chronological period, but its geographic distribution was confined to the coastal areas of Hokkaido and Sakhalin facing the Okhotsk Sea (cf. Beru and Chard 1964).

Japanese nation. The life to the north, on the other hand, continued to be based upon the hunting and gathering of natural resources from land and water.

The introduction of metal goods around 100 B.C. into these nonagricultural areas, however, changed the lives of the people. This change is reflected archaeologically as a new period called Post-Jomon. Some elements in this culture are suggestive of Ainu affinity, although not conclusively. For example, the Post-Jomon people used a bear motif in decorations on pottery and bone implements. Skeletal material at some Post-Jomon sites is interpreted to show a close affinity to the Ainu in northeastern Hokkaido. Around A.D. 700–800, this Post-Jomon culture developed into what is called the Satsumon culture, which shows more striking resemblances to Ainu culture (Okada 1950:126, 133). Similarities between the two cultures include the use of semisubterranean pits, hearths, cooking fires, and mode of burial, as well as the aforementioned Naiji pottery. We have thus been able to trace the Ainu through the archaeological sequence on Hokkaido up to the Post-Jomon period. In other words, there is an indication that all these peoples (Post-Jomon, Satsumon, and Ainu) may represent one population whose subsistence economy consisted of hunting and fishing along the coasts and in rivers and lakes (for further details, see Fujimoto 1971; Sakurai 1967).

Because the Jomon culture precedes the Post-Jomon culture, it is tempting to assume that the Ainu should have derived ultimately from at least a segment of the former Jomon population. Unfortunately, at this moment the link between the Post-Jomon and the Jomon remains tenuous. Therefore, the relation of Ainu to Jomon culture too remains a promising hypothesis.

Returning to the archaeological developments on the main island, there is little doubt among scholars of Japanese prehistory that a continuity in culture, physical type, and language may be traced from the beginning of the agricultural (Yayoi) period to the present. In other words, scholars agree that the Yayoi agricultural population in southwestern Japan was ancestral to the present-day Japanese. The relation of the Yayoi population to that of the Jomon, however, remains somewhat uncertain.

Thus we see a parallel both in Hokkaido and Honshu archaeology. The relationship between the Post-Jomon and the Jomon in Hokkaido and the relationship between the Yayoi and the Jomon on Honshu both remain tenuous. Theoretically, there are four possibilities for the identity of the Jomon people: they are the ancestors of the Ainu, of the Yayoi population and hence of the contemporary Japanese, both, or neither. The three-way comparison of the Ainu, Japanese, and Jomon remains is not an easy task, because scholars are increasingly aware that the Jomon population was not monolithic.

In order to get to the finer points in the issue, let me now introduce interpretations of a few scholars. A significant contribution to the study of the Ainu in recent years resulted from the excavations in 1959 at the Onkoromanai site at the northern tip of Hokkaido and the Bozuyama site near Sapporo. These excavations were carried out by the Department of Cultural Anthropology of the University of Tokyo. An analysis of the skeletal material has been published by Yamaguchi (1961, 1963a, 1963b). Using the shape distance method of Penrose, Yamaguchi compared the five Post-Joman skeletons at the Onkoromanai site and the six skeletons at the Bozuyama site with skeletons from other sites. The skeletons compared included: the Sakhalin Ainu, the Hokkaido Ainu, the Kurile Ainu, the Yakumo Ainu, Japanese of the Hokuriku region, and the Tsukumo Shell Mound (Jomon) people. Yamaguchi concludes that the Onkoromanai type of the Post-Jomon population shows the closest affinity to the Ainu in northeastern Hokkaido and those on the Kuriles, the Jomon people on the Japanese mainland, and the Cro-Magnon of western Siberia, whereas they are furthest away from the Mongoloid peoples of northeast Asia. The Sakhalin Ainu, the Yakumo Ainu, and the recent Japanese are intermediate between these two groups. The Onkoromanai people are clearly different from the Okhotsk people. Although they possess characteristics of both the recent Ainu and the Jomon people on the mainland, the Ainu characteristics are slightly more dominant. Thus, Yamaguchi believes that the carriers of the Post-Jomon culture at these sites were the ancestors of the recent Ainu. Although Yamaguchi's conclusions are highly significant, they are based on the analysis of a limited number of skeletons, and we may infer that they are still applicable only to the Onkoromanai people. Nevertheless, it suggests that the Post-Jomon culture on Hokkaido was carried by the ancestral population of recent Ainu and that there is a possible linkage between the Jomon people and the ancestors of the Ainu. Yamaguchi's opinion carried weight not only among Japanese scholars but also among Western authorities such as W. W. Howells and C. S. Chard.

Howells published the result of his own discriminant analysis of Japanese and Ainu crania in 1966 (Howells 1966). His material for analysis included the Ainu, recent Japanese, Japanese during the Kamakura period (the fourteenth century), Yayoi people, and Jomon people (Howells 1966:28). He concludes that the Ainu are one surviving population who were the carriers of the Jomon culture. The historic Japanese populations, except those of the Kamakura period, are clearly different from both the Ainu and Jomon populations, and they derive from the populations who arrived as immigrants in western Japan with the agricultural Yayoi culture at the beginning of the Yayoi period (Howells 1966:3, 38).

A conclusion based on dental evidence by C. Turner (1976) is also concordant. Working closely with Hanihara, who specializes in Ainu dentition, Turner sees a correlation between the Ainu and the prehistoric Jomon people, on the one hand, and the ancient Chinese and modern Japanese, on the other. In addition, his analysis indicates that "the dentition of the Anyang Chinese and the Jomon are similar enough to conclude that both populations were derived from an earlier proto-Mongoloid gene pool in eastern Asia" (Turner 1976:913).

Chard believes that the Ainu represent a genetic remnant and refers to Howells's opinions just discussed. He further thinks that like other so-called genetic remnants of the world, the Ainu probably have neither a distinctive culture nor a language of their own, although they may possibly retain a few older beliefs (Chard 1967).

M. Yoshizaki expounded his view in 1962 that the ancestors of the Ainu came from the general region of the maritime provinces of the Soviet Union, Mongolia, and north China in successive small waves. These areas on the Asian continent have the same ecological conditions as northern Japan. He thinks that the ancestral population of the historic Japanese, on the other hand, came from the area of central and south China to Kyushu and later moved north. Yoshizaki believes that the ancestral populations of both groups were already present at the beginning of the Jomon period and intermixed, engaging in similar cultural activities during the Jomon period. A sharp distinction between these two groups started to form with the introduction of the Yayoi agricultural culture from the Asian continent. The Yayoi agricultural technique rapidly penetrated the warm southern areas of the Japanese archipelago, changing the ecological basis of the population in this area from the gathering economy of the Jomon period to food production. The agricultural techniques, however, did not reach the northern parts of Japan inhabited by the ancestral population of the Ainu, who retained a gathering economy until recently. The difference in the ecological conditions that began in the Yayoi period increased the difference between these two populations, which had separate origins in the first place (Yoshizaki 1962).

To recapitulate, an interpretation of Ainu identity that seems to be receiving increasing support among scholars is that the Ainu are the descendants of one segment of the Jomon population. However, opinions among scholars at present are too varied to suggest any type of consensus.

The genetic affiliation of the Ainu language too has been discussed by a number of scholars, such as Austerlitz (1970), Hattori (1956), Kindaichi (1960:267), Ono (1966:36–50, 206), and Street (1962). In his suggestion for the reconstruction of the Proto-North-Asiatic, Street speculates that Korean, Japanese, and Ainu are most likely to be found interrelatable, and that the three may be the descendants of a possible sister language of the Proto-Altaic (Street 1962:94–5).

Hattori applied the lexicostatistical method to a comparison of the Japanese and Ainu languages (Hattori 1956). He concluded that the Japanese and Ainu are of the same stock, but that they separated around 7,000–10,000 B.P. (Hattori 1956:130). He also considers the present Japanese language to be derived from the language of the Yayoi people who migrated to the Japanese islands and replaced the Jomon people, who, he believes, spoke a different language (Hattori 1956:121–2).

Hattori's postulated linkage between the Japanese and Ainu languages may suggest a different interpretation of the relationship of the two peoples and cultures from that of Howells and Chard. However, the language of a people may take a different course from that of the people and other aspects of their culture; for example, there have been cases in which a people replaced their own language with another. Hence, the ethnic relationships of the Japanese and the Ainu cannot be conclusively established on the basis of language alone. More importantly, lexicostatistics as a method has too much built-in uncertainty and arbitrariness. Because it is based on assumptions that have not been well tested, the meaning of the separation date is still very questionable (Bergsland and Vogt 1962, and comments following the article; Hymes 1960:32–3).

However, it should be noted that Hattori's proposed date for the separation of the Ainu and Japanese languages coincides roughly with the proposed date of the beginning of the Jomon period at about 9,000 B.P. (For a controversy over the Jomon dating, see T. Kobayashi, ed., 1977:192–3.)

Appendix E

The history of the Sakhalin Ainu

Although documented history does not trace the Sakhalin Ainu to the earliest date of their presence on the island of Sakhalin, it is possible, as noted in the text, that they settled there as early as the first millennium A.D. and definitely were there by the thirteenth century. They had long been in contact with the so-called native populations both on Sakhalin and along the Amur River, such as the Gilyaks primarily in the western area of northern Sakhalin, the Oroks primarily in the east, and various other less numerous peoples.

The history of these native populations had been largely one of intensive attempts at colonization by the neighboring populations – the Chinese, Russians, and Japanese. Although some scholars, especially those in the Soviet Union, seem to hold a view that the Russians were the first to reach Sakhalin, many others think that it was the Chinese, whose influence reached the island probably by the first millennium A.D. and was intensified during the thirteenth century, when northern Sakhalin submitted to Mongol suzerainty after the Mongol conquest of China. The period between 1263 and 1320 saw Mongol colonization and the "pacification" of the Gilyaks and the Ainu. The Sakhalin Ainu fought valiantly until 1308, when they too finally submitted to the sovereignty of the Yuan dynasty, the Mongolian dynasty that ruled China, to whom the Ainu started to pay tribute. The tribute system, together with trade with other peoples along the way, merged with the Japanese–Hokkaido Ainu trade during the fifteenth century. As a result, Japanese ironware reached the Manchus, and, conversely, Chinese brocade and cotton made their way to Osaka in western Japan.

This trade reached its height during the eighteenth century. During this period, the Manchus, who had conquered the Chinese, coerced all the natives along the Amur and on Sakhalin in sending tribute missions to Manchu posts on the Amur River. The Sakhalin Ainu presented the Manchus with fur, especially marten, and eagle feathers, dried fish, and other products of their own, as well as Japanese ironware. In return they received from the Manchus brocade, beads, cotton material, pipes, and needles, some of which they traded to the Japanese. The Ainu received

213

from the Japanese rice, rice wine, tobacco, and ironware. The trade was carried out in stages involving all the native populations in the area, many of whom served as middlemen. Not only the Manchus and Japanese took advantage of the Ainu in this trade; even the other peoples who acted as middlemen exploited them. The Gilyaks were said to have been especially cruel to the Ainu, enslaving those who failed to pay their debts. (For details of the trade, see Harrison 1954; Takakura 1939.)

Toward the end of the eighteenth century, Manchu control over Sakhalin dwindled rapidly, and at the beginning of the nineteenth century the tribute system was discontinued. By then, however, both the Japanese and the Russians were rapidly approaching Sakhalin, each racing to take political control of the island and monopolize its natural resources. There followed a century and a half of territorial conflict between the two countries, and the fate of the Sakhalin Ainu fell under the control of these two nations.

To its credit, however, in 1809 the Japanese government paid all the debts that the Ainu owed to others who served as middlemen in the trade system and assumed all responsibility for the Ainu. The Japanese government was motivated by self-interest. It resorted to this action believing that the exploitation of the Ainu by others would lead to Manchu control, because these middlemen were supposedly official Manchu government representatives whose duty it was to collect tribute. At any rate, the action by the Japanese government alleviated the Ainu situation considerably.

With the establishment of the Meiji government in Japan in 1868, the impact of the Japanese on the Ainu was intensified. Waves of Japanese immigrants were sent to southern Sakhalin to exploit its resources. The Ainu came under Russian control in 1875 when southern Sakhalin was taken by Russia, only to be regained by the Japanese in 1905. During these decades, there were numerous events with devastating effects upon the Ainu and their way of life. In particular, the move between 1912 and 1914 by the Japanese government to place the Ainu on reservations uprooted the Sakhalin Ainu, and their way of life, needless to say, was drastically altered as a result. With the conclusion of World War II, southern Sakhalin again was reclaimed by the Soviet Union, and most of the Ainu were resettled in Hokkaido. (Sakhalin north of 50°N had remained under Soviet control all this time.)

What are the effects of these major events in history upon the lives of the Sakhalin Ainu of the northwest coast? The northwest coast of southern Sakhalin referred to in this book includes an area between Rayčiska and the former Russo-Japanese border (see Figure E.1). Situated to the south of the Gilyak territory in northern Sakhalin, the Ainu in the northernmost

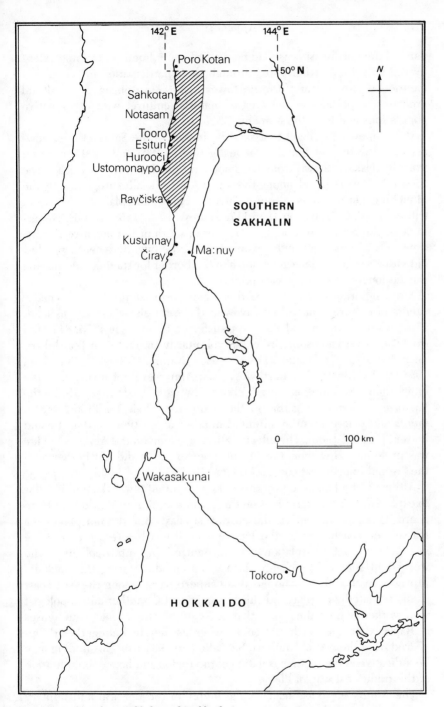

Figure E.1. Southern Sakhalin and Hokkaido.

parts of the northwest coast had no doubt been influenced to some extent by the Gilyaks. Furthermore, through their participation in the above-mentioned Santan trade, the northwest coast Ainu engaged in cultural exchange, especially in the area of material culture, with other native populations and with the Manchu Chinese.

It is somewhat difficult to assess the impact of the Santan trade, however. At the time of Mamiya's investigation in 1808 and 1809, one Ainu from Rayčiska and two from Ustomonaypo on the northwest coast (see Figure E.1) were listed among the seven Ainu officially designated by the Manchu government as *kashinta* ("district chief") and placed in charge of tribute missions (Harrison 1955:117; Mamiya 1943 [1855]:100–1). Nevertheless, the centers of trading were to the south of the northwest coast, especially at Kusunnay and Nayoro. During the twentieth century, a few individuals seem to have gone north of the border for trading, and trading was no longer intensively carried on.

Most importantly, the Ainu in this region were exempt from two major agents of culture change that involved the Ainu elsewhere in Sakhalin. First, when southern Sakhalin was transferred to Russia in 1875, 843 Ainu from the eastern and southern coasts voluntarily emigrated to Tsuishikari, near Sapporo, Hokkaido (Dixon 1883; Natori 1959:81–2; Takakura 1958:69–91, 135–8). The northwest coast Ainu were not involved in the emigration. Second, as noted above, between 1912 and 1914, the Japanese government gathered the Ainu from their traditional settlements and placed them in a limited number of locations so that it could better "protect" them. The effect of this relocation on the Ainu way of life was profound. However, the Japanese government did not bother with the "remote northwest coast" (Kodama 1972a:14).

Although the Japanese progressively penetrated into Sakhalin in order to exploit the natural resources on the island and, during World War II, to guard its northern frontier, the northwest coast Ainu did not perceive a massive encroachment by the Japanese until just before the end of the war. Their relative isolation was recognized by anthropologists who worked in southern Sakhalin. T. Yamamoto, director of the Sakhalin Museum in the 1940s, who has done superb work among the east coast Ainu, repeatedly emphasized this fact to me. Ito, another anthropologist who worked in Sakhalin, notes that he found two traditional Ainu houses at Rayčiska on the northwest coast, whereas they had altogether disappeared from the rest of southern Sakhalin (Ito 1935:13). This finding may be indicative of the relative isolation of the region and hence the retention of the traditional way of life.

The Ainu were once again at the mercy of the political and military struggle between their neighbors when southern Sakhalin was claimed by the Soviet Union at the end of World War II. As the Soviets were already coming down from the border to southern Sakhalin toward the end of the war, many Ainu, who were Japanese citizens, crossed the Soya Strait in fishing boats to settle in Hokkaido, and others waited until the two governments arranged their relocation after the war. Their way of life on their homeland was thus abruptly and brutally terminated. The Japanese government placed the Ainu, together with Japanese settlers returning from Sakhalin, in underdeveloped areas of Hokkaido so that they themselves could exploit the natural resources. The Ainu were provided with free housing, land, and capital to start their new life.

Most of the Sakhalin Ainu chose to settle in coastal areas to make fishing their occupation. Most of these areas, however, were not as rich in fish and other food resources as they were in Sakhalin. In addition, during the years after the relocation, catches of herring, salmon, and other fish declined drastically, making life quite difficult for the Ainu. Many of their young men now seek employment at more prosperous fishing ports and during the nonfishing season obtain jobs as lumberjacks or as crew members in ocean fishing boats. Women, especially young women, also seek employment in the cities, primarily those of Hokkaido but also some on Honshu, because their small fishing communities provide no jobs for them.

Yakovlev (1947) supposedly found 1,200 Sakhalin Ainu in Sakhalin in 1946. A Soviet source cited by Stephan (1971:193) reports that 600 Sakhalin Ainu remained on the island in 1967, and that they are now organized into fishing cooperatives in eight settlements in the southern part of Sakhalin. This population figure seems rather high, but I have no way of checking its accuracy.

The Ainu as a minority group in Japanese society, the Japanese government's effort to alleviate the difficult conditions of the Ainu, and Ainu efforts to promote their causes and to assert their own identity are important subjects. They are not discussed here, because the Sakhalin Ainu constitute only a small segment of the Ainu population in Hokkaido and have not been actively involved in the recent movements, and these matters do not directly relate to the theme of this book.

Notes

1. Introduction

1 In this book I use the term *perception* in the most general sense of identifying the object or a phenomenon in the external world, rather than as strictly sensory perception. Basically, the sense image, concept, and sound images of a linguistic label are inseparable, and their presence in the mind of the onlooker provides the mechanism that enables the identification to be made. Once a lion, for example, is culturally identified, it can acquire further symbolic meaning, such as the King of Beasts (see Chapters 8 and 10).

2 Although these statements by Sahlins are meant to characterize the bourgeois and tribal societies, respectively, I think the importance of kinship is found in other industrialized societies, such as those of Japan and even Western Europe.

2. The Ainu

1 This seasonal movement was discontinued around the turn of the century. The introduction of the Russian-style log cabin then enabled the Ainu to stay in their summer houses on the shore, thus eliminating the necessity to move inland for the winter.

3. The ethnomedical approach

1 *Nuhča – Ledum palustra* L. var. *dilatatum* Wahlb. (Chiri 1953:53).

2 Spruce – *sunku* in Ainu. *Picea jezoensis* Carr (Chiri 1953:236-7).

3 Willow – *susu* in Ainu. *Salix sachalinensis* Fr. Schm. (Chiri 1953:190).

4 As with the relationships among the English terms *illness*, *sickness*, and *disease*, the precise semantic relation between *araka* and *ikoni* is somewhat ambivalent. During my 1969 fieldwork, it was explained that the term *ikoni* is synonymous with *araka*, except that *araka* belongs to the language of the young, whereas *ikoni* belongs to a special set of lexical and grammatical structures used exclusively by male and female elders (called *onne itah* – language of the elders; for its linguistic description, see Hattori 1957). During my 1973 fieldwork, however, it was explained that the two terms are not exactly identical. *Ikoni* refers to serious illnesses, as in the phrase *ikoni aynu* (*aynu* means a person or human being), which is used by elders in referring to someone mortally ill. Another kind of distinction became apparent when two terms denoting labor pain, *honi araka* and *tuye ikoni*, were compared. *Honi araka* (abdomen aches) is a general term, whereas *tuye ikoni* (guts-pain) is a descriptive term expressing the recurring nature of labor pain. Chiri (1954:220; 340-1) and B. Wada (in K. Wada 1964:103-4) state that although *araka* and *ikoni* are both used to denote pain, *araka* refers to a temporary pain, *ikoni* to a chronic one; thus, *sapa-arka* [*sic*] denotes a temporary headache, whereas *sapa-koni* [*sic*] denotes a chronic headache (Chiri 1954:220). These scholars note that both terms are also

used to mean illness in a generic sense; in Ainu there is singular and dual distinction, but no distinction between singular and plural. Chiri further notes that among the Hokkaido Ainu *ikoni* is an archaic term, appearing only in the oral tradition and in compound words (1954:340, 341). The other lexeme for pain, *tasum*, in the northwest coast dialect refers to a particularly acute pain. Thus, *poni tasum araka* is a general term for illnesses characterized by acute pain in the bones (*poni* = bone; *tasum* = acute pain; *araka* = illness). Chiri (1954:340) translates *tasum* as a chronic pain. Some dialectical differences, as well as changes in the meaning of these terms through time, are involved here.

4. Habitual illnesses

1 *nuhča* – *Ledum palustre* L. var. *dilatatum* Wahlb. (Chiri 1953:53). *kito* – leek. *Allium Victorialis* L. var. *platyphyllum* Makino (Chiri 1953:195–6).

5. Body-part and skin illnesses

1 *hewnay* in Ainu. *Actiniaria* (Chiri 1962:135). Chiri records the pronunciation as *heun-nay*.
2 *Lysichiton camtschatense* Schott var. *japonicum* Makino (Chiri 1953:216).
3 *Impatiens Noli-tangere* L. (Chiri 1953:81).

6. Metaphysical illnesses

1 Historical accounts of specific incidents of smallpox epidemics among various Ainu groups are given in Kubodera and Chiri (1940:124–58), Sekiba (1966:12–14), and B. Wada (1941:98–9).
2 The demons are called *wen kamuy* (evil deity), *wen araka kamuy* (evil illness deity), or *wen kamiasin* (evil deity). The inclusion of the term *kamuy* (deity) in these designations stems from an Ainu belief that deferential treatment of a demon may prevent its destructive deeds toward humans. These demons may be more bluntly referred to as *wen oyasi* (evil demons) or, in the case of those responsible for influenza, *onke oyasi* (coughing demons).
3 *Sikataro kina* – An unidentifiable plant, probably of the *Allium* family, with white bell-shaped flowers that are supposed to turn blue when stepped on.
4 alder – *kene* in Ainu. *Alnus hirsuta* Rupr. (Chiri 1953:179–80).
   elder – *osokoni* or *sokoni* in Ainu. *Sambucus Buergeriana* Bl. var. *Miquelij* Nakai (Chiri 1953:28–30).
   white birch – *tahni* in Ainu. *Betula Tauschii* Koidz. (Chiri 1953:183–4).
   juniper – *uyta:ni* in Ainu. *Juniperus conferta* Parl (Chiri 1953:232–3).
   sedge grass – *pehsamus* in Ainu. *Carex dispalata* Boott (Chiri 1953:217).
5 *Osokoni* – *osokoni* = *osikoni*; *o* = buttocks; *si* = excrement; *kor* = to have; *ni* = tree (Chiri 1953:28–30).
6 Various small figurines in human form are made from this tree and are worn regularly as personal charms against demons and evil spirits. This type of charm, as well as chopsticks made of elder, is considered an effective corrective for stuttering, which is caused by evil spirits. An elder charm called *ranka:rari* in Ainu is worn as a belt by individuals with heart trouble.
7 The charm belt discussed in note 6 also contains a figurine made from white birch, and various other charms for daily use are often made from this tree. Thin layers of its bark provide an equivalent to our bandages and are used in the treatment of cuts and burns, but symbolic meaning does have a role in this medical use. The Ainu consider white

birch a poor wood material and use it only to make sleds, baskets, and infant carriers.

8 It is considered effective for *kemasinke* (blood-spitting illness) and for all the *nius araka* – a group of illnesses characterized by a sudden attack of sharp pain with multiple loci (see Appendixes A and F).

9 Red box mosses – *hu:re nupoto* in Ainu. *Sphagnum* spp. esp. S. *cymbifollium* Warnst. and S. *girgensonii* Russ. (Takeda 1949:12).

10 Influenza victims are also urged to drink a lot of water, lest their stomachs burn out, because this illness too is accompanied by high fever. Influenza epidemics too have afflicted the Ainu a number of times and are also believed to be spread by demons.

11 Detailed descriptions of the Hokkaido Ainu beliefs concerning smallpox are provided by Chiri (1973a:20–1, 325–38), Kubodera (1937:25–7), and Kubodera and Chiri (1940). Kubodera's report (1937) on the beliefs and practices of the Hokkaido Ainu differs from Kubodera and Chiri's report (1940) on several significant points. For example, Kubodera (1937:25) explicitly states that it is the smallpox deities, and not demons, that are responsible for this illness, whereas in Kubodera and Chiri (1940) they are referred to as demons. Kubodera and Chiri (1940) is reprinted in Chiri (1954:355–85).

In all of these publications by Chiri, by Kubodera, and by both, it is reported that the Hokkaido Ainu believe that the demons that spread smallpox are a certain kind of migratory bird, or appear to humans in that form. The northwest coast Sakhalin Ainu also believe in half-human and half-bird creatures, which they refer to as *sikataro kamuy;* they are thought to be birds, resembling ducks, when in the air but are transformed into human figures when they come down to the ground. Seals being their favorite food, these birds in human form ask people for a boat to hunt for seals and a pot to cook their meat. If obliging, the people will be treated to a piece of seal meat left behind in the borrowed pan. The pan should be reused by the humans without washing. If cooperative, the humans will be protected, but if not, they may be killed. These activities are conducted only at night.

Although the northwest coast Sakhalin Ainu do not relate these birdlike creatures to smallpox, there may have been some such link in the past. The plant they hang in the upper corner of the doorway is called *sikatorke kamuy* (*si* = excretion; *kat* = from; *or* = place; *kamuy* = demon/deity – "demon who has excretion"), which is a designation for the smallpox demon among the Horobetsu Ainu of Hokkaido (Chiri 1954:354). Kindaichi (1923:293) lists *shikatoroke* [sic] as a term for an illness, cold, or some other illness accompanied by fever, and B. Wada surmises that among the east coast Sakhalin Ainu this term denotes a category of serious contagious illnesses accompanied by fever (K. Wada 1964:109).

12 As the definition of this illness clearly indicates, in the Ainu social code a verbal attack, even on one's own family members, is considered a very serious offense, sometimes more serious than an actual physical attack. This belief is echoed in the Ainu legal code. If A utters harsh words to or about B, who in turn commits suicide, A is then regarded as a murderer and is tried, just like a person who physically commits a murder.

13 When my informant, Husko, was still a young girl, one afternoon she suddenly experienced an acute pain and felt as if she could no longer breathe. Her mother not only immediately identified the illness as *aymawko ahun* but also diagnosed the cause to be the harsh words uttered by her (the mother's) brother, who lived next door and had been having trouble with his wife. Soon after Husko started to suffer, her mother went next door to reaffirm her diagnosis; she learned then that the man had indeed quarreled with his wife and was ready to commit a violent action, but was prevented by Husko's mother's visit. Husko was cured by the use of ritual shreddings and a decoction, which put her into a deep sleep.

14 Although the northwest coast Ainu do not emphasize the metaphysical nature of otters, Chiri (1962:148), without specifying from which group of Ainu he obtained the informa-

tion, reports that because otters are believed to be forgetful, one becomes forgetful or enters a trance if one eats the meat from an otter's head. Chiri speculates that the Ainu term for otter, *esaman,* may have originated from a Tungic term, *saman,* which of course is the source of our anthropological term *shaman.* In view of the influence of the Tungic-speaking neighbors on Ainu shamanism, especially on the east coast of Sakhalin, Chiri suspects that, because a skull of an otter is used in divination, the Tungic term *saman,* for shaman, eventually became a label for this animal (Chiri 1952:74–6; 1962:148). To my knowledge, the northwest coast Sakhalin Ainu engage in divination, but not with otter skulls. On the other hand, sleepiness or excessive sleeping, which is the symptomatic criterion for the identification of this illness, may very well have once been related to the condition of trance.

15 Wormwood – *noya* in Ainu. *Artemisia vulgaria* var. *yezoana* Kudo (Chiri 1953:1–8).
16 Yesso spruce – *sunku* in Ainu. *Picea jazoensis* Carr (Chiri 1953:236–7).
    Larch – *kuy* in Ainu. *Larix dahurica* Turcz (Chiri 1953:237).
    Nuhča is identified as *Ledum palustre* var. *dilatatum* Wahlb. (Chiri 1953:53).
    Leek – *kito* in Ainu. *Allium Victorialis* var. *platyphyllum* Makino (Chiri 1953:195).
17 Tangle – *ruru kina* in Ainu. *Laminaria ochotensis* Miyabe (Chiri 1953:253–4). The "neck part" (the part next to the root) is used for this purpose.
18 Musk deer *–opokay* in Ainu. *Moschus moschiferus* L. (Chiri 1962:173).
    The plant *raramani* is identified as *Taxus cuspidata* Sieb et Zucc. (Chiri 1953:238).
19 The literal meaning of this term is not clear. *Kosimpu* [sic] is also the term applied to shamans' spirits by the Sakhalin Ainu on the east coast around the turn of the century (Pilsudski 1961:184). Among the Horobetsu Ainu of Hokkaido, Chiri (1954:96) learned that *kosimpk* [sic] had originally referred to the deities who enter the body of shamans, but by the time of his investigation, the term had come to apply to evil spirits with pale faces who reside in the mountains and the sea. Among the Saru Ainu of Hokkaido, *kosimpu* [sic] are also a group of evil spirits with pale faces residing in the mountains and the sea, possession by which is considered to cause insanity (Chiri 1954:143–5).
20 grasshopper = *pahtaki;* crow = *etuhka;* raven = *ačawre;* crane = *nuhka;* duck = *kopeča.*
21 Many scholars of the Ainu, most of whom worked among the Hokkaido Ainu, report that their group of Ainu define their deities more broadly. For example, Watanabe (1973:81) equates Ainu deities with everything in nature, whereas Sternberg (1906:425–7) equates them with beasts. Chiri (1954:359; Chiri and Oda 1956:235–6) includes not only animals but also plants and objects such as boats and anchors among the deities. Kindaichi (1944:244–306) includes an equally wide range of phenomena in the class of deities. The differences in interpretation of Ainu deities should be largely attributed to regional differences and to changes in Ainu concepts over time. On the other hand, the extensive use of the term *kamuy* (deity) to refer to nondeities out of respect may also exist among other Ainu groups.
22 It is not clear whether these evil shamans as perceived by the northwest coast Ainu correspond to *pauchi* – female witches who cast spells – who appear in an epic poem of the east coast Sakhalin Ainu as recorded by Kindaichi (1914:36; no Ainu phonemes are provided for the term *pauchi,* which is written in Japanese as *kana*).
23 The kite is identified as *Milvus migrans lineatus* (Gray) (Chiri 1962:202).
24 Regional variation is extremely well developed in the shamanistic practices of the Ainu. This book focuses on the practices and beliefs of the Ainu of the northwest coast of southern Sakhalin. However, a brief reference to the shamanistic complex of other Ainu and sources of information may be useful to some readers. First, the most significant differences occur between the shamanism of the Sakhalin Ainu and that of the Hokkaido Ainu; among the latter, shamanism is little developed and occupies a much less significant place in their culture (Kindaichi 1944:299; Hanihara et al. 1972:178).

Some scholars attribute the more elaborate nature of the Sakhalin Ainu shamanism to influences from the shamanism of the Siberian peoples (e.g., Hanihara et al. 1972:178; Kindaichi 1944:33; Pilsudski 1961:183). The Sakhalin Ainu of the east coast had more contact with the Oroks and Gilyaks, and their shamanism seems to reflect that influence. For example, in contrast to the northwest coast shamans, whose paraphernalia for the performance is relatively simple, the east coast shamans have elaborate attire (cf. Chiri and Wada 1943; Kubodera 1960:104) that resembles that of the Gilyak and Orok shamans. Shamans' spirits among the east coast Ainu also seem to differ. For example, foxes, which are deified among the northwest coast Ainu but do not play a prominent role in their culture, are not only intimate figures in the east coast Ainu mythology (Pilsudski 1912) but are believed to possess shamans. A shaman at the Wakasakunai settlement, where part of my fieldwork was carried out, was from Tarantomari in the southern part of Sakhalin and was often possessed by a fox. Kubodera notes that among the east coast Sakhalin Ainu the shaman's spirits take the form of a snake (1960:104). The best published source of information on the east coast Sakhalin Ainu shamanism is Pilsudski (1961), who worked at Aihama and other settlements on the east coast. Kubodera (1960) carried out his fieldwork in 1935 at the Niitoi settlement, and Chiri and Wada's work (1943) was done during the early 1940s at the Shirahama settlement.

Despite these regional differences among the Sakhalin Ainu, all share some important features. Common to all is that shamanism is not an insignificant cultural practice, both men and women can be shamans, and a drum is an important ingredient in shamanistic performances. In contrast, among the Hokkaido Ainu shamanism receives much less cultural value, shamans are all women, and the drum is not used in their rituals. The implication of these differences is presented in Chapter 8.

Perhaps because shamanism was not as well developed among the Hokkaido Ainu as it was among the Sakhalin Ainu, even the best-qualified scholars of the Hokkaido Ainu discuss shamanism only in passing or allocate to it only a small portion of their work, often in the context of exorcism and divination in general. For example, Kindaichi, the father of Ainu studies in Japan, devotes less than one page to the subject in his 1961 work and only thirteen pages (pp. 288–300) in his 1925 work (Kindaichi 1944), which consists primarily of quotations from Hokkaido Ainu epics in which shamans "from outside of Hokkaido" (i.e., Sakhalin and the Kuriles) are described. The impressive work of Munro (1963) on the Nibutani Ainu of Hokkaido discusses shamanism in a single paragraph (p. 104) in the general context of exorcism, although it includes some important texts of the shaman's invocations in an appendix. An intensive study of the Saru Ainu of Hokkaido carried out by a group of competent scholars (Nihon Minzokugaku Kyokai, ed., 1952) does not include a specific section on shamanism (one of the scholars is H. Watanabe, author of a superb ecological study published in English in 1973). Some discussion of Hokkaido Ainu shamanism is also found in Batchelor (1927), Chiri (1973b:23–9), Hanihara et al. (1972), Hilger (1971), Murdock (1934), and Yoshida (1912). But Batchelor's information is often inaccurate (see a detailed analysis of his work in Chiri 1956:237–53), and Hilger's work is aimed at the general public and insufficiently reflects her anthropological training. Sarashina, whose publications on the Hokkaido Ainu of various regions are insightful but are aimed at the general public, notes that many of the spirits are major deities of the Ainu pantheon (1968:188); however, he does not specify the source of information, and there are not enough details to evaluate his statement.

7. Metaphysical illnesses and healing rituals

1　The sucking-paw story is found not only among the Sakhalin Ainu but also among the Kurile Ainu (Torii 1919:255), with whom the Sakhalin Ainu have apparently had no contact, at least in the recent past. In his well-known study on bear ceremonialism in the Northern Hemisphere, Hallowell (1926:27–31) pointed out that the elaborate bear ceremonies and the sucking-paw story are found only among a limited number of peoples and that the Ainu is one of them. For more details of the sucking-paw story, see Ohnuki-Tierney (1969a:166–7).

2 I always felt somewhat uncomfortable that whenever I arrived after a period of separation from my Ainu friends they would ask me if I came with "lots and lots of presents." Likewise, their farewell remarks were accompanied by requests for many presents upon my return. Until my third fieldwork session, I did not realize that I was interpreting their remarks within my Japanese framework of cultural conditioning. What my Ainu friends wanted was my goodwill toward them, because in their culture gifts represent the genuine goodwill of the visitor.

3 Ainu data on the transcendental nature of shamanism provides both a parallel and a contrast to the generalization presented by Eliade, a major contributor to the study of shamanism. For this purpose, the Ainu spatial conception of the universe is briefly discussed here. Eliade (1972:510–11) is perceptive in pointing out how shamans transcend ordinary time and space; however, the major spatial configuration of the universe as presented by Eliade seems too narrowly perceived. The universe he presents emphasizes verticality: World Tree, World Pillar, and the shaman's celestial ascent from and descent to the underworld. In both Christianity and Buddhism, heaven, earth, and hell are vertically arranged, and the spatial orientation of the people whose shamanism Eliade examined stresses verticality. However, to assume the universality of the vertical arrangement of these three worlds, or to assume the presence of all three in the first place, is ethnocentric and risks a superimposition of the investigator's own vision of the universe on the culture being studied. Although shamanistic practice is found everywhere, the universe can have a different configuration for different people. For instance, the universe of the Totonac Indians looks like half of an orange (Nida 1964:93). The Ainu universe looks something like a layer cake. The Ainu expression of their vertical sphere is *iwan kanto wenka us:* literally translated, six skies piled on top of one another. However, I interpret this expression to mean many, rather than six, layers. In Ainu, 1 to 5 are the basic numbers and 6 is the first derived number. Therefore, 6 is often used to denote "many" or "great quantity," rather than literally signifying six; many days are expressed as six days and six nights, and many years are six cold seasons and six warm seasons.

Each of these many layers consists of a layer of ground, a layer of sky, and the space between. No great depth is assigned to the layer of ground (*toy*); only the surface of the ground, called *itaru*, is significant to the Ainu. The space between the ground and the sky is called *between* (*uturukehe*) and is assigned no special meaning. The Ainu term for sky (*kanto*) refers to the bluish part of the sky. The Ainu picture of the vertical plane, then, consists of many identical layers like this, with the Ainu world belonging to the bottom layer and many others on top of it. A more realistic picture, however, is that the Ainu collectively consider whatever is above to be "the above" (*kanna*), characterized by the presence of various deities, in contrast to the ground, "the below" (*pohna*), where they reside. To the Ainu, the most dominant beings of the above are the Goddess of Sun and Moon and the Dragon Deities. (For further details of the vertical plane of the Ainu universe, see Ohnuki-Tierney 1972.)

My description of the Ainu vertical plane brings to light two major points in reference to Eliade's interpretation of the universe. First, the Ainu universe is quite different from the universe characterized by the heaven above, the underworld below, and the earth in between, with great depth to each. Neither world tree nor world pillar exists in the Ainu universe. Second, Ainu shamanism has little reference to the vertical plane. The world of the deities is located in the mountains, not in the sky. Although height is perhaps the most important defining feature of the English term *mountains*, the most important defining feature of *nupuri*, which I translate as *mountains*, is to the Ainu the distance from the shore. Thus, there are two types of elevated land in Ainu topography: *kipiri* (hills), which are closer to the shore, and *nupuri* (mountains; holiness), which are farther away from the shore. The fact that hills are shorter and mountains are taller is simply a corollary to the primary feature of these two types of elevated land; the mountains are situated farther inland and hence are taller than hills. Furthermore, there is a conspicuous lack of involvement of the deities who reside in the above. Thus, the Goddess of Sun and Moon, an otherwise important deity in the Ainu pantheon, has no role in shamanistic rites, nor do any of the other deities of the above. Similarly, the world of the dead Ainu is not located deep down below, as in Christianity or Buddhism, but on the opposite side of the mountains. Thus it constitutes a mirror image of the Ainu settlement, with a dark horizontal tunnel going through the mountain connecting the two worlds.

To recapitulate, Ainu shamanism is characterized by spatiotemporal transcendence, as with shamanism in many other societies. There is a complete lack of emphasis on the vertical transcendence of space, however. The Ainu universe does have a vertical dimension, but it consists of layers rather than vertical space. In Ainu shamanism the past, present, and future merge, and the shamans and their spirits move between the worlds of living humans, dead humans, and the deities, all located on the same horizontal plane.

4 Even this practice is observed only by the courageous, and thus many do not participate. The bear's tongue, heart, and often the brain are cooked and consumed by males. To eat these parts of the bear is taboo for women. Sarashina (1968:209–10) reports more extensive use of raw food among the Hokkaido Ainu; however, because he does not specify the location of his investigation, it is hard to evaluate whether or not this practice is due to Japanese influence.

5 The Ainu justification for their attitude toward the Oroks is of special interest when one knows that both the Oroks and the Gilyaks, so-called primitive populations on Sakhalin, joined the Chinese, Russians, and Japanese in exploiting the Ainu in the Santan trade. But although the Ainu demonstrate much antagonism toward the Tungic-speaking Oroks, whose lifestyle as reindeer herders is very different from that of the Ainu, they are much more favorable toward the Gilyaks, who have adopted a hunting-fishing-gathering economy and who they believe are similar in their customs and facial features to the Ainu.

6 Yamamoto (1944:197–201) recorded a tale very similar to this one about how the war started between the Ainu of the Rayčiska settlement and the Oroks from the Tarayka region of the east coast of southern Sakhalin. Similar stories about the origin of the Ainu-Orok War are recorded by several other scholars (Chiri 1944:122–3; Ishida 1910:476–7; Nonaka 1933:173–8; Pilsudski 1912:66–76). In all these tales, there are two common themes: the war takes place at Tarayka instead of at Rayčiska, as in the tale I recorded, and the Ainu mistake what the Oroks offer them to eat, usually intestines of reindeer, as something related to the human female reproductive organ, such as a uterus or an afterbirth. Ainu anger over this starts the war. In Pilsudski's story, the Oroks offer the Ainu reindeer stomach stained with human excrement. Of course, the Oroks too have their version of the war with the Ainu (cf. Sekiguchi 1940).

8. Symbolic studies and the Ainu data

1 In formulating this typology of anomaly, I am indebted to Professor Jan Vansina of the University of Wisconsin, who first suggested the necessity to distinguish several types of anomaly and suggested the first three. (From Ohnuki-Tierney, 1980a:139.)

9. Modes of perception

1 S. Kodama, a physical anthropologist with a medical degree, attributes this factor to the "toughness" of their skin against insect bites and cold (1972b:484). Sekiba (1966:58) also reports on the low frequency of skin diseases among the Hokkaido Ainu. My limited and nonprofessional observation parallels their conclusion. During my stay among the Sakhalin Ainu, I saw very few skin infections of any kind, and the Ainu appeared virtually immune to the flea bites that were a constant source of irritation and infection to me.

11. Illness, the individual, and society

1 The pattern, however, is not a conscious one on the part of the Ainu, and I was not aware of it in my earlier publication (1973a).

References

Ackerknecht, Erwin H. 1946. Natural diseases and rational treatment in primitive medicine. *Bulletin of the History of Medicine* 19:467-97.

Ardener, Edwin. 1971. The new anthropology and its critics. *Man* 6(3):449-67.

——— 1972. Belief and the problem of women. In *The Interpretation of Ritual*, J. S. La Fontaine, ed. London: Tavistock. pp. 135-58.

——— 1975. The 'problem' revisited. In *Perceiving Women*, Shirley Ardener, ed. London: Malaby Press. pp. 19-27.

Austerlitz, Robert. 1970. Agglutination in northern Eurasia in perspective. In *Studies in General and Oriental Linguistics*, Roman Jakobson and Shigeo Kawamoto, eds. Tokyo: TEC Company. pp. 1-5 (on offprint).

Babcock, Barbara. 1978. Introduction. In *The Reversible World*, Barbara Babcock, ed. Ithaca, N.Y.: Cornell University Press. pp. 13-36.

Baelz, E. 1883. Die Koeperlichen Eigenschaften der Japaner. *Mittheilugen der Deutschen Gesellschaft fur Natur und Volkerkunde Ostasiens* 3:330-59.

Bailey, F. G. 1970. *Stratagems and Spoils*. Oxford: Blackwell.

Barnouw, Victor. 1973. *Culture and Personality*. Homewood, Ill.: Dorsey Press.

Barthes, Roland. 1979. *Elements of Semiology*. New York: Hill and Wang.

Batchelor, John. 1927. *Ainu Life and Lore*. Tokyo: Kyobunkan.

Batchelor, J., and K. Miyabe. 1893. Ainu economic plants. *Transactions of the Asiatic Society of Japan* 21:198-240.

Beattie, John. 1977. Spirit mediumship as theatre. *Royal Anthropological Institute News No. 20* (June):1-16.

Beattie, J., and J. Middleton, eds. 1969. *Spirit and Mediumship and Society in Africa*. London: Routledge & Kegan Paul.

Befu, Harumi, and Chester S. Chard. 1964. A prehistoric maritime culture on the Okhotsk Sea. *American Antiquity* 30(1):1-18.

Beidelman, T. O. 1963. Kaguru omens: an east African people's concepts of the unusual, unnatural and supernormal. *Anthropological Quarterly* 36(1):43-59.

——— 1964. Pig (Guluwe): an essay on Ngulu sexual symbolism and ceremony. *Southwestern Journal of Anthropology* 20:359-92.

——— 1966. Swazi royal ritual. *Africa* 36(4):373-405.

Bergsland, Kneut, and Hans Vogt. 1962. The validity of glottochronology. *Current Anthropology* 3(2):115-53.

Berlin, Brent. 1967. Categories of eating in Tzeltal and Navaho. *International Journal of American Linguistics* 33:1-6.

——— 1976. The concept of rank in ethnobiological classification: some evidence from Aquaruna folk botany. *American Ethnologist* 3(3):381-99.

Berlin, Brent, Dennis E. Breedlove, and Peter H. Raven. 1968. Covert categories and folk taxonomy. *American Anthropologist* 70:290-9.

——— 1974. *Principles of Tzeltal Plant Classification*. New York: Academic Press.

Berlin, Brent, and Paul Kay. 1969. *Basic Color Terms*. Berkeley, Calif.: University of California Press.

Bidney, David. 1963. So-called primitive medicine and religion. In *Man's Image in Medicine and Anthropology*, I. Galdston, ed. New York: International Universities Press. pp. 141–56.

Birdsell, Joseph B. 1951. The problem of the early peopling of the Americas as viewed from Asia. In *(Papers on the) Physical Anthropology of the American Indian*, William S. Laughlin, ed. New York: Viking Fund. pp. 1–68, 68a.

Bourguignon, Erika. 1973a. Introduction: a framework for the comparative study of altered states of consciousness. In *Religion, Altered States of Consciousness, and Social Change*, E. Bourguignon, ed. Columbus, Ohio: Ohio State University Press. pp. 3–35.

　1973b. An assessment of some comparisons and implications. In *Religion, Altered States of Consciousness, and Social Change*, E. Bourguignon, ed. Columbus, Ohio: Ohio State University Press. pp. 321–39.

Buchbinder, Georgeda, and Roy A. Rappaport. 1976. Fertility and death among the Maring. In *Man and Woman in the New Guinea Highlands*, Georgeda Buchbinder and Paula Brown, eds. Washington, D.C.: American Anthropological Association. pp. 13–35.

Bulmer, Ralph. 1967. Why is the cassowary not a bird? a problem of zoological taxonomy among the Karam of the New Guinea highlands. *Man (N.S.)* 2:5–25.

Buxton, Jean. 1973. *Religion and Healing in Mandari*. London: Oxford University Press.

Carstairs, G. M. 1977. Medical anthropology. *Royal Anthropological Institute News No. 22* (October):1–2.

Chard, Chester S. 1967. Lecture on the Ainu delivered in the course "Topics on Old World Archaeology." Spring Semester, Department of Anthropology, University of Wisconsin, April 13.

　1968. A new look at the Ainu problem. *Proceedings of the Eighth International Congress of Anthropological and Ethnological Sciences*. Vol. III. Tokyo: Science Council of Japan. pp. 98–9.

Chiñas, Beverly L. 1973. *The Isthmus Zapotecs – Women's Roles in Cultural Context*. New York: Holt, Rinehart & Winston.

Chiri, Mashio. 1942. Ainugo Goho Kenkyu - Karafuto Hogen o Chushin to shite [Research on the Ainu language - primarily on the Sakhalin Ainu dialects]. *Karafuto Hakubutsu-kan Hokoku* 4(4):51–172.

　1944. Karafuto Ainu no Setsuwa [Folktales of the Sakhalin Ainu]. *Karafutocho Hakubu-tsukan Iho* 3(1):1–145.

　1952. Jushi to Kawauso [The magician and the otter]. *Hoppo Bunka Kenkyu Hokoku* 7:47–80.

　1953. *Bunrui Ainugo Jiten* [*Classified Dictionaries of the Ainu Language*]. Vol. I: *Shokubutsuhen* [*Plants*]. Tokyo: Nihon Jomin Bunka Kenkyujo.

　1954. *Bunrui Ainugo Jiten* [*Classified Dictionaries of the Ainu Language*]. Vol. III: *Ningenhen* [*Humans*]. Tokyo: Nihon Jomin Bunka Kenkyujo.

　1956. *Ainugo Nyumon* [*Introduction to the Ainu Language*]. Tokyo: Nire Shobo.

　1960. *Kamui Yukara – Ainu Jojishi Nyumon* [*Kamuy Yukaru – Introduction to Ainu Epic Poems*]. Sapporo: Aporo Shoten.

　1962. *Bunrui Ainugo Jiten* [*Classified Dictionaries of the Ainu Language*]. Vol. II. *Dobutsuhen* [*Animals*]. Tokyo: Nihon Jomin Bunka Kenkyujo.

　1973a. *Chiri Mashio Chosakushu* [*Collected Works of Mashio Chiri*], Vol. 2. Tokyo: Heibonsha.

　1973b. *Chiri Mashio Chosakushu* [*Collected Works of Mashio Chiri*], Vol. 3. Tokyo: Heibonsha.

　1973–76. *Chiri Mashio Chosakushu* [*Collected Works of Mashio Chiri*]. Tokyo: Heibonsha.

Chiri, Mashio, and Kunio Oda. 1956. *Yukara Kansho* [*Ainu Epic Poems and Their Values*]. Tokyo: Gengensha.

Chiri, Mashio, and Bunjiro Wada. 1943. Karafuto Ainu-go ni okeru Jintai Kankei Meii [Body terms in the Sakhalin Ainu dialect]. *Karafutocho Hakubutsukan Hokoku* 5(1):39–80.

Chomsky, Noam. 1968. *Language and Mind*. New York: Harcourt, Brace and World.

Cohen, A. 1974. *Two-Dimensional Man: An Essay on the Anthropology of Power and Symbolism in Complex Societies*. London: Routledge & Kegan Paul.

Colby, B., and M. Cole. 1973. Culture, memory and narrative. In *Modes of Thought*, R. Horton and R. Finnegan, eds. London: Faber & Faber. pp. 63–91.

Conklin, Harold C. 1955. Hanunoo color categories. *Southwestern Journal of Anthropology* 11:339–44.

    1971. Comment on C. O. Frake's "The ethnographic study of cognitive systems." In *Anthropology and Human Behavior*, T. Gladwin and W. C. Sturtevant, eds. Washington, D.C.: Anthropological Society of Washington. Second edition. pp. 86–93.

de Beauvoir, Simone. 1974. *The Second Sex*. New York: Random House. Vintage Books.

Dixon, J. M. 1883. The Tsuishikari Ainos. *Transactions of the Asiatic Society of Japan* XI:39–50.

Douglas, Mary. 1966. *Purity and Danger*. London: Routledge & Kegan Paul.

    1973. *Natural Symbols*. London: Barrie & Jenkins.

    1975. *Implicit Meanings*. London: Routledge & Kegan Paul.

    1978. *Cultural Bias*. London: Royal Anthropological Institute of Great Britain and Ireland.

Durkheim, Emile. 1965. *The Elementary Forms of the Religious Life*. New York: Free Press. (First published in 1915.)

Durkheim, Emile, and Marcel Mauss. 1963. *Primitive Classification*. Chicago: University of Chicago Press. (Originally published in *Année Sociologique* 1901–2 [1903].)

Eliade, Mircea. 1961. *The Sacred and the Profane*. New York: Harper & Row. Torchbooks.

    1971. *Patterns in Comparative Religion*. New York: World. Meridian Book.

    1972. *Shamanism – Archaic Techniques of Ecstasy*. Princeton, N.J.: Princeton University Press. (Original publication in French in 1951, English translation in 1964.)

Elliott, Alan J. A. 1955. *Chinese Spirit Medium Cults in Singapore*. London: London School of Economics.

Fabrega, Horacio, Jr. 1970. On the specificity of folk illness. *Southwestern Journal of Anthropology* 26(3):305–14.

    1972. Medical anthropology. In *Biennial Review of Anthropology, 1971*, B. Siegel, ed. Stanford, Calif.: Stanford University Press. pp. 167–229.

    1974. *Disease and Social Behavior*. Cambridge, Mass.: MIT Press.

    1975. The need for an ethnomedical science. *Science* 189:969–75.

Fabrega, Horacio, Jr., and Daniel B. Silver. 1973. *Illness and Shamanistic Curing in Zinacantan: An Ethnomedical Analysis*. Stanford, Calif.: Stanford University Press.

Faithorn, Elizabeth. 1976. Aspects of female life and male-female relations among the Kafe. In *Man and Woman in the New Guinea Highlands*, Georgeda Buchbinder and Paula Brown, eds. Washington, D.C.: American Anthropological Association. pp. 86–95.

Finnegan, Ruth. 1973. Literacy versus non-literacy: the great divide? In *Modes of Thought*, R. Horton and R. Finnegan, eds. London: Faber & Faber. pp. 112–44.

Firth, Raymond. 1966–67. Ritual drama in Malay spirit mediumship. *Comparative Studies in Society and History* IX:190–207.

Flannery, Kent V. 1968. Archaeological systems theory and early mesoamerica. In *Anthropological Archaeology in the Americas*, B. J. Meggers, ed. Washington, D.C.: Anthropological Society of Washington. pp. 67–78.

Forde, D., and M. Douglas. 1967. Primitive economics. In *Tribal and Peasant Economics*, G. Dalton, ed. New York: Natural History Press. pp. 13–28.

Foulks, Edward. 1972. *The Arctic Hysterias.* Washington, D.C.: American Anthropological Association.

Frake, Charles O. 1961. The diagnosis of disease among the Subanun of Mindanao. *American Anthropologist* 63:113–32.

——— 1971. The ethnographic study of cognitive systems. In *Anthropology and Human Behavior*, T. Gladwin and W. C. Sturtevant, eds. Washington, D.C.: Anthropological Society of Washington. pp. 72–85.

Freedman, Maurice. 1969. Geomancy. *Proceedings of the Royal Anthropological Institute of Great Britain and Ireland for 1968.* London: Royal Anthropological Institute of Great Britain and Ireland. pp. 5–15.

Fujita, Kiyonobu. 1930. *Karafuto Ainu Kumamatsuri no Kaisetsu* [Sakhalin Ainu bear ceremony]. Toyohara, Sakhalin: Keimosha.

Fukuyama, Koreyoshi, and Sennosuke Nezu. 1942. Karafuto no Shokuyo Yaso [Edible plants in Sakhalin]. *Karafutocho Hakubutsukan Sosho. No. 7.* Toyohara: Karafutocho.

Geertz, Clifford. 1973. *The Interpretation of Cultures.* New York: Basic Books.

Gluckman, Max. 1965. *Politics, Law and Ritual in Tribal Society.* New York: New American Library. A Mentor Book.

Gonzalez, Nancie S. 1966. Health behavior in cross-cultural perspective: a Guatemalan example. *Human Organization* 25:122–5.

Good, Byron J. 1977. The heart of what's the matter: the semantics of illness in Iran. *Culture, Medicine and Psychiatry* 1(1):25–58.

Goodenough, Ward H. 1956. Componential analysis and the study of meaning. *Language* 32:195–216.

——— 1957. Cultural anthropology and linguistics. In *Report of the Seventh Annual Round Table Meeting on Linguistics and Language Study*, Paul L. Garvin, ed. Monograph Series on Language and Linguistics, No. 9. Washington, D.C.: Georgetown University Press. pp. 167–73.

Haddon, A. C. 1925. *The Races of Man and their Distribution.* New York: Macmillan.

Hall, Edward T. 1969. *The Hidden Dimension.* New York: Doubleday. Anchor Books. (Originally published in 1966.)

Hallowell, A. Irving. 1926. *Bear Ceremonialism in the Northern Hemisphere.* Philadelphia: University of Pennsylvania Press.

——— 1963. Ojibwa world view and disease. In *Man's Image in Medicine and Anthropology*, Iago Galston, ed. New York: International Universities Press. pp. 258–315.

——— 1964. Ojibwa ontology, behavior, and world view. In *Primitive Views of the World*, S. Diamond, ed. New York: Columbia University Press. pp. 49–82.

Hanihara, Kazuro, Hideo Fujimoto, Toru Asai, Masakazu Yoshizaki, Motomichi Kono, and Yoichi Nyui. 1972. *Shimpojumu Ainu [Symposium on the Ainu].* Sapporo: University of Hokkaido Press.

Hanihara, K., T. Masuda, T. Tanaka, and M. Tamada. 1975. Comparative studies of dentition. In *Anthropological and Genetic Studies on the Japanese*, S. Watanabe, S. Kondo, and E. Matsunaga, eds. Tokyo: University of Tokyo Press. pp. 256–62.

Harrison, John A. 1954. The Saghalien trade: a contribution to Ainu studies. *Southwestern Journal of Anthropology* 10(3):278–93.

——— 1955. Kita Yezo Zusetsu or a description of the island of northern Yezo by Mamiya Rinzo. *Proceedings of the American Philosophical Society* 99(2):93–117.

Hasebe, Kotondo. 1956. Nihonjin no Sosen [The ancestors of the Japanese]. In *Zusetsu Nihon Bunkashi Taikei*, K. Kodama, ed. Vol. 1. Tokyo: Shogakukan. pp. 94–105.

Hattori, Shiro. 1956. Nihongo no Keito [The genetic affiliation of the Japanese language]. In *Zusetsu Nihon Bunkashi Taikei*, K. Kodama, ed. Vol. 1. Tokyo: Shogakukan. pp. 117–30.

——— 1957. Ainugo ni okeru Nenchoshaso Tokushugo [A special language of the older generations among the Ainu]. *Minzokugaku Kenkyu* 21(3):38–45.

1961. Ainugo Karafuto Hogen no "Ninsho Setsuji" ni tsuite [Personal affixes in the Sakhalin dialect of Ainu]. *Gengo Kenkyu* 39:1–20.

Hattori, Shiro, ed. 1964. *Ainugo Hogen Jiten [An Ainu Dialect Dictionary]*. Tokyo: Iwanami Shoten.

Hertz, Robert. 1960. *Death and the Right Hand*. Glencoe, Ill.: Free Press. (Originally published in 1907 and 1909.)

Hilger, M. I. 1971. *Together with the Ainu*. Norman, Okla.: University of Oklahoma Press.

Hoijer, Harry. 1968. The Sapir–Whorf hypothesis. In *Readings in Anthropology*, M. H. Fried, ed. Vol. 1. New York: Thomas Y. Crowell. pp. 404–17.

Hopper, Kim. 1979. Of language and the sorcerer's appendix: a critical appraisal of Horacio Fabrega's *Disease and Social Behavior*. *Medical Anthropology Newsletter* 10(3):9–14.

Hora, Tomio. 1956. *Karafutoshi Kenkyu [Research on the History of Sakhalin Island]*. Tokyo: Shinjusha.

Howells, William W. 1966. Craniometry and multivariate analysis: the Jomon population of Japan. *Papers of the Peabody Museum of Archaeology and Ethnology*. Vol. LVII, no. 1. Cambridge, Mass.: Peabody Museum, pp. 1–43.

Hsu, Francis L. K. 1973. Prejudice and its intellectual effect in American anthropology: an ethnographic report. *American Anthropologist* 75(1):1–19.

Hymes, Dell H. 1960. Lexicostatistics so far. *Current Anthropology* 1:3–34.

Ishida, Shuzo. 1910. Orokko to Ainu no Senso Monogatari [Stories about wars between the Orok and the Ainu]. *Jinruigaku Zasshi* 25(294):476–7.

Ito, Nobuo. 1935. Karafutocho Hakubutsukan no Dozoku Kokohitsu [Ethnographic and archaeological exhibitions at the Sakhalin Museum]. *Dorumen* 4(3):10–15.

Jakobson, Roman, G. Fant, and M. Halle. 1967. *Preliminaries to Speech Analysis*. Cambridge, Mass.: MIT Press.

Jakobson, Roman, and M. Halle. 1956. *Fundamentals of Language*. The Hague: Mouton.

Jimbo, Saburo. 1901. Imbakko ni tsuite [About the Imbakko]. *Tokyo Igakukai Zasshi* XV(4):1–15.

Jung, Carl G. 1971. *The Portable Jung*, R. F. C. Hull, trans. New York: Viking Press.

Kajima, Seisaburo. 1895. *The Ainu of Japan*. Tokyo: Genrokukan.

Kapferer, Bruce. 1979. Mind, self, and other in demonic illnesses: the negation and reconstruction of self. *American Ethnologist* 6(1):110–33.

Katz, Fred, and Marlene Dobkin de Rios. 1971. Hallucinogenic music. *Journal of American Folklore* 84:320–7.

Keesing, Roger M. 1972. Paradigms lost: the new ethnography and the new linguistics. *Southwestern Journal of Anthropology* 28(4):299–332.

1975. *Kin Groups and Social Structure*. New York: Holt, Rinehart & Winston.

1976. *Cultural Anthropology: A Contemporary Perspective*. New York: Holt, Rinehart & Winston.

Kennedy, John. 1973. Cultural psychiatry. In *Handbook of Social and Cultural Anthropology*, John Honigmann, ed. Chicago: Rand McNally. pp. 1119–98.

Kenny, Michael G. 1978. Latah: the symbolism of a putative mental disorder. *Culture, Medicine and Psychiatry* 2(3):209–31.

Kiev, Ari. 1964. The study of folk psychiatry. In *Magic, Faith and Healing*, A. Kiev, ed. New York: Free Press. pp. 3–35.

Kindaichi, Kyosuke. 1914. *Kita Ezo Koyo Ihen [An Epic Poem of Northern Ezo]*. Tokyo: Kyodo Kenkyusha.

1923. *Ainu Seiten [The Sacred Epics of the Ainu]*. Tokyo: Sekai Bunko Kankokai.

1944. *Ainu no Kenkyu [The Study of the Ainu]*. Tokyo: Yashima Shobo. (Originally published in 1925.)

1960. *Ainugo Kenkyu [A Study of the Ainu Language]*. Tokyo: Sanseido.

1961. *Ainu Bunkashi* [*A History of Ainu Culture*]. Tokyo: Sanseido.

Kiyono, Kenji. 1925. *Nihon Genjin no Kenkyu* [*Research on the Aborigines of Japan*]. Tokyo: Oka Shoin.

1949. *Kodai Jinkotsu no Kenkyu ni motozuku Nihonjinshuron* [*Theory on the Racial Classification of the Japanese on the Basis of Research on Skeletal Material of Prehistoric Peoples*]. Tokyo: Iwanami Shoten.

Kleinman, Arthur M. 1974. Medicine's symbolic reality: on a central problem in the philosophy of medicine. *Inquiry* 16:206-13.

1977. Lessons from a clinical approach to medical anthropological research. *Medical Anthropology Newsletter* 8(4):11-15.

1978a. Concepts and a model for the comparison of medical systems as cultural systems. *Social Science and Medicine* 12:85-93.

1978b. The need for ethnomedical understanding of clinical categories and praxis: on Stein and Hippler. *Medical Anthropology Newsletter* 9(2):29-30.

Kobayashi, Hiroshi. 1952. Saru Ainu no Ketsuekigata ni tsuite [On the blood groups of the Saru Ainu]. *Minzokugaku Kenkyu* 16(3-4):93-5.

Kobayashi, Tatsuo, ed. 1977. *Nihon Genshi Bijutsu Taikei* [*Archaeological Treasures of Japan*]. Vol. 1: *Jomon Doki* [*Jomon Pottery*]. Tokyo: Kodansha. pp. 192-3.

Kodama, Sakuzaemon. 1972a. Ainu no Bunpu to Jinko [The distribution and demography of the Ainu]. In *Ainu Minzokushi*, Ainu Bunka Hozon Taisaku Kyogikai, ed. Tokyo: Daiichihoki Shuppan. pp. 3-25. (Originally published in 1970.)

1972b. Ainu no Byoki no Igakuteki Kansatsu [Medical observations of disease among the Ainu]. In *Ainu Minzokushi*, Ainu Bunka Hozon Taisaku Kyogikai, ed. Tokyo: Daiichihoki Shuppan. pp. 483-5. (Originally published in 1970.)

Koganei, Ryozo. 1927. Aino Minzoku sono Kigen Narabini Taminzoku tono Kankei [The origin of the Ainu people and their relationship to other peoples]. *Jinruigaku Zasshi* 42(5):159-62.

Kubodera, Itsuhiko. 1937. Ainu no Hososhin *Pakoro Kamuy* ni tsuite [On the Ainu smallpox deity, *Pakoro Kamuy*]. *Tokyo Jinruigakukai Nihon Minzokugakukai Rengo Kiji* 2:25-7.

1960. Karafuto Ainu no Shamanisumu [The shamanism of the Sakhalin Ainu]. *Nihon Jinruigakukai Nihon Minzokugakukai Rengo Taikai*, 15th Session, pp. 103-6.

Kubodera, Itsuhiko, and Mashio Chiri. 1940. Ainu Hososhin Pakoro Kamui ni tsuite [On the *Pakoro Kamuy* or the smallpox deity of the Ainu]. *Jinruigaku Zasshi* 55(3):124-58 and 55(4):169-99.

Kuhn, Thomas S. 1962. *The Structure of Scientific Revolutions*. Chicago: University of Chicago Press.

Kumasaka, Y. 1964. A culturally determined mental reaction among the Ainu. *Psychiatric Quarterly* 38:733-9.

La Fontaine, J. S. 1972. Ritualization of women's life-crises in Bugisu. In *The Interpretation of Ritual*, J. S. La Fontaine, ed. London: Tavistock. pp. 159-86.

Landar, Herbert. 1964. Seven Navaho verbs of eating. *International Journal of American Linguistics* 30:94-6.

Leach, Edmund R. 1963. Two essays concerning the symbolic representation of time. In *Rethinking Anthropology*. London: Athlone Press. pp. 124-36. (Originally published in 1961.)

1967a. Introduction. In *The Structural Study of Myth and Totemism*, E. Leach, ed. London: Tavistock. pp. vii-xix.

1967b. Magical hair. In *Myth and Cosmos*, J. Middleton, ed. New York: Natural History Press. pp. 77-108.

1967c. Genesis as myth. In *Myth and Cosmos*, J. Middleton, ed. New York: Natural History Press. pp. 1-13.

1968. Anthropological aspects of language: animal categories and verbal abuse. In *New Directions in the Study of Language*, E. Lenneberg, ed. Cambridge, Mass.: MIT Press. pp. 23–63. (Originally published in 1964.)

1970. *Claude Lévi-Strauss*. New York: Viking Press.

1976. *Culture and Communication*. Cambridge: At the University Press.

Lebra, William P. 1964. The Okinawan shaman. In *Ryukyuan Culture and Society*, Allan H. Smith, ed. Honolulu: Unive:sity of Hawaii Press. pp. 93–8.

1969. Shaman and client in Okinawa. In *Mental Health Research in Asia and the Pacific*, William Caudill and Tsung-Yi Lin, eds. Honolulu: East-West Center Press. pp. 216–22.

Lee, Richard B. 1968. What hunters do for a living, or how to make out on scarce resources. In *Man the Hunter*, R. B. Lee and I. DeVore, eds. Chicago: Aldine. pp. 30–48.

Leslie, Charles. 1976. Introduction. In *Asian Medical Systems: A Comparative Study*, C. Leslie, ed. Berkeley, Calif.: University of California Press. pp. 1–12.

Levin, M. G. 1963. Ethnic origins of the peoples of northeastern Asia. In *Arctic Institute of North America. Anthropology of the North, Translations from Russian Sources, No. 3*, H. N. Michael, ed. Toronto: University of Toronto Press.

Lévi-Strauss, Claude. 1966. *The Savage Mind*. Chicago: University of Chicago Press. (Originally published in French in 1962.)

1967. *Structural Anthropology*. New York: Doubleday. (Originally published in French in 1958 and in English in 1963.)

1969a. *The Elementary Structures of Kinship*. London: Eyre & Spottiswoode. (Originally published in French in 1949.)

1969b. *The Raw and the Cooked: Introduction to a Science of Mythology*. Vol. 1. New York: Harper Torchbooks. (Originally published in French in 1964.)

1973. *From Honey to Ashes: Introduction to a Science of Mythology*. Vol. 2. New York: Harper & Row. (Originally published in French in 1966.)

Lewis, Ioan M. 1971. *Ecstatic Religion*. Harmondsworth: Penguin Books.

Loudon, J. B. 1975. Stools, mansions and syndromes. *Royal Anthropological Institute News, No. 10.* (September/October):1–5.

Mair, Lucy. 1969. *An Introduction to Social Anthropology*. New York: Oxford University Press. (Originally published in England in 1965.)

Mamiya, Rinzo. 1943. *Kita Ezo Zusetsu [A Description of the Island of Northern Ezo]*. Toyohara: Karafutocho. (Originally published in 1855; see Harrison 1955 for the English translation.)

Marriott, McKim. 1955. Western medicine in a village of northern India. In *Health, Culture and Community: Case Studies of Public Reactions to Health Programs*, B. D. Paul, ed. New York: Russell Sage Foundation. pp. 239–68.

Martin, M. K., and B. Voorhies. 1975. *Female of the Species*. New York: Columbia University Press.

McLuhan, Marshall. 1964. *Understanding Media*. New York: New American Library. Signet Books.

Mitsuhashi, Hiroshi. 1976. Medicinal plants of the Ainu. *Economic Botany* 30:209–17.

Miyabe, Kingo. 1939. Ainu no Yakuyo Shokubutsu ni tsuite [About the medicinal plants of the Ainu]. *Hokkaido Yakugaku Koenkaishi* 5:1–17.

Miyabe, Kingo, and Tsutome Miyake. 1915. *Karafuto Shokubutsushi [Plants in Sakhalin]*. Toyohara: Karafutocho.

Molony, Carol H. 1975. Systematic valence coding of Mexican "hot" – "cold" food. *Ecology of Food and Nutrition* 4(2):67–74.

Munro, Neil Gordon. 1963. *Ainu Creed and Cult*. New York: Columbia University Press. n.d. Manuscripts intended for his *Ainu Past and Present* (in ten folders); photographs;

miscellaneous letters written by and to Munro. MS #249 of the Royal Anthropological Institute of Great Britain and Ireland.

Murdock, George P. 1934. *Our Primitive Contemporaries.* New York: Macmillan.

1960. Cognatic form of social organization. In *Social Structure in Southeast Asia,* G. P. Murdock, ed. Viking Fund Publications in Anthropology, No. 29. Chicago: Quadrangle Books. pp. 1–14.

1967. *Ethnographic Atlas.* Pittsburgh: University of Pittsburgh Press.

Murphy, H. B. M. 1976. Notes for a theory on latah. In *Culture-Bound Syndromes, Ethnopsychiatry, and Alternate Therapies,* W. P. Lebra, ed. Honolulu: East-West Center Press. pp. 3–21.

Nagano, Toshimitsu, Mikio Ishibashi, and Shuzo Nakagawa. 1966. Hoppo Minzoku (Hokkaido Ainu, Karafuto Ainu, Giriyaku, Orokko no Shamanisumu ni Kansuru Hikakuteki Kenkyu) [A comparative study of shamanism and other magical behavior of northern peoples]. *Nihon Jinruigakukai Nihon Minzokugakukai Rengo Taikai (20) (Kenkyu Happyo Shoyaku).* pp. 14–17.

Natori, Takemitsu. 1959. Karafuto Chishima Ainu no Inau to Itokupa [The Inaw and Itokpa of the Sakhalin and Kurile Ainu]. *Hoppo Bunka Kenkyu Hokoku 14:*79–114.

Needham, Rodney. 1963. Introduction. In *Primitive Classification* by Emile Durkheim and Marcel Mauss. Chicago: University of Chicago Press. pp. vii–xlvii.

1972. *Belief, Language, and Experience.* Chicago: University of Chicago Press.

1973. Right and left in Nyoro symbolic classification. In *Right and Left,* R. Needham, ed. Chicago: University of Chicago Press. pp. 109–27.

1975. Polythetic classification: convergence and consequences. *Man 10*(3):349–69.

1976. Nyoro symbolism: the ethnographic record. *Africa 46*:(3):236–45.

1979. *Symbolic Classification.* Santa Monica, Calif.: Goodyear.

Nida, Eugene. 1964. Linguistics and ethnology in translation problems. In *Language in Culture and Society,* Dell Hymes, ed. New York: Harper & Row. pp. 90–100.

Nihon Minzokugaku Kyokai, ed. 1952. Saru Ainu Kyodo Chosa Hokoku [Report of the joint research on the Saru Ainu]. Presented to Dr. Kyosuke Kindaichi on his seventieth birthday. *Minzokugaku Kenkyo 16*(3–4):1–101.

Nonaka, Fumio. 1933. *Kita-Ezo Hibun – Karafuto Ainu no Sokuseki [Confidential Stories of Northern Ezo – Traces of the Sakhalin Ainu].* Toyohara: Hokushindo Shoten.

Obeyesekere, Gananath. 1970a. Ayurveda and mental illness. *Comparative Studies in Social History 12*:292–6.

1970b. The idiom of demonic possession: a case study. *Social Science and Medicine 4*:97–111.

Ohnuki-Tierney, Emiko. 1968. A northwest coast Sakhalin Ainu world view. Ph.D. dissertation. Department of Anthropology, University of Wisconsin–Madison.

1969a. Sakhalin Ainu folklore. *Anthropological Studies No. 2.* 183 pp. Washington, D.C.: American Anthropological Association.

1969b. Concepts of time among the Ainu of the northwest coast of Sakhalin. *American Anthropologist 71*(3):488–92.

1972. Spatial concepts of the Ainu of the northwest coast of southern Sakhalin. *American Anthropologist 74*(3):426–57.

1973a. The shamanism of the Ainu of the northwest coast of southern Sakhalin. *Ethnology XII*(1):15–29. Abstracted in *Human Behavior* (June):54–5.

1973b. (With Hideo Fujimoto.) Mashio Chiri – Ainu scholar of Ainu culture and professor of linguistics. *American Anthropologist 75*:868–76.

1973c. Sakhalin Ainu time reckoning. *Man 8*(2):285–99.

1974a. *The Ainu of the Northwest Coast of Southern Sakhalin.* New York: Holt, Rinehart & Winston.

1974b. Another look at the Ainu. *Arctic Anthropology* XI(Supplement):189–95.

1976a. Regional variation in Ainu culture. *American Ethnologist* 3(2):297–329.

1976b. Shamanism and world view – case of the Ainu of the northwest coast of southern Sakhalin. In *The Realm of the Extra-Human: Ideas and Actions. World Anthropology*, A. Bharati, ed. Paris: Mouton. pp. 175–200.

1977a. An octopus headache? a lamprey boil? multi-sensory perception of 'habitual illness' and world view of the Ainu. *Journal of Anthropological Research* 33(3):245–57.

1977b. The classification of the 'habitual illnesses' of the Sakhalin Ainu. *Arctic Anthropology* XIV(2):9–34.

1980a. Ainu illness and healing – a symbolic interpretation. *American Ethnologist* 7(1):132–51.

1980b. Shamans and *Imu*: among two Ainu groups – toward a cross-cultural model of interpretation. *Ethos* 8(3):204–28.

In press. Phases in human perception, conception and symbolization process – cognitive anthropology and symbolic classification. *American Ethnologist* 8(3) (August, 1981).

Okada, Hiroaki. 1950. Ainu Bunkashi ni Kansuru Ichi Kosatsu [Some notes on the history of Ainu culture]. Masters thesis, Department of Cultural Anthropology, University of Tokyo.

Omoto, Keiichi. 1974. Blood protein in polymorphism and the problem of the genetic affinities of the Ainu. *Paper presented at the Ninth International Congress of Anthropological and Ethnological Sciences, Chicago, 1973*. The Hague: Mouton.

Ong, Walter. 1969. World view and world as event. *American Anthropologist* 71(4):634–47.

Ono, Susumu. 1966. *Nihongo no Kigen [The Origin of the Japanese Language]*. Tokyo: Iwanami Shoten.

Ortiz, Alfonso. 1969. *The Tewa World: Space, Time, Being and Becoming in a Pueblo Society*. Chicago: University of Chicago Press.

Ortner, Sherry B. 1974. Is female to male as nature is to culture? In *Woman, Culture and Society*, M. Z. Rosaldo and L. Lamphere, eds. Stanford, Calif.: Stanford University Press. pp. 67–87.

Peabody, Robert L. 1968. Authority. In *International Encyclopedia of the Social Sciences*, D. L. Sills, ed. Vol. 1. New York: Macmillan and Free Press. pp. 473–7.

Pilsudski, Bronislov. 1911. Karafuto-to ni okeru Senjumin [The aborigines of Sakhalin] (trans. by Ryuzo Torii). *Jinruigaku Zasshi* 27(2):83–9; 27(3):163–7; 27(4):226–32. (Originally published as Die Urberwohner von Sachalin, 1909, *Globus* 96[27]:325–30.)

1912. *Materials for the Study of the Ainu Language and Folklore*. Cracow: Spółka Wydawnicza Polska.

1915. Na medvedž 'em prazdnik ajnov o. Sachalina. *Zhivaia Starina* 23(1–2) [1914]:67–162. (Petrograd 1915.)

1961. Karafuto Ainu no Shamanisumu [Shamanism of the Sakhalin Ainu] (trans. by Kan Wada). *Hoppo Bunka Kenkyo Hokoku*. No. 16:179–203. (Originally published as Der Schamanismus bei den Ainu-Stämmen von Sachalin, 1909, *Globus* xv-4:261–74; xvi-2:117–32.)

Porkert, Manfred. 1974. *The Theoretical Foundations of Chinese Medicine: Systems of Correspondence*. Cambridge, Mass.: MIT Press.

Raun, Alo, David Francis, C. F. Voegelin and F. M. Voegelin, eds. 1965. Language of the world: Boreo-Oriental fascicle one. *Anthropological Linguistics* 7(1):143 pp.

Redfield, Robert. 1959. *The Primitive World and Its Transformations*. Ithaca, N.Y.: Cornell University Press. (Originally published in 1953.)

Rosaldo, Michelle Zimbalist. 1974. Woman, culture and society: a theoretical overview. In *Woman, Culture and Society*, M. Z. Rosaldo and L. Lamphere, eds. Stanford, Calif.: Stanford University Press. pp. 17–42.

Rosaldo, Michelle Zimbalist, and Jane Monnig Atkinson. 1975. Man the hunter and woman: metaphors for the sexes in Ilongot magical spells. In *The Interpretation of Symbolism*, Roy Willis, ed. New York: Halsted Press. pp. 43-75.

Rubel, Arthur J. 1964. The epidemiology of a folk illness: *Susto* in Hispanic America. *Ethnology III*(3):268-83.

Sacks, Karen. 1974. Engels revisited: women, the organization of production, and private property. In *Woman, Culture and Society*, M. Z. Rosaldo and L. Lamphere, eds. Stanford, Calif.: Stanford University Press. pp. 207-22.

Sahlins, Marshall D. 1960. Political power and the economy in primitive society. In *Essays in the Science of Culture*, G. E. Dole and R. L. Carneiro, eds. New York: Thomas Y. Crowell. pp. 390-415.

   1976a. *Culture and Practical Reason*. Chicago: University of Chicago Press.

   1976b. *The Use and Abuse of Biology*. Ann Arbor, Mich.: University of Michigan Press.

Sakurai, Kiyohiko. 1967. *Ainu Hishi* [*The Hidden History of the Ainu*]. Tokyo: Kadokawa Shoten.

Sanday, Peggy R. 1974. Female status in the public domain. In *Woman, Culture and Society*, M. Z. Rosaldo and L. Lamphere, eds. Stanford, Calif.: Stanford University Press. pp. 189-206.

Sapir, Edward. 1964. Conceptual categories in primitive language. In *Language in Culture and Society*, Dell Hymes, ed. New York: Harper & Row. p. 128. (Originally published in 1931.)

Sapir, Edward, and M. Swadesh. 1964. American Indian grammatical categories. In *Language, Culture and Society*, Dell Hymes, ed. New York: Harper & Row. pp. 101-11.

Sarashina, Genzo. 1968. *Ainu no Shiki* [*The Four Seasons of the Ainu*]. Tokyo: Tanko Shinsha.

Segall, Marshall H., D. T. Campbell, and M. J. Herskovits. 1966. *The Influence of Culture on Visual Perception*. Indianapolis: Bobbs-Merrill.

Segawa, Kiyoko. 1972. *Ainu no Konin* [*Marriage among the Ainu*]. Tokyo: Miraisha.

Sekiba, Rido. 1966. *Sekiba Rido Senshu* [*Selected Writings of Rido Sekiba*]. Tokyo: Kanehara Shuppan.

Sekiguchi, Ryushi. 1940. Orokko Soga Monogatari [Orok war stories]. *Karafuto Jiho* 38:62-7.

Serizawa, Chosuke. 1963. *Sekki Jidai no Nihon* [*The Stone Age of Japan*]. Tokyo: Tsukiji Shokan. Third edition.

Sigerist, Henry E. 1951. *Primitive and Archaic Medicine. A History of Medicine*. Vol. 1. New York: Oxford University Press.

Simpson, George Gaylord. 1961. *Principles of Animal Taxonomy*. New York: Columbia University Press.

Siskind, Janet. 1973. *To Hunt in the Morning*. New York: Oxford University Press.

   1974. Special hunt of the Sharanahua. *Natural History* 83(8):73-9.

Smith, Michael G. 1960. *Government in Zazzau*. London: Oxford University Press.

Smith, W. Robertson. 1972. *The Religion of the Semites*. New York: Schocken Books. (Originally published in 1889.)

Southall, Aidan. 1972. Twinship and symbolic structure. In *The Interpretation of Ritual*, J. S. La Fontaine, ed. London: Tavistock. pp. 73-114.

Sperber, Dan. 1976. Dirt, danger and pangolins - review of M. Douglas: *Implicit Meanings*. *Times Literary Supplement*, No. 3,868 (April 30):502-3.

Spiro, Melford E. 1965. Religious systems as culturally constituted defense mechanisms. In *Context and Meaning in Cultural Anthropology*, M. E. Spiro, ed. New York: Free Press. pp. 100-13.

   1977. *Burmese Supernaturalism*. Philadelphia: Institute for the Study of Human Issues. Expanded edition.

Spuhler, J. N. 1966. Numerical taxonomy and the Ainu problem. *Paper presented at the United States-Japan Cooperative Science Program Seminar, Sapporo, Japan.*

Stein, Howard F. 1977. Commentary on Kleinman's "Lessons from a clinical approach to medical anthropological research." *Medical Anthropology Newsletter* 8(4):15–16.

Steiner, Franz. 1967. *Taboo.* Middlesex: Penguin Books. (Originally published in 1956.)

Stephan, John J. 1971. *Sakhalin – A History.* London: Oxford University Press.

Sternberg, Leo. 1906. The Inau cult of the Ainu. In *Boas Anniversary Volume.* New York: Stechert. pp. 425–37.

——— 1929. The Ainu problem. *Anthropos* 24:755–99.

Strathern, Andrew, and Marilyn Strathern. 1968. Marsupials and magic: a study of spell symbolism among the Mbowamb. In *Dialectic in Practical Religion,* E. R. Leach, ed. London: Cambridge University Press. pp. 179–202.

Street, John C. 1962. Review of *Vergleichende Grammatik der altaischen Sprachen,* by Von Nikolaus Poppe (1960). *Language* 38(1):92–8.

Suwa, N., S. Morita, K. Yamashita, T. Kuroda, and M. Ishigane. 1963. Imu ni tsuite – Saikin no Chosa ni yoru Chiken [Imu – its recent findings]. *Seishin Igaku* 5(5):397–403.

Takakura, Shinichiro. 1939. Kinsei ni okeru Karafuto o Chushin to shita Nichiman Koeki [The Japanese-Manchurian trade on Sakhalin in the recent past]. *Hoppo Bunka Kenkyu Hokoku,* No. 1:163–94.

——— 1958. *Embetsu no Tanjo [The Birth of Embetsu].* Embetsu: Embetsu City Office.

——— 1960. The Ainu of northern Japan: a study in conquest and acculturation. Translated and annotated by John A. Harrison. In *Transactions of the American Philosophical Society,* N.S. Vol. 50, Part 4. Philadelphia: American Philosophical Society.

Takeda, H. 1949. *Systematic List of Economic Plants in Japan.* Report #121 (October). General Headquarters Supreme Commander for the Allied Powers, Natural Resources Section.

Tambiah, S. J. 1969. Animals are good to think and good to prohibit. *Ethnology* VIII(4):423–59.

Torii, Ryuzo. 1903. *Chishima Ainu [The Kurile Ainu].* Tokyo: Yoshikawa Kobunkan.

——— 1919. Etudes Archéologiques et Ethnologiques: Les Ainou de Îles Kouriles. *Journal of the College of Science, Tokyo Imperial University* 42, Article 1. 337 pp.

Tsuboi, Shogoro. 1889. Ainu no Fujin [Ainu women]. *Tokyo Jinruigakukai Zasshi,* No. 42:453–9.

Tsunoda, Tadanobu. 1971. The difference of the cerebral dominance of vowel sounds among different languages. *Journal of Auditory Research* 11:305–14.

——— 1974. Nihonjin to Seiyojin no Bunkagata to Onninshiki [Culture patterns and sound perception between Japanese and Westerners]. *Gengo* 3(6):510–17.

Turner, Christy G., II. 1976. Dental evidence on the origins of the Ainu and Japanese. *Science* 193 (September):911–13.

Turner, Victor. 1967. *The Forest of Symbols.* Ithaca, N.Y.: Cornell University Press.

——— 1969. *The Ritual Process.* Chicago: Aldine.

——— 1975. Symbolic studies. In *Annual Review of Anthropology,* B. J. Siegel, A. R. Beals, and S. A. Tyler, eds. Vol. 4. Palo Alto, Calif.: Annual Reviews. pp. 145–61.

Uchimura, Y. 1935. "Imu" – a malady of the Ainu. *Lancet CCXXVIII,* Vol. 1:1272–3.

Uchimura, Y., H. Akimoto, and T. Ishibashi. 1938. Ainu no Imu ni tsuite [Imu of the Ainu]. *Senshin Shinkeigaku Zasshi* 42(1):1–69.

Umesao, Tadao. 1960. *Nihon Tanken [Explorations of Japan].* Tokyo: Chuokoron.

van Gennep, Arnold. 1961. *The Rites of Passage.* Chicago: University of Chicago Press. Phoenix Book. (Originally published in 1909.)

Vansina, Jan. 1969. The Bushong poison ordeal. In *Man in Africa,* M. Douglas and O. M. Kaberry, eds. London: Tavistock. pp. 245–60.

Vygotsky, Lev Semenovich. 1970. *Thought and Language*. Cambridge, Mass.: MIT Press. (Originally published in Russian in 1934.)

Wada, Bunjiro. 1941. Karafuto Ainu Nagushi Monogatari – Karafuto Ainu no Chibyojutsu [Curing methods of the Sakhalin Ainu]. *Karafuto Jiho* 50:90–107.

1956. Ainugo Byomei to sono Igi [Ainu terms of illness and their meaning]. *Nihon Iji Shimpo*, No. 1969:43–5.

Wada, Kan. 1964. Ainugo Byomei ni tsuite – Wada Bunjiro Iko (1) [Names of illnesses in Ainu – manuscripts left by the late Bunjiro Wada (1)]. *Minzokugaku Kenkyu* 29(2):99–112.

1965a. Ainugo Byomei Shiryo – Wada Bunjiro Iko (2) [Data on the names of illnesses in Ainu – manuscripts left by the late Bunjiro Wada (2)]. *Minzokugaku Kenkyu* 30(1):47–67.

1965b. *Imu* ni kansuru Jakkan no Mondai [Some problems of *Imu*]. *Minzokugaku Kenkyu* 29(3):263–71.

1971. Ainu no shamanizumu [Ainu shamanism]. *Shunju*, No. 127:17–21.

Walker, Willard. 1965. Taxonomic structure and the pursuit of meaning. *Southwestern Journal of Anthropology* 21(3):265–75.

Wallace, Anthony F. C. 1970. *Culture and Personality*. New York: Random House. Second edition.

1972. Mental illness, biology and culture. In *Psychological Anthropology*, Francis L. K. Hsu, ed. Cambridge, Mass.: Schenkman. New edition. pp. 363–402.

Washburn, Sherwood L., and C. S. Lancaster. 1972. The evolution of hunting. In *Man the Hunter*, Richard B. Lee and Irven Devore, eds. Chicago: Aldine. pp. 293–303.

Watanabe, Hotoshi. 1973. *The Ainu Ecosystem*. Seattle: University of Washington Press. (Originally published in 1964.)

Watanabe, S., S. Kondo, and E. Matsunaga, eds. 1975. Anthropological and genetic studies on the Japanese. *JIBP Synthesis*. Vol. 2. (Japanese Committee for the International Biological Program.) Tokyo: University of Tokyo Press.

Weber, Max. 1947. *The Theory of Social and Economic Organization*. New York: Free Press.

Whorf, Benjamin L. 1952. *Collected Papers on Metalinguistics*. Washington, D.C.: Department of State, Foreign Service Institute.

Wilson, Monica. 1957. *Rituals of Kinship among the Nyakusa*. London: Oxford University Press for the International African Institute.

Wilson, P. J. 1967. Status ambiguity and spirit possession. *Man* 2(3):366–78.

Winiarz, W., and J. Wielawski. 1936. Imu – a psychoneurosis occurring among Ainus. *Psychoanalytic Review* 23:181–6.

Wittgenstein, Ludwig. 1968. *Philosophical Investigations*. New York: Macmillan. Third edition.

Wolf, Margery. 1974. Chinese women: old skills in a new context. In *Woman, Culture and Society*, M. Z. Rosaldo and L. Lamphere, eds. Palo Alto, Calif.: Stanford University Press. pp. 157–72.

Worsley, Peter. 1967. Groote Eylandt totémism and *Le Totémisme aujourd'hui*. In *The Structural Study of Myth and Totemism*, Edmund Leach, ed. London: Tavistock. pp. 141–59.

1968. *The Trumpet Shall Sound*. New York: Schocken.

Yakovlev, N. 1947. A visit to the Ainu in southern Sakhalin. *Asiatic Review* 43 (July):276–9.

Yalman, Nur. 1967. The raw: the cooked::nature:culture – observations on *Le Cru et le Cuit*. In *The Structural Study of Myth and Totemism*, Edmund Leach, ed. London: Tavistock. pp. 71–89.

Yamaguchi, Bin. 1961. Soya-misaki Onkormanai Shutsudo Jinkotsu [Human skeletal material excavated at the Onkoromanai site at Soya]. Nihon *Jinruigakukai Nihon Min-zokugakukai Rengo Taikai Kiji*, No. 15:99–101.

1963a. Soya-misaki Onkoromanai Kaizuka Shutsudo Jinkotsu [Human skeletal material at the Onkoromanai shell mound in northern Hokkaido]. *Jinruigaku Zasshi* 70(3–4):131–46.

1963b. Embetsu-gun Tsuishikari Bozuyama Iseki Jinkotsu [Human skeletal material at the Bozuyama site, Tsuishikari, Embetsu]. *Jinruigaku Zasshi* 71(2):55–71.

Yamamoto, Toshio (Yuko). 1944. Karafuto Ainu Giriyakku Orokko no Setsuwa [Folktales of the Sakhalin Ainu, Gilyaks and Oroks]. *Karafutocho Hakubutsukan Iho* 3(1):147–211.

1968. *Hoppo Shizen Minzoku Minwa Shusei* [*An Anthology of the Folktales of the Peoples of the North*]. Tokyo: Sagami Shobo.

1970. Karafuto Ainu Jukyo to Mingu [*The Dwellings and Artifacts of the Sakhalin Ainu*]. Tokyo: Sagami Shobo.

Yang, C. K. 1969. *Chinese Communist Society: The Family and the Village*. Cambridge, Mass.: MIT Press. (Originally published in 1959.)

Yoshida, Iwao. 1912. Ainu no Bokuzei Kinatsu [Ainu divination and taboo]. *Jinruizaku Zasshi* 28(6):314–28.

Yoshizaki, Masakazu. 1962. *Seminar on Japanese Prehistory*. Department of Anthropology, University of Wisconsin–Madison.

1963. Prehistoric culture in southern Sakhalin in the light of Japanese research. *Arctic Anthropology* 1(2):131–58.

Index

abnormalities not considered illnesses by
    Ainu, 36, 41
Ackerknecht, Erwin H., 136
Ainu
    Hokkaido Ainu, 22
    identity, 1–2, 21, 204–212
    Kurile Ainu, 22
    northwest coast Ainu, *see* northwest coast
      Ainu
    population estimates, 24
    Sakhalin Ainu, 22–4
Alder, 64–5, 91
ambiguity, distinguished from anomaly, 123
anomaly, 6–7
    decay, 125
    defined in anthropology, 119–21
    defined by author, 121–3
    defined by Douglas, 120–1
    demonic, 87–8, 103
    distinguished from ambiguity, 123
    formlessness, 121, 124–5
    illness causation, 88–9
    lack of identity, 87, 121
    medical symbols, 92–3
    out of place, 87–8, 121
    power, 123, 125–9
    taxonomic as opposed to symbolic, 124
    unclassifiable, 6–7, 15
    see also blood (old blood); demons;
      menstrual blood; women
anthropological interpretation, individual
    in, 16–17
Ardener, Edwin, 14, 118, 119, 130
Atkinson, Jane Monnig, 117

Babcock, Barbara, 119
Batchelor, John, 174
bear ceremony, 76
    political function, 84–5
    see also bears (deities)

bear headache, 49, 51, 52
bears (deities), 37, 45, 67, 77, 83
    injury by, 41
Beauvoir, Simone de, 112, 115, 117
behavior, 13–15
Beidelman, T. O., 148
Berlin, Brent, 124, 153
binary opposition
    in Ainu classification, 136–7, 141–3
    in anthropology, 9, 141–4
    relationship to taxonomic classification,
      144
biomedicine, 2, 11
    distinguished from Western medicine,
      32–3
blood (old blood), 43–4
    see also menstrual blood; parturient
      blood
bodily dirt
    symbolic meaning, 126–7
    see also excrement, symbolic use;
      menstrual blood; urine
body, Ainu classification, 40
body-part illnesses, 39–40, 183–195
    see also habitual illnesses
boils, 5, 12, 48, 53–5
    aquatic animal boils, 53–5
    classification, 53–5
    description, 41–2
    diagnosis, 53–5
    land animal boils, 53–5
    pain, 53, 55
    remedies, 44, 196–7
    and spatial classification of the universe,
      53, 55
    and temporal classification, 55
bone illnesses
    description, 39, 40–1
    treatment, 46
    see also habitual illnesses

239

Bourguignon, Erica, 179
Breedlove, Dennis E., 124, 154
bruises, 36, 41
Bulmer, Ralph, 120, 124
burns, 36, 41

chill
 chill/nonchill opposition, 59
 as diagnostic criterion, 49–52, 57–9, 62
Chiñas, Beverly L., 166
Chiri, Mashio, 23, 77, 173
 association between *imu*: and shamanism,
 176
 interpretation of Ainu animal deities, 84
Chomsky, Noam, 14, 156
classificatory systems, 4, 7
 binary oppositions, 141–3
 inversions, 6–7 (*see also* anomaly)
 monothetic, 144
 nonstructural, 145
 polythetic, 145
 principles of, 9, 11, 12
cognitive anthropology, *see* ethnosemantics
cognitive dimension of human perception
 and behavior, 8
conceptual forms
 evidence for their presence, 151–7
 meaning, 158
Conklin, Harold C., 154, 155
cooking
 ingredients in shamanistic ritual, 91
 symbolic meaning, 98–9, 106
cosmopolitan medicine, *see* biomedicine
covert categories, *see* ethnosemantics,
 covert categories
culture
 equated with Ainu men, 104
 equated with Ainu women, 103–4
 see also nature:culture
culture-bound syndromes, see *imu*:
cures
 arrowhead or spearhead in, 66
 description, 183–95, 196–7
 efficacy, 46
 multiplicity, 46–7
 see also materia medica; illnesses
cuts, 36, 41

dead human's soul, entrance by, 66
deities, 83–4
 language, 75, 86
 punishment by, 67

 see also bears (deities); foxes (deities);
 Grandmother Hearth; owls (deities);
 seals (deities); wolves (deities)
demons
 exorcism, 64–5, 70
 as illness pathogens, 63–4, 70
 symbolic meaning, 87–8, 96–7, 103, 122
dogs, 28, 45, 49, 67
 in materia medica, 39, 45
domestic domain, 84–5, 112–113, 129–131
Douglas, Mary
 anomaly, 7, 119–21, 123, 125, 127
 nature:culture:: uncontrolled: controlled,
 115
 reference to Judeo-Christian concept of
 God, 109–11
dreams, 68
drum, 75, 100
Durkheim, Emile, 143–4
 emotion, 8, 147
 sacred and profane, 109, 141

elder (plant), 64–5, 91
elders
 language of, 75, 85
 male, 86
Eliade, Mircea, 124
emic view, 31, 153
emotive dimension of human perception
 and behavior, 8, 147–8
empiricist approach, 33–4
epidemics, 63–5
 influenza, 63
 measles, 41
 prevention, 63–5
 smallpox, 41, 63, 65
ethnomedicine, 3, 13, 31
 illness and disease contrasted, 32
ethnoscience, *see* ethnosemantics
ethnosemantics, 10, 14
 compared with symbolic classification,
 152, 157
 covert categories, 14, 38, 153–4
etic approach, 32
etiologies, Ainu, 5–6
exchange system, 85
excrement, symbolic use, 65, 91–4
exorcism rites, 64–5, 90–1

Fabrega, Horacio, Jr.
 adaptive function of medical systems, 17

emotions and illness, 136, 147
illness and disease, 32, 168
fir, 70, 79, 91
fluid as a diagnostic criterion, 57-9, 62
folk medicine, 32
   see also non-Western medicine,
     philosophical basis
food, cultural valuation of, 116-17
fox, 53, 55
foxes (deities), 30, 67
Frake, Charles O., 136, 140, 152
funerals, 68
   for nonhumans, 68

gallbladder trouble, 45-6
Geertz, Clifford, 8, 11, 17, 133
Goddess of Hearth, *see* Grandmother
   Hearth
Goddess of Sun and Moon, 30, 92
Good, Byron J., 13, 16, 171
Goodenough, Ward H., 153
grammatical categories, and illness
   classification, 60-2
   see also Sapir-Whorf hypothesis
Grandmother Hearth, 30, 81, 107
   anomalous, 94
   help in curing, 34-5, 74
   as mediator, 76, 83, 92
group rituals
   contrasted with shamanistic rituals, 101-4
   expression of formalized ideology, 102
   rules for performance, 101-3

habitual illnesses, 5, 37, 39, 183-95, 196-7
   classification, 55-6, 60, 62, 135-40
   contrasted with metaphysical illnesses,
     135-40
   cures, 44
   and world view, 135-7
   see also body-part illnesses; boils; bone
     illnesses; headaches
Hall, Edward T., 9, 148
Hallowell, A. Irving, 136
headaches, 5, 39
   aquatic animal headaches, 51, 55
   classification, 49-52
   cures, 44
   diagnostic criteria, 51
   land animal headaches, 51, 55
   pain, 49, 52
   symptom of other illness, 48

healing rituals, 5, 73-8, 103
   symbolic interpretation, 88-94
health, Ainu concept of, 34-5
hearth, 74
Hertz, Robert, 108
Hoijer, Harry, 159
humoral element in medical systems, 149
humoral medicine, 59
hunter-gatherers, 1
hunting, cultural valuation of, 117

illnesses
   aquatic vs. land animal illnesses, 59
   araka (Ainu illness, pain), 35-6, 37
   arrow intrusion illness, 66
   blood-spitting illness, 11, 42-3, 44, 48
   causation, 134, 138-9
   crab illnesses, 60
   vs. disease, 32 (*see also* non-Western
     medicine)
   domain of, 34-8, 134-5
   emotions causing, 69, 147
   eye illnesses, 56
   eye illnesses, remedies, 44
   hana, 12, 42-4, 48
   heart illness, remedies, 45, 47
   ikoni (Ainu illness, pain), 35-6
   labels, 58, 134
   lamprey illnesses, 60
   mouth illnesses, 56
   otter punishment illness, 66
   purification rites, 89
   subclassifications, 134-5, 140
   throat illnesses, 56
   see also mental illnesses; metaphysical
     illnesses; pathogens; skin illnesses
imu:, 10, 175-8, 198-203
   and other culture-bound syndromes,
     177-8
   and the socially marginal, 177-8, 180
   and women, 177, 198-203
influenza, 63

juniper, 64-5

Kapferer, Bruch, 89
Keesing, Roger M., 116, 145, 154, 156
Kennedy, John, 175
kinship organization, 84
kite (bird), 79
Kleinman, Arthur M., 13, 31-2, 139-40,
   180

Kubodera, Itsuhiko, 164
Kuhn, Thomas S., 157

labor pains, 47
La Fontaine, J. S., 114-15
language and cognition, 5, 10
larch, 74, 91
Leach, Edmund R., 119-20, 125, 127, 129
  classification, 143
  criticism of Lévi-Strauss, 115-16
  sacred:profane, 108-9
leek, 74, 91, 98
Lévi-Strauss, Claude
  contrasted with Turner, 106
  exogamy, 115-16
  healing power of a shaman, 168
  mediation, 7, 128
  nature:culture, 110-16, 148
  and rationalist tradition, 8, 147
  structure of the human mind, 133
  unconscious nature of symbolic referent,
    128
Lewis, Ioan, 177, 178-9

McLuhan, Marshall, 9, 149
materia medica, 39, 183-95
  bears, 45
  chosen by analogy, 44-5
  dogs, 45
  leek, 46
  metaphysical value, 45
  practical efficacy, 46
  resin, 46
  ritual value, 45-6
Mauss, Marcel, 8, 143, 144, 147
measles, 41
mediation, 7, 128
  see also Lévi-Strauss, Claude, mediation
mediation, Ainu
  in healing rites, 90-1
  symbols of, 94-5
  see also Grandmother Hearth; Goddess of
    Sun and Moon; shamans
medical anthropology, 13, 17
men, 27, 84-7, 100-1
  equated with culture, 104
  role in hunting and fishing, 84
  role in political arena, 84
  role in religion, 84
  see also sex roles, Ainu
men:women::nature:culture, see nature:
  culture::men:women

men:women::public:domestic, see public:
  domestic::men:women
menstrual blood, 8, 64, 67, 91-3, 128
  anomalous, 93-4
  antidote to smallpox, 65
  dual meaning, 103
  symbolic meaning, 130
  see also anomaly; women
menstrual cramps, 47
mental aberrations, minor, 73
mental illnesses, Ainu, 69-73
  attitudes toward, 70-1
  causation, 69-70
  classification, 69-70
  cures by exorcism, 70
  delusions, 69
  diagnosis by shaman, 70
  patient confined, 69, 71
  physical violence, 69
metaphysical illnesses, 5, 35-7, 65-7
  bear injury, 41
  contrasted with habitual illness, 135
  demons as cause, 80
  human misconduct as cause, 80
  shamanistic curing rites, 63
  somatic, afflicting only individuals, 65-7
  see also shamanistic healing; shamanistic
    rites
Munro, Neil Gordon, 176

nature, in Ainu world view, 109-10
nature:culture, 7, 110
  Ainu, 98-100
nature:culture::men:women, 111-18
  childbearing/rearing, 112
  controlled:uncontrolled, 115
  cooking, 116-17
  decay, 113-14
  defloration, 114
  economic roles, 117-18
  exogamy, socialization, and cooking,
    113-14
  hunting, 116-17
  incest taboos, 113, 116
  inversion of, 112-13
Needham, Rodney
  anomaly, 119
  classification, 9, 133, 141, 143-5
  conceptual forms, 157-8
  ordering, 3
  Whorfian hypothesis, 157
nonbiomedical traditions, 11-12

see also non-Western medicine,
    philosophical basis
non-Western medicine
    philosophical basis, 33
    systems, 2–3
northwest coast Ainu
    bear ceremony, 29–30
    deities, 29–30
    economic activities, 26–8
    political structure, 26
    population, 25
    settlement pattern, 25
    social structure, 25
nuhča (tea), 35, 74, 91

Obeyesekere, Gananath, 177, 178
Ortiz, Alfonso, 15, 143
Ortner, Sherry B., 112–13, 115–17, 118
otter, 66, 68
owls (deities), 30

pain, 49, 51
    accompanying boils, 53–4
    as classificatory principle, 60, 62
    tasum, 35, 36
    see also illnesses
parturient blood, 64, 93
pathogens, 5–6, 47–8
    see also metaphysical illnesses; sorcery;
    souls
physical characteristics of Ainu, 19–21
Pilsudski, Bronislov, 77, 163
politically powerful:politically peripheral,
    131
    see also public:domestic::men:women;
    shamans
Porkert, Manfred, 139
possession trance, 178–9
"processual symbology," 13
profane, *see* sacred:profane
profane, Ainu, 82–7, 92, 108, 110
psychotherapy, *see* shamanistic healing
public domain, 84
public:domestic::men:women, 129–31
punishment by the wrath of a deity, 67
purification rites, 89–91

rationalist approach, 33
red bog moss, 65
religions, established vs.
    noninstitutionalized, 109

ritual shavings, in curing, 66
Rosaldo, Michelle Zimbalist, 117, 129

sacred, in Ainu symbolic classification, 83–7
    see also deities
sacred:profane
    Ainu, 6, 86, 100, 108–10
    in anthropological interpretation, 7–8,
        108–10
sacred:profane::nature:culture, 110–11
Sahlins, Marshall, D., 17, 85
Sapir, Edward, 156
Sapir-Whorf hypothesis, 4, 10, 60–2, 156–7
science in non-Western cultures, 32
scientific medicine, 32
    see also biomedicine
seals (deities), 77
senses, use in perception, 97–8
sensory dimension of human perception and
        behavior, 8–9, 148–9
settlement pattern, 85
sex roles, 84, 99–100
    childbearing/rearing, 118
    cooking, 117
    cultural interpretations, 115
    formalized and nonformalized, 166
    see also nature:culture::men:women;
        public:domestic::men:women
shamanism, 30
    cultural valuation in the past, 173–4, 175
    means of social control, 170
    professional role for women, 172
shamanistic healing
    communal nature, 168
    as psychotherapy, 168
shamanistic rites, 73–6, 78, 91
    amnesia following trance, 75
    contrasted with group rituals, 101–4
    cooking, 91. 98
    for curing sick bears, 76
    drum, 74–5, 97
    expression of nonformalized ideology, 102
    and fertility and sex, 81
    mediation, 90–1
    rules for performance, 73–4, 101–2
    shaman's spirits, 76–9
shamans
    individual personalities, 175–9
    mental disorder, 178–9 (see also *imu:*)
shamans, Ainu, 10
    anomaly, 95
    assistants, 75–6

shamans, Ainu (*continued*)
career, 162–3
as covert politicians, 169–71
cultural valuation of, 162
diagnosis of social ills, 169–70, 180
formalized roles, 167
healing rites, 73–6 (*see also* shamanistic rites)
as health care specialists, 167–8
and *imu:*, 175–6
and intersettlement communication, 171
male/female shamans, 73, 164, 166
as mediators, 92, 180
mental aberrations, 73 (see also *imu:*)
multiple roles, 166–8
nonformalized power, 172
nonformalized roles, 167
among other Ainu societies, 173–4
paraphernalia, 75
and the politically peripheral, 172
possession trance, 168
as religious specialists, 167
as social analysts, 170
social identity, 163–4
spirit possession, 78–9
as theatrical performers, 167
shaman's spirits, Ainu
deities distinguished from, 77
evil spirits in bird form, 79
exorcism of evil spirits, 79
guardian deities, 78
mediation, 92
relationship to shaman, 78
symbolic interpretation, 94
skin illnesses, 41–2, 56
see also boils
smallpox, 41, 63, 65
Smith, W. Robertson, 108–9, 119, 129
snakes, 77
society
legal code, 80
stratification, 85–6, 102
sorcery, 43, 78–9
soul loss, 67, 73
souls, 68–9
concepts of, 87–8
as illness pathogen, 68, 69
shaman's, 68
spatial classification, 87, 101
Sperber, Dan, 123
spirit possession, 74–5
see also shamanistic rites

Spiro, Melford E., 175, 177, 178
spruce, 35, 74, 91
structural approaches in anthropology, 6, 12, 145
structure, *see* classificatory systems
supernatural illnesses, *see* metaphysical illnesses
symbolic belief systems, multiplicity of
Ainu, 8, 100–2
general, 8, 129
symbolic classification, 6, 10
compared with ethnosemantics, 152
symbolic structure, formalized:nonformalized, 8, 129–31
Ainu, 12, 102
symbols
emotive dimension, 8, 17, 147–8
function, 17, 127
interpretation of referents, 105–8
multivocal, 106
sensory dimension, 8–9, 17, 148–9
symbols, Ainu
meaning at structural level, 107
multivocal, 106–7, 131

Tambiah, S. J., 120–1, 127
tangle (seaweed), 74, 91
taxonomic classification, 5, 86
taxonomy, *see* classificatory systems
temporal concepts, 61–2
traditional medicine, *see* non-Western medicine
Turner, Victor
anomaly, 7, 123, 125
emotive dimension of human perception, 8, 147
Ndembu headaches, 136–7
"processual symbology," 13
sensory dimension of human perception, 148
symbolic meaning of hunting, 117
symbols, multivocal, 105–7, 159
twins, 100

Uchimura, Y., 176
universe
classification, 88
codified, 82–3
society of, 84
urine, 93
see also bodily dirt

van Gennep, Arnold, 6, 119
Vansina, Jan, 89
Vygotsky, Lev Semenovich, 144–5

Wada, Bunjiro, 16, 44, 77, 176
Wada, Kan, 176
Western scientific medicine, *see*
    biomedicine
white birch, 64–5
Whorf, Benjamin L., 4, 156–7
Whorfian hypothesis, *see* Sapir-Whorf
    hypothesis
willow, 79
Wittgenstein, Ludwig, 157
wolves (deities), 34
women, 28, 84–7, 100–1
  in classification of humans, 84–7, 100–1

equated with domestic domain, 117
and *imu:*, 177, 198–203
mediating role, 92 (*see also* mediation,
    Ainu)
reproduction, 99–100
role as food gatherer, 161
role in medical system, 161
sex roles, 85, 99–100
as shamans, 172
symbolic representation, 99, 106
women:men, *see* nature:culture; public:
    domestic::men:women
world view, 34, 62, 92
wormwood, 70, 91
Worsley, Peter, 145

Yalman, Nur, 158